Internet of Things in Biomedical Sciences

Challenges and applications

Online at: https://doi.org/10.1088/978-0-7503-5311-3

IPEM–IOP Series in Physics and Engineering in Medicine and Biology

About the Series

The series in Physics and Engineering in Medicine and Biology will allow the Institute of Physics and Engineering in Medicine (IPEM) to enhance its mission to 'advance physics and engineering applied to medicine and biology for the public good'.

It is focused on key areas including, but not limited to:

- clinical engineering
- diagnostic radiology
- informatics and computing
- magnetic resonance imaging
- nuclear medicine
- physiological measurement
- radiation protection
- radiotherapy
- rehabilitation engineering
- ultrasound and non-ionising radiation.

A number of IPEM–IOP titles are being published as part of the EUTEMPE Network Series for Medical Physics Experts.

A full list of titles published in this series can be found here: https://iopscience.iop.org/bookListInfo/physics-engineering-medicine-biology-series.

Internet of Things in Biomedical Sciences

Challenges and applications

Edited by
Varun Bajaj and Irshad Ahmad Ansari
Indian Institute of Information Technology, Design and Manufacturing, Jabalpur, India

IOP Publishing, Bristol, UK

ISBN 978-0-7503-5311-3 (ebook)
ISBN 978-0-7503-5309-0 (print)
ISBN 978-0-7503-5312-0 (myPrint)
ISBN 978-0-7503-5310-6 (mobi)

DOI 10.1088/978-0-7503-5311-3

Version: 20230601

IOP ebooks

British Library Cataloguing-in-Publication Data: A catalogue record for this book is available from the British Library.

Published by IOP Publishing, wholly owned by The Institute of Physics, London

IOP Publishing, No.2 The Distillery, Glassfields, Avon Street, Bristol, BS2 0GR, UK

US Office: IOP Publishing, Inc., 190 North Independence Mall West, Suite 601, Philadelphia, PA 19106, USA

Dedicated to my father Late Mahendra Bajaj and Family members.

—Varun Bajaj

Dedicated to my better half and strength 'Nuzra'

—Irshad Ahmad Ansari

Contents

Preface

Nowadays, the biomedical domain is heavily dependent on technology. Connectivity is a much sought after trait in biomedical devices. Telemedicine is an age-old idea but it has got momentum due to the introduction of Internet of Things (IoT). The effect of IoT is ubiquitous. The combination of IoT with the biomedical domain has created an entirely new area of research called IoMT (Internet of Medical Things). It is a niche area of research. Therefore, the idea behind this book is to bring forward the latest research happening in this multidisciplinary field of biomedical science and IoT. The intervention of IoT in the biomedical field has led to the development of numerous medical devices. Therefore, the aim of this book is to assess the impact and effect of IoT in the biomedical and telemedicine domain. This book features diverse research in the field of IoMT. It can act as a knowledge sharing resource for academicians, professionals and even beginners to get an idea about this area. The primary subject of this edited book is healthcare and medicine. It is a crucial area of research and it has a very positive affect on the quality of human life. It can certainly be called one of the most important areas of research given the present scenario.

Telemedicine is the most prominent area where a combination of IoT and biomedicine is significant. Telemedicine, as the name suggests, deals with treatment even when doctor and patients are far away from each other. It is helpful for remote areas where healthcare facilities are scarce. In telemedicine, patient consultation, data sharing, diagnosis, management, etc, are done through various electronics devices over a communication network. The opportunities in telemedicine are endless and it is a boon for patients. Introduction of remote surgeries based on robotics has phenomenal potential. There will be no need of the physical presence of a surgeon. Surgeons with a certain set of skills can operate on their patient from any part of the world. What felt impossible previously has become a reality with the introduction of technologies like IoT.

Wireless and wearable medical devices are important for monitoring patients in telemedicine applications. These devices are the main parts of point-of-care (POC) systems. These types of devices are important in monitoring diseases like type 1 diabetes. In type 1 diabetes, continuous monitoring of sugar level is required. Similarly, continuous monitoring of heart and brain activities is required in various diseases. These devices collect vital information from subjects. There is a grooming industry that is involved in research and production of wearable medical devices. This data can help in early detection and rapid diagnosis of the ailment. Wearable devices are a wonderful step in minimizing the gap between the advent of a medical condition and its diagnosis. Design of such devices, their management, power requirement, etc becomes an active area of research.

Data acquisition is fairly important in IoT-based telemedicine applications. Various sensors are required to record accurate data. The recorded data is either processed in the wearable device itself or sent to cloud servers and processed there. A large amount of medical data is generated from sensors, it requires signal processing algorithms to analyze the data. Therefore, signal processing is another major research area in IoMT. The main purpose of IoT based wearable medical devices is data logging of the subject. This historical data of the subject is required to predict future medical conditions or early onset of diseases. The prediction is done on the basis of a large amount of medical data collected from IoT based devices. The machine learning (ML) and artificial learning (AI) algorithms can be employed for predictions. Deep learning is also specialized in working with a large amount of raw data from sensors. Introduction of ML in IoT based medical devices is developing a whole new area called Intelligent IoMT (IIoMT). Apart from wearable devices, IoT plays an important role in management of hospitals. In hospitals IoT can be seen in many devices beyond patient monitoring devices. Hospitals are full of equipment like MRI, x-ray machines, ventilators, etc. IoT can create a single point of control for all these devices. Using IoT-based devices doctors can store and access a patient's data from any location. Hospitals are now capable of remote surgeries thanks to technologies like IoT.

A large amount of data handling is required in medical devices and hospitals. In this case, the security of data becomes an important task. The patient data is regularly transmitted over a network and stored in cloud-based storage systems. Various data protection techniques like encryption and watermarking are required to safeguard the medical data. Blockchain-based data security mechanisms are also currently gaining traction. The chapter-wise description of this book is as follows.

Chapter 1 provides an IoT-based wearable cardiac healthcare system to prevent cardiovascular diseases (CVDs) using continuous monitoring of electrocardiogram (ECG) signals and heart rate. **Chapter 2** presents an overview of the state-of-the-art of IoT, architectures in health care, and their applications in biomedical devices. **Chapter 3** demonstrates the fundamental concept of IoT, AI and ML in medical devices. Interoperability is the major function of AI and IoT to maintain the track of happenings on the devices and to react according to it. It involves a transformation towards an active patient who can be monitored in real time and a more complicated data management strategy. **Chapter 4** develops a system that includes a number of volatile organic compound (VOC) sensors, electronic signal conditioning circuits for signal extraction from the sensor, a data-transferring unit for instituting with IoT, a server for data collection, and software for data analysis and better prediction of lung cancer with high accuracy. **Chapter 5** presents the role of IoT in wearable technology; wearables with IoT capabilities offer people the data they need to improve their health. **Chapter 6** explores the integration of IoT-enabled devices with chatbots and ML. With the integration of IoT-enabled devices with chatbots and ML, we can easily reduce the number of cancer deaths throughout the world. **Chapter 7** introduces present IoT as a potential solution for controlling antimicrobial resistance (AMR) via its ability in improving diagnosis, treatment, and surveillance of AMR. **Chapter 8** proposes a novel IoT-based framework to detect heart valve disorders (HVDs) in humans using an amplitude and frequency modulated (AFM) signal decomposition model. **Chapter 9** offers a review study revolving around IoT and AI applications in biomedical systems in biomedical wearables, diagnostic devices, connected hospital machinery/devices, POC technologies, etc. **Chapter 10** discusses IoMT in detail. IoMT has various applications like medical devices, wearable sensors, communication systems, and mobile user interfaces.

Chapter 11 discuses experiences in the care of cardiac patients through three specific examples: a cardiac event recorder derived from a Holter system, a device to follow-up cardiac arrhythmias and an assistive device for elderly patients who remain alone in their homes for long durations. **Chapter 12** provides dissemination of clinical research findings and medical evidence through electronic medical records, direct insights, and virtual clinical trial datasets that are viewed as a major driver for delivering valuable scientific findings to patients and clinicians. **Chapter 13** presents a detailed state-of-the-art analysis on IoT and biomedical systems, followed by the major issues related to the implementation of IoT along with the significance and various applications of IoT in the biomedical system. The **chapter 14** proposed study presents an automatic detection of leg movements (LMs) and periodic leg movements (PLMs) by developing a model based on ML and signal processing techniques.

Acknowledgements

Dr Bajaj expresses his heartfelt appreciation to his mother Prabha, wife Anuja, daughter Avadhi, for their wonderful support and encouragement throughout the completion of this important book *IoT in Biomedical Sciences: Challenges and applications*. His deepest gratitude goes to his mother-in-law and father-in-law for their constant motivation. This book is an outcome of sincere efforts that could be given to the book only due to great support of the family.

Dr Ansari expresses his gratitude and sincere thanks to his wife, family members and teachers for their constant support and motivation. I really appreciate my wife for all the time that she has given me to work on this book, while she took care of everything.

We sincerely thank Professor Bhartendu K Singh, Director of PDPM IIITDM Jabalpur for his support and encouragement. We would like to thank all our friends, well-wishers and all those who keep us motivated in doing more and more; better and better. We sincerely thank all contributors for writing relevant theoretical background and applications of this book.

We express our humble thanks to Mr Michael Slaughter and all editorial staff of IOP for great support, necessary help, appreciation and quick responses. We also wish to thank IOP for giving us this opportunity to contribute on this relevant topic with a reputed publisher. Finally, we want to thank everyone, in one way or another, who helped us editing this book.

Dr Bajaj especially thanks his family, who encouraged him throughout the time of editing this book. This book is heartily dedicated to his father who took the lead to heaven before the completion of this book.

Last but not least, we would also like to thank God for showering us his blessings and strength to do this type of novel and quality work.

Varun Bajaj
Irshad Ahmad Ansari

Editors' biographies

Varun Bajaj

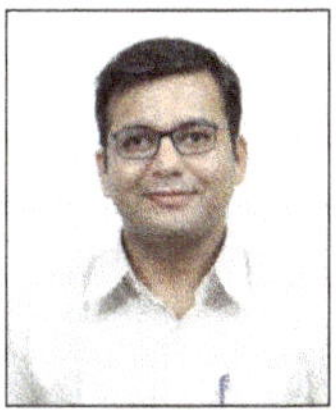

Varun Bajaj (PhD, SMIEEE20) has been working as an Associate Professor in the discipline of Electronics and Communication Engineering, at Indian Institute of Information Technology, Design and Manufacturing (IIITDM) Jabalpur, India since July 2021. He worked as Assistant Professor in IIITDM Jabalpur from March 2014 to July 2021. He also worked as a visiting faculty in IIITDM Jabalpur from September 2013 to March 2014. He worked as Assistant Professor at Department of Electronics and Instrumentation, Shri Vaishnav Institute of Technology and Science, Indore, India during 2009–10. He received his PhD degree in the discipline of electrical engineering, at Indian Institute of Technology Indore, India in 2014. He received an MTech degree with Honors in Microelectronics and VLSI design from Shri Govindram Seksaria Institute of Technology and Science, Indore, India in 2009, BE degree in Electronics and Communication Engineering from Rajiv Gandhi Technological University, Bhopal, India in 2006.

He is an Associate Editor of *IEEE Sensor Journal* and Subject Editor-in-Chief of IET *Electronics Letters*. He served as a Subject Editor of IET *Electronics Letters* from November 2018 to June 2020. He has been a Senior Member IEEE since June 2020, MIEEE 16-20, and also contributes as an active technical reviewer of leading international journals of IEEE, IET, Elsevier, etc. He has 156 publications which include journal papers (100), conference papers (32), books (11), and book chapters (13). He has also been granted two international patents and published two Indian patents. The citation impact of his publications is around 5238 citations, h index of 38, and i10 index of 101 (Google Scholar March 2023). He has guided seven (5 completed and 3 in process) PhD Scholars, Eight MTech scholars. He has been listed as the world's top 2% researchers/scientists by Stanford University, USA (October 2020 and October 2021). He has worked on research projects funded by DST and CSIR. He is a recipient of various reputed national and international awards. His research interests include biomedical signal processing, AI in healthcare, brain–computer interface, pattern recognition and ECG signal processing.

Irshad Ahmad Ansari

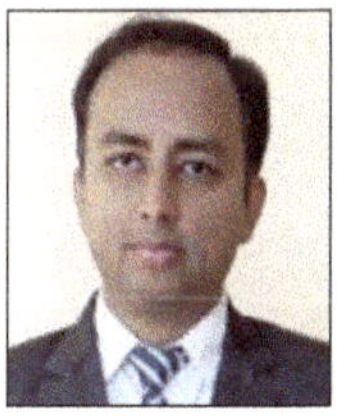

Irshad Ahmad Ansari (PhD, SMIEEE20) has been working as faculty in the discipline of Electronics and Communication Engineering, at PDPM Indian Institute of Information Technology, Design and Manufacturing (IIITDM) Jabalpur, India since 2017. He received a BTech degree in electronics and communication engineering from Gautam Buddh Technical University (formally UPTU), Lucknow, India in 2010, MTech degree in control and instrumentation from Dr B R Ambedkar

National Institute of Technology Jalandhar, Punjab, India in 2012. He completed his PhD from IIT Roorkee with MHRD teaching assistantship, and subsequently joined Gwangju Institute of Science and Technology, South Korea as a Postdoctoral fellow. His major research interests include signal and image processing, brain–computer interface and machine learning. He contributes as an active technical reviewer of leading international publishers like IEEE, IOP, Elsevier, and Springer etc. He has more than 55 publications which include journal papers (25), conference papers (26), books (3), and book chapters (4). The citation impact of his publications is around 752 citations, h index of 14, and i10 index of 17 (Google Scholar September 2022). He has guided three (two submitted and one in process) PhD scholars, 13 MTech scholars.

List of contributors

Ifti Akib Abir
University of Dhaka, Dhaka, Bangladesh

Mehedi Uddin Ahmed
University of Dhaka, Dhaka, Bangladesh

Irshad Ahmad Ansari
PDPM IIITDM Jabalpur, India

Mohammad Arif
Department of Electrical and Computer Science Engineering, Institute of Infrastructure, Technology, Research and Management (IITRAM), Ahmedabad, India

Kushagra Asthana
Department of Electrical and Computer Science Engineering, Institute of Infrastructure, Technology, Research and Management (IITRAM), Ahmedabad, India

Varun Bajaj
PDPM IIITDM Jabalpur, India

Mohan Bansal
School of Electronics Engineering, VIT-AP University, Amaravati, India

Nitesh Singh Bhati
Delhi Technical Campus, Greater Noida, India

Sama Bolog
University of Basel, Basel, Switzerland

Arjun Chaudhary
Centre for cyber security, Sardar Patel University of Police Security and Criminal Justice Jodhpur, India

Pushpa Choudhary
JSS Academy of Technical Education, Noida, India

Adiba Tabassum Chowdhury
University of Dhaka, Dhaka, Bangladesh

Ajay Dagar
School of Electronics Engineering, VIT-AP University, Amaravati, India

Ngoc Tung Dang
International University, Vietnam National University of Ho Chi Minh City, Ho Chi Minh City, Vietnam

Roopa Golchha
National Institute of Technology, Raipur, Chhattisgarh, India

René Iván Gonzalez-Fernandez
Cuban Center for Neurosciences, La Habana, Cuba

Kapil Gupta
PDPM IIITDM Jabalpur, India

José Luis Hernandez-Caceres
Cuban Center for Neurosciences, La Habana, Cuba

Ruby Jain
SAGE University, Indore, India

Daniel Jimenez-Gonzalez
COMBIOMED Medical Devices, La Habana, Cuba

Apoorv Joshi
National Institute of Technology, Raipur, Chhattisgarh, India

Samyak Kothari
Ahmedabad University, Pravesh, Ghatlodia, Ahmedabad, India

Alejandro Lopez-Reyes
COMBIOMED Medical Devices, La Habana, Cuba

Bhoumik Mahajan
SAGE University, Indore, India

Anto Manuel
School of Electrical Sciences, IIT Goa, Farmagudi, Ponda, Goa, India

Gisela Montes de Oca-Colina
COMBIOMED Medical Devices, La Habana, Cuba

Abu Jaffor Morshedul Abedin
University of Dhaka, Dhaka, Bangladesh

Margarita Lucía Mulet-Cartaya
COMBIOMED Medical Devices, La Habana, Cuba

Cuong Nguyen
Institute of Information Technology, Vietnam Academy of Science and Technology, Hanoi, Vietnam

Thi Thu Hoai Nguyen
International University, Vietnam National University of Ho Chi Minh City, Ho Chi Minh City, Vietnam

Anand Pandey
G L Bajaj Institute of Technology and Management, Greater Noida, India

Nikhil Kumar Parida
National Institute of Technology, Raipur, Chhattisgarh, India

Antonio Pesqueira
ISCTE, Lisboa, Portugal

Bidhan Pramanick
School of Electrical Sciences, IIT Goa, Farmagudi, Ponda, Goa, India

Mehedi Hasan Raju
Texas State University, San Marcos, TX, USA

Mridu Sahu
National Institute of Technology, Raipur, Chhattisgarh, India

Palanivel Rajan Selvakumaran
M. Kumarasamy College of Engineering (Autonomous), Anna University, Thalavapalayam, Karur, India

Hiba Shakeel
Delhi Technical Campus, Greater Noida, India

Hiral Shah
Ahmedabad University, Pravesh, Ghatlodia, Ahmedabad, India

Jash Shah
Ahmedabad University, Pravesh, Ghatlodia, Ahmedabad, India

Manan Shah
Pandit Deendayal Energy University, Raisan, Gandhinagar, India

Manish Sharma
Department of Electrical and Computer Science Engineering, Institute of Infrastructure, Technology, Research and Management (IITRAM), Ahmedabad, India

Priya Sharma
Delhi Technical Campus, Greater Noida, India

Rajeev Sharma
School of Electronics Engineering, VIT-AP University, Amaravati, India

Arun Singh
G L Bajaj Institute of Technology and Management, Greater Noida, India

Uday Pratap Singh
National Institute of Technology, Raipur, Chhattisgarh, India

Abirami Tamilarasu
M. Kumarasamy College of Engineering (Autonomous), Anna University, Thalavapalayam, Karur, India

Ashish Tripathi
G L Bajaj Institute of Technology and Management, Greater Noida, India

Contributors' biographies

Ifti Akib Abir

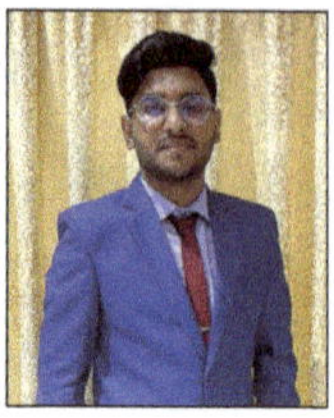

Ifti Akib Abir has recently completed a BSc engineering degree in electrical and electronic engineering from University of Dhaka, Bangladesh. Currently, he is an Operations Expert (DevOps) at Red.Digital Limited, a subsidiary of Robi Axiata Limited. He was awarded prizes in several International and National competitions (second in MIT Solveathon 2021, third in MIT App Inventor Hackathon 2020, Top 12 in New Normal Hackathon 2020). His research interests include cyber security, Internet of Things (IoT), machine learning.

Mosabber Uddin Ahmed

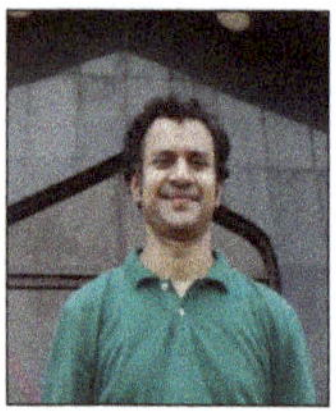

Dr Mosabber Uddin Ahmed is currently a professor in the Department of Electrical and Electronic Engineering (EEE) at University of Dhaka. He received BSc (Hons) and MSc degrees from the Department of Applied Physics and Electronics, University of Dhaka in 1998 and 1999, respectively. He received a second MSc degree in communications and signal processing and PhD degree in signal processing from Imperial College London (ICL), UK in 2006 and 2012, respectively. From 2015 to 2016, he was a postdoctoral fellow in EEE Department of ICL. To date, he has authored more than 40 research articles that are published in refereed journals, books, and conference proceedings. Dr Ahmed, a senior member of IEEE, has also co-edited a book titled *Signal Processing Techniques for Computational Health Informatics* published by Springer Nature. He has won several fellowships and research grants including the Commonwealth Academic Fellowship, Commonwealth Scholarship, Charles Wallace Bangladesh Trust (CWBT) grant, Mirza Samsul Huda and Mahmuda Begum Memorial Trust Gold Medal, Roushan Innas Ali Welfare Trust Gold Medal, and the Taylor & Francis Commonwealth Scholar Highly Commended Journal Article Prize. His research interests include signal processing, time–frequency analysis, multivariate time series analysis, complexity analysis, multiscale entropy analysis, embedded system design, Internet of Things (IoT), information security and machine intelligence.

Mohammad Arif

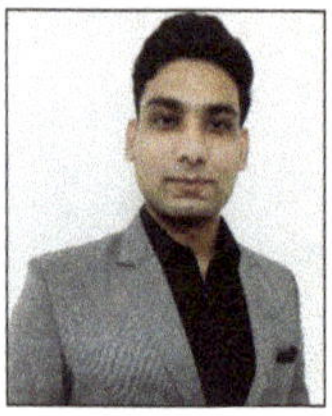

Mr Mohammad Arif received his BTech in electrical engineering from institute of infrastructure technology research and management in 2022. He completed his research on sleep stage classification and a periodic leg moment detector as a part of his final year BTech project under the guidance of Dr Manish Sharma (Assistant Professor, IITRAM, Ahmedabad).

Kushagra Asthana

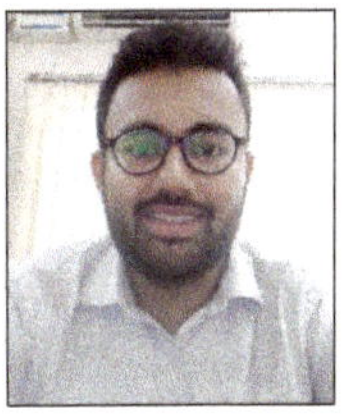

Mr Kushagra Asthana completed his BTech in electrical engineering from Institute of Infrastructure, Technology, Research and Management, Ahmedabad, India in 2022. In his BTech project, he worked on two projects, automated sleep stage classification and automated periodic leg movement detector under the guidance of Dr Manish Sharma (Assistant Professor Dr Manish Sharma). He joined Adapt Ideations, a Hyderabad based company as an embedded design engineer after graduation. Currently, he is an SiB Shine fellow (School of International Biodesign—Synergizing Healthcare Innovation and Entrepreneurship). SiB Shine is a joint venture between King George's Medical University, Lucknow and IIT Kanpur to identify healthcare needs and innovation in medical devices. His expertise lies in electronic product development.

Mohan Bansal

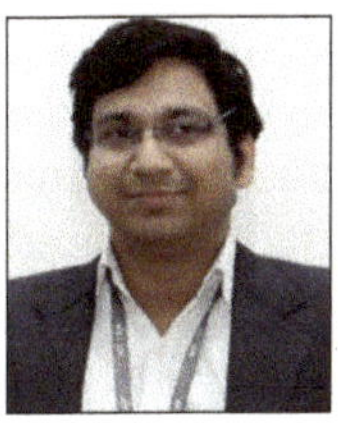

Dr Mohan Bansal, received his BE degrees in electronics and communication engineering from RGPV Bhopal, India in 2008 and MTech from National Institute of Technology (NIT) Kurukshetra, India in 2011. He received the PhD degree in Electrical Engineering Department, Indian Institute of Technology (IIT) Kanpur, India in 2020. He is currently working as Sr Assistant Professor in the School of Electronics Engineering (SENSE) at VIT-AP University at Amaravati, AP India. His research interests include digital signal processing, speech signal processing, parametric modeling of the signal, machine learning and deep learning.

Nitesh Singh Bhati

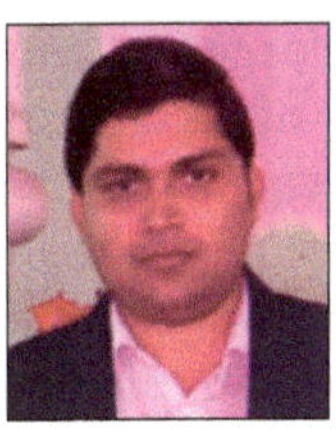

Dr Nitesh Singh Bhati received his doctorate from GGISP University, Delhi. He obtained his MTech in CSE and BTech in Computer Science and Engineering from the G.G.S.I.P. University Delhi. He is an Assistant Professor in the Department of Computer Science and Engineering of Delhi Technical Campus, UP, India. He has published various research papers in international journals and conferences. His current research area is information security.

Sama Bolog

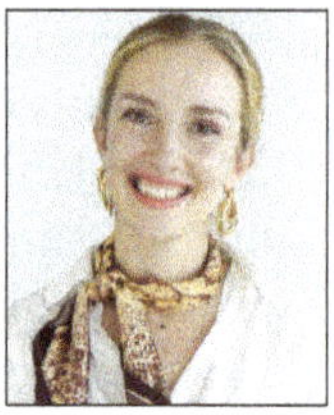

Sama Bolog has a background in law and holds two Master of Law Degrees. After graduating from the University of Basel with a magna cum laude, she pursued an LLM specializing in intellectual property and technology law at IE Law School in Madrid. This international background has enabled her to look beyond jurisdictions and offer broad legal advice. Besides her studies she worked for the IE Legal Clinic drafting an opinion for the Inter-American Court of Human Rights defending the rights of the indigenous people of Ecuador. Her passion for the law comes from her true desire to help others, especially in this fast developing digital world. She is particularly interested in protecting IP rights and personal data in a digital environment.

Arjun Chaudhary

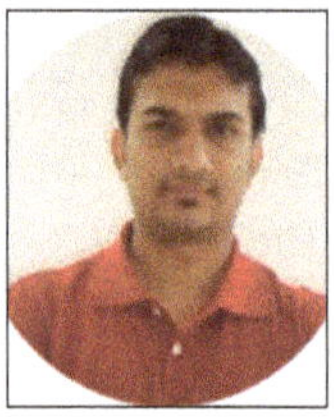

Lt Arjun Chaudhary has been an Assistant Professor with the Department of Cyber Security, Sardar Patel University of Police. He is Deputy Director at the Centre of Cyber Security, Sardar Patel University of Police, Security and Criminal Justice. His current research interests include cloud computing, web apps, and digital forensics. He has organized various international and national training programs for law enforcement agencies. He also has (co-) authored many journal/conference papers and book chapters.

Pushpa Choudhary

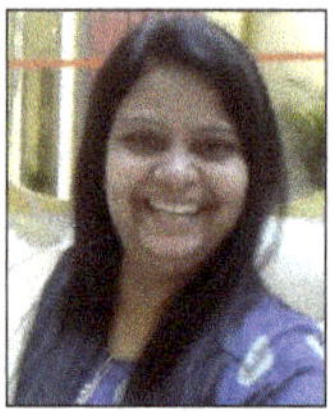

Professor Pushpa Choudhary received her PhD (in computer science) from MNNIT Allahabad in 2015, and an MTech (CS) from UPTU, Lucknow in 2007 along with an MCA degree in 2002 from Allahabad University. Currently, she is working as Professor and Head in the MCA Department of JSS Academy of Technical Education, Noida. She has worked as Professor and Head in various engineering colleges in computer science and information technology departments with more than 20 years of rich experience in teaching and research. She has published more than 50 research papers in international and national conferences and journals. She has organized many international conferences and technical events at institute levels.

Adiba Tabassum Chowdhury

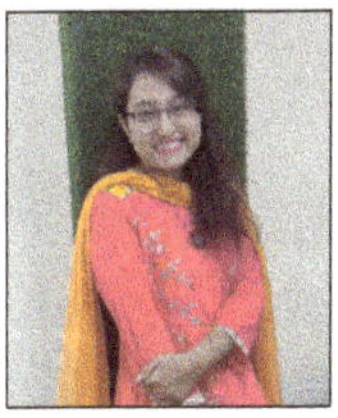

Adiba Tabassum Chowdhury has recently pursued a BSc in engineering from the Department of Electrical and Electronic Engineering at the University of Dhaka, Bangladesh. Her major was computers and the minor field she chose was communication. She is working full-time at Shikho Technologies, Bangladesh, and continues research work simultaneously. She would like to introduce herself as a communication and technology enthusiast. Her research fields are artificial intelligence (AI), IoT, machine learning, mobile cellular networks, etc. She has worked on several research projects with the collaboration of FabLab, University of Dhaka as a research assistant there. She was one of the ten representatives of Bangladesh in the Huawei Seeds for the Future 2020 program. She received training in AI, cloud computing, 5G technology, and HMS technology in that program. She always looks forward to taking part in competitions and challenging herself, as well as, improving herself with time.

Ajay Dagar

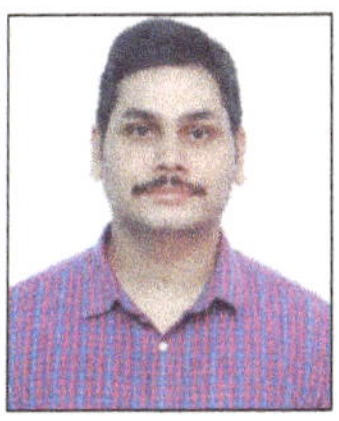

Dr Ajay Dagar, received his BTech in electronics and communication engineering from UPTU Lucknow, India in 2010 and an MTech in digital communication from IIITM Gwalior, India in 2012. He received his PhD in electrical engineering from the Department of Electrical Engineering, IIT Kanpur, India in July 2021. He is currently working as an Assistant Professor in the School of Electronics Engineering at VIT-AP University, Amaravati, India, having started in May 2022. Before joining VIT-AP, he was associated as Visiting Assistant Professor with the IIIT Sonepat, India from December 2021 to April 2022 and as an Assistant Professor with LPU Jalandhar, India from 2013 to 2014. His current research interests include acoustic signal processing, spatial audio processing and multi-zone sound reproduction methodologies in shared environments.

Ngoc Tung Dang

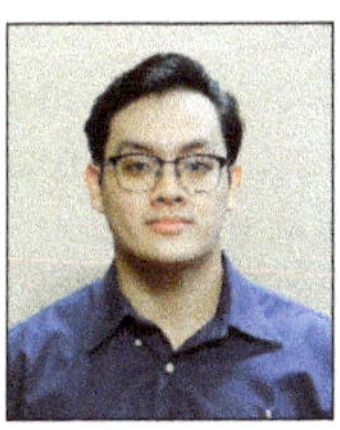

Mr Ngoc Tung Dang received his Bachelor in Biotechnology from International University, Vietnam National University of Ho Chi Minh City in 2022. Since 2019, he has been a member of the International University Medical Microbiology group, working in the field of nanomaterials against antimicrobial resistance. He is currently working at the microbiology laboratory in CJ Food Vietnam Food Safety Center.

Roopa Golchha

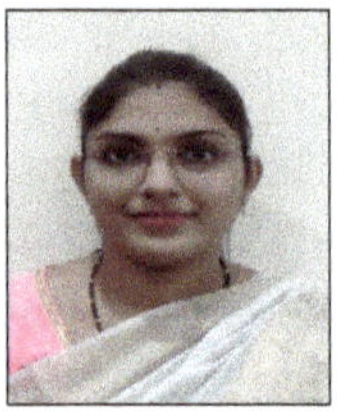

Mrs Roopa Golchha is pursuing a Master's in Information Technology from National Institute of Technology, Raipur, Chhattisgarh, India. She has completed her Bachelors in engineering in computer science and engineering from Bhilai Institute of Technology, Durg, Chhattisgarh, India, in 2013. Her main research interests are in the area of quantum computing, cryptography, Internet of Things, and information security.

René Iván González-Fernández

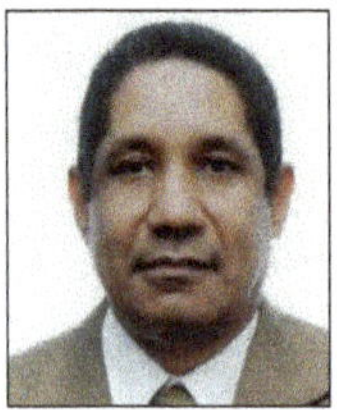

Professor René Iván González-Fernández received his BSE, MSc and PhD degrees from Technological University of Havana, Cuba, in 1982, 1986 and 1996, respectively. He joined Cuban Center for Neurosciences, 2018, and was designated as the Head of the Department of Neurostimulation. From March 1983 to April 2018, his scientific progress was remarkable, working as a researcher, head of projects, head of department and director of the Research Division at the Central Institute for Digital Research; obtaining highlighted results in software and medical devices development, mainly for cardiology and vital signs monitoring. Simultaneously, he was working as professor at the Informatics and Automation faculties of the Technological University of Havana, combining lecturing with the advising of PhD and MSc theses. He was honored as Academician of Merit of the Academy of Sciences of Cuba in 2018. His research interests include biomedical signal processing, development of medical devices, neurostimulation and new materials and technologies. Professor Gonzalez-Fernandez has authored/co-authored 102 publications in peer-reviewed scientific journals, book chapters and international conferences. He has been a member of the scientific committee of multiple pan American and world congress on biomedical engineering congresses. He is a member of the CORAL-IFMBE group, The Cuban Society of Bioengineering, the International Society of Electrophysiology and the Cuban Society of Bioengineering.

Kapil Gupta

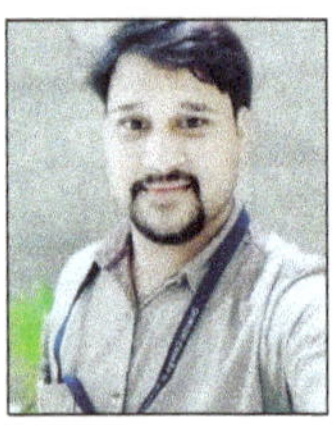

Kapil Gupta received his BE (Hons) degree in electronics and communication engineering from the Oriental Institute of Science and Technology, Bhopal, India, in 2011, and his MTech degree in nanotechnology from the School of Nanotechnology, Rajiv Gandhi Proudyogiki Vishwavidyalaya, Bhopal, in 2013. He is pursuing a PhD degree with the PDPM Indian Institute of Information Technology, Design, and Manufacturing (IIITDM), Jabalpur, Jabalpur, India. He was an Assistant Professor with the Oriental College of Technology, Bhopal, from 2013 to 2020. His research interests include biomedical signal processing, pattern recognition, machine learning, deep learning, time-frequency analysis, artificial intelligence, cardiovascular systems, and brain–computer interfaces. Mr Gupta is serving as an Active and Potential Technical Reviewer for IEEE, Elsevier, Springer, and several other reputed journals and conferences.

José Luis Hernández-Cáceres

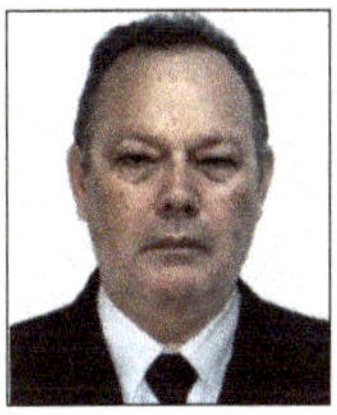

Professor José Luis Hernández-Cáceres received his BSc, MSc in Physico-Mathematical Sciences (Biophysics) from Moscow 'Lomonosov' University in 1979. His PhD dissertation on non-linear qEEG analysis was defended on 1996 at Havana University. He is a Senior Researcher at the Cuban Center for Neurosciences and a Full Professor at Havana Medical University. His experimental work includes, enzyme kinetics analysis of the Na, K-ATPase electrophysiological studies on isolated, perfused single neurons as well as with different experimental epilepsy models. His theoretical studies include a resonant recognition model for protein interactions, Hodgkin–Huxley-based modeling of membrane currents, epilepsy modeling, heart rate variability analysis, nonlinear analysis of photoplethysmography signals, nonlinear EEG and ECG analysis, as well as epidemic prediction, and modeling athletes' physical performance. He received six Cuban National Awards and Medals, and was appointed Professor at the Walter Sisulu university (South Africa, 2001–4) and at the University of The Gambia (2012–5). He was Associate Member (1995–2000) and Senior Associate (2004–7) of the International Center for Theoretical physics in Trieste (Italy). He is author/coauthor of more than 100 scientific papers (h-index = 14 with a total of 879 citations; and Research Interest Score = 374.7). He is a Member of the Steering Board of the Cuban Society for Neurosciences, and a Member of the Physiological Society of Southern Africa, as well as a Member of the Cuban Society for Medical Informatics.

Ruby Jain

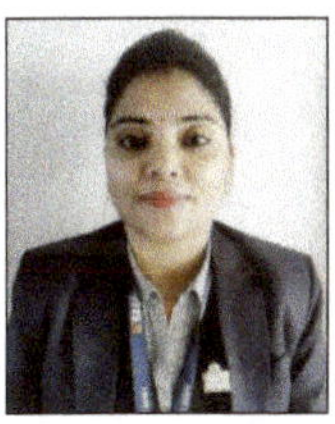

Mrs Ruby Jain, has an MTech received in VLSI design from RGPV University, a BE in electronics and communication engineering from RGPV University, in 2017 and 2011, respectively. She joined Malwa Institute of Science and Technology as a lecturer in 2012, working there between 18 April 2012 and 22 July 2019. She was faculty of engineering and after that she joined SAGE University, Indore in July 2019 as an Assistant Professor to date. Her research areas are in IoT and VLSI design, and she has published many research papers in high impact factor journals and has two Indian patents published and one copyright. She is a member of IFERP.

Daniel Jesus Jimenez-Gonzalez

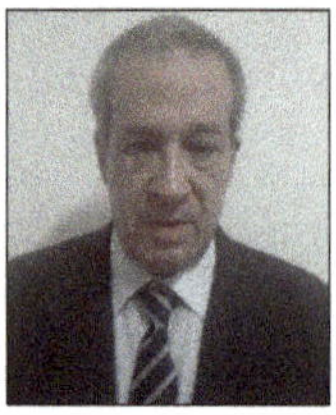

Professor Daniel Jesus Jimenez-Gonzalez received his BSE and MSc degrees from Technological University of Havana, and Medical Sciences University of Havana, in 1988 and 2014, respectively. He has been at Central Institute for Digital Research, from 1988 to the present, and was designated as the Head of the Department of Cardiology in 2021. Since September 1988, his scientific progress has been remarkable, working as a researcher, head of projects, head of department and Director of the Production Division at the Central Institute for Digital Research; obtaining highlighted results in hardware and firmware for medical devices developing, mainly for cardiology and vital signs monitoring. His research interests include biomedical signal processing, data compression algorithms for ECG signal, development of hardware for medical devices and development of very low power devices. Eng. Jimenez-Gonzalez has authored/co-authored seven publications in peer-reviewed scientific journals, book chapters and international conferences. He is a member of the CORAL-IFMBE group, and The Cuban Society of Bioengineering.

Apoorv Joshi

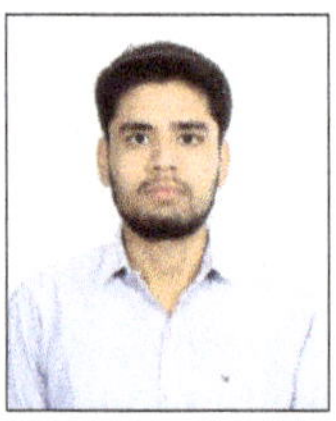

Mr Apoorv Joshi is pursuing a Master's in information technology from National Institute of Technology, Raipur, Chhattisgarh India. He received a BTech in Computer Science and Engineering from SDCET, Muzaffarnagar, UP, India, in 2019. His main research interests are in the area of blockchain, cyber security, Internet of Things and AI.

Samyak Kothari

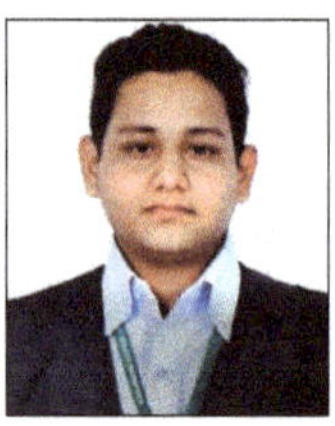

Mr Samyak Kothari, is currently a student pursuing his BTech in computer science and engineering from School of Engineering and Applied Sciences, Ahmedabad University, Ahmedabad, India, and will complete his graduation in the year 2023. He has completed his secondary (10th) from Mount Carmel High School, Gandhinagar and higher secondary education (12th) from Sahajanand School of Achiever, Gandhinagar in the years 2017 and 2019, respectively.

Alejandro Manuel López Reyes

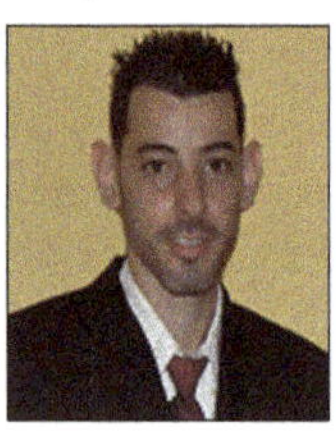

Mr Alejandro Manuel López Reyes, received his BSE from Technological University of Havana, Cuba, in 2013. Since September 2013, he has worked as a researcher at the Central Institute for Digital Research; obtaining highlighted results in software developing, mainly for cardiology and vital signs monitoring. His research interests include biomedical signal processing, development of medical software and new software technologies. Mr López Reyes has co-authored six publications in peer-reviewed scientific journals and international conferences. He is a member of the CORAL-IFMBE and the Cuban Society of Bioengineering

Bhoumik Mahajan

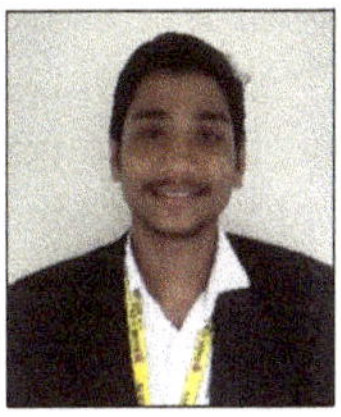

Mr Bhoumik Mahajan is currently pursuing a BTech in electronics and communication engineering from sage university Indore India. I have been a member of the institute of electronics and telecommunication engineers. And I also compete in national level athletics games.

Anto Manuel

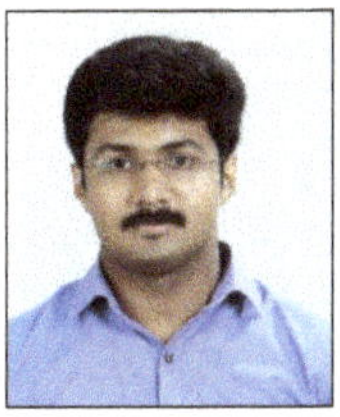

Mr Anto Manuel is a doctoral student at the Indian Institute of Technology Goa. After earning his MTech from the same university in 2015 with a focus on VLSI and embedded systems, he started working with Simstream India Pvt Ltd as a research and development officer. In 2016, he joined Electronics and Communication Engineering Department at St. Joseph's College of Engineering and Technology in Palai, Kerala, India as an assistant professor. His research interests are biosensors, wearable tech, the Internet of Things, biomedical system advancements, real-time instrumentation systems, sensor design, biological actuators, telemetry, AI in biomedical applications, and VLSI design.

Gisela Montes de Oca Colina

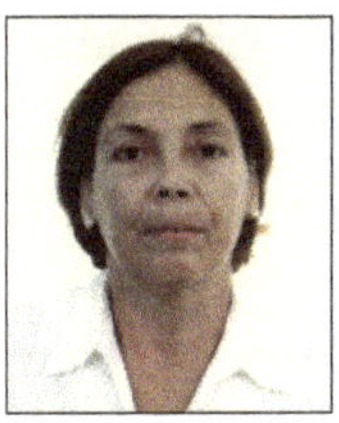

Mrs Gisela Montes de Oca-Colina received her BSE degree from University of Havana, Cuba in 1986, and MSc degree from Medical Sciences University of Havana, Cuba, in 2014. Since September 1983, she has worked as a researcher and project leader developing for medical systems and devices, most of them related to cardiology, at the Central Institute for Digital Research. Her research interests include biomedical signal processing, embedded Linux-based systems, development of medical devices and telemedicine. Her work results were selected as scientific achievements of the Cuban Academy of Sciences. Montes de Oca-Colina has authored/co-authored 24 publications in peer-reviewed scientific journals and international conferences. She is a member of the CORAL-IFMBE group and the Cuban Society of Bioengineering.

Abu Jaffor Morshedul Abedin

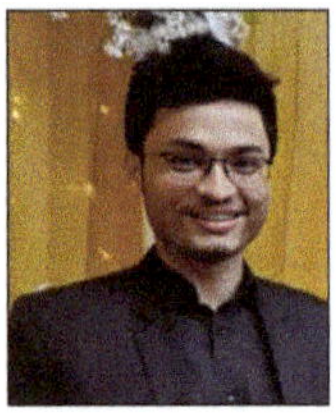

Abu Jaffor Morshedul Abedin has lately received a BSc in engineering from the Department of Electrical and Electronic Engineering, University of Dhaka, Bangladesh. He chose computing as a major and power as a minor while studying engineering. Having a keen interest in technology, his research interests lie in machine learning, artificial intelligence, and IoT-based intelligent systems. He has worked on a few research projects based on machine learning, and IoT while studying in the final year where some of those were in collaboration with FabLab, University of Dhaka. He received a professional certificate from Coursera in DeepLearning.AI TensorFlow Developer Professional Certificate and is currently pursuing a professional certificate in Google UX Design Professional Certificate and IBM software development. He always awaits the opportunity to participate in competitions and exert himself along with flourishing steadily.

Margarita Lucia Mulet-Cartaya

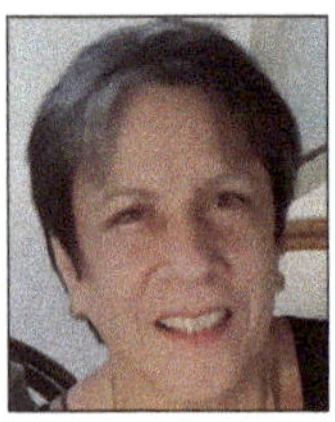

Professor Margarita Lucia Mulet-Cartaya received his BS and MSc degrees from University of Havana, Cuba, in 1984 and 1999, respectively. She has been working for the Central Digital Research Institute since she was graduated. Her main activities have been as a researcher and head of research project in groups focused on process automation and development of medical devices, mainly for vital signs monitoring. Simultaneously, she has been working as professor at the University of Informatics Sciences of Havana, advising graduated theses and researching projects. Her research interests include biomedical signal processing, development of medical devices and telemedicine systems. Professor Mulet-Cartaya has authored/co-authored 46 publications in peer-reviewed scientific journals, book chapters and international conferences. She is a member of the CORAL-IFMBE group and the Cuban Society of Bioengineering.

Cuong Nguyen

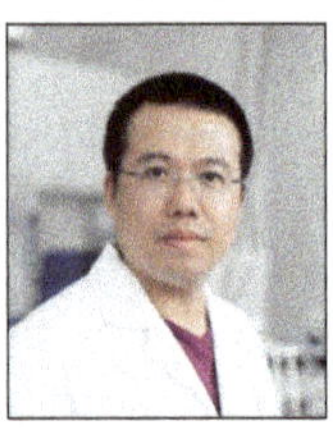

Dr Cuong Nguyen received his PhD degree in physics from Chungbuk National University, Cheongju, Korea in 2009. He joined the SnM department of the Institute of Information Technology (IoIT), Vietnam Academy of Science and Technology (VAST) as a researcher in 2009. In 2013, he moved to the Institute of Biotechnology, VAST, and established a Bioinformatic Laboratory where he is the head. In 2017, he moved to the private sector and established a new Bioinformatic Laboratory of Vinmec Healthcare system, the biggest private healthcare system in Vietnam. After four years, he moved back to IoIT, VAST where he is currently a main investigator. Dr Cuong Nguyen has authored/co-authored 23 publications in peer-reviewed journals. Dr Cuong Nguyen served as General Chair of the Organization Committee of The 2nd and 3rd Vinmec International Conference on Cell and Gene Therapy (VCGT2018 and VCGT2019). He is a member of the Vietnam Medical Genetic Association, Vietnam Stem Cell Therapy Association.

Thi Thu Hoai Nguyen

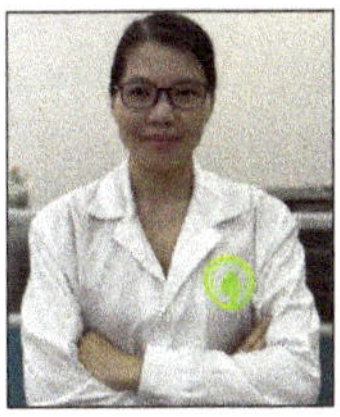

Professor Thi Thu Hoai Nguyen obtained her PhD degree from Greifswald University, Germany in Biomedical Sciences in 2008 and did her postdoctoral research in Louvain Drug Research Institute, UCL, Belgium and National Institute of Allergy and Infectious Diseases, NIH, USA. Professor Hoai Nguyen is working in the field of antimcrobial resistance and vaccine development. She is author/co-author of more than 60 national and international publications. Professor Hoai Nguyen is now Vice Director of the Research Center for Infectious Diseases, International University, Vietnam National University of Ho Chi Minh City.

Anand Bhushan Pandey

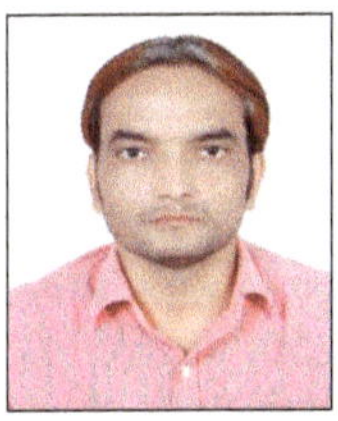

Professor Anand Bhushan Pandey has an MTech in computer science and engineering and a BTech in information technology. He has a 12+ years of teaching experience in different reputed engineering institutes. Currently, he is working as an Assistant Professor in the Department of Information Technology at G L Bajaj Institute of Technology and Management, Greater Noida, India. His current research is concerned with artificial intelligence, machine learning and Internet of Things.

Nikhil Kumar Parida

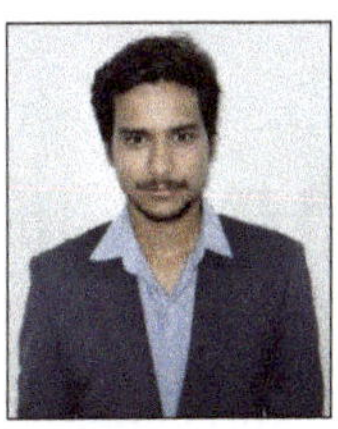

Mr Nikhil Kumar Parida, is an MTech scholar from Department of IT, NIT Raipur, he has received his BTech in computer science engineering, from Amity School of Engineering and Technology, Delhi affiliated to GGSIPU University. He has published a paper on hyper spectral imaging, and is currently working in many different interesting areas of computer science. He has immense research interest in the field of quantum computing, blockchain, data structures and complexity theory.

Antonio Miguel Pesqueira

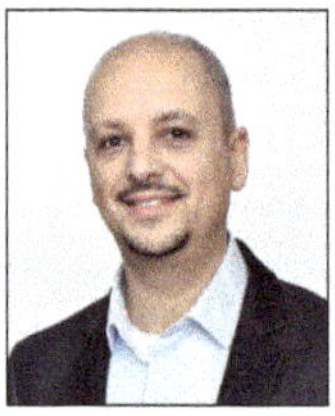

Antonio Miguel Pesqueira (MSc in Innovation Management), a healthcare commercial leader specializing in life sciences, is a university professor and a research fellow at ISCTE/IUL. The current areas of his research interest are digital technologies, healthcare data management, and blockchain, as well as innovation and business management. Being the last chair of the Pharmaceutical Supply Chain and Security World Forum and a regular keynote speaker at the Pharma Track and Trace, Serialization and Labeling Summit are among his other activities.

In addition to co-authoring more than 20 articles and book chapters, Antonio has published in several scientific journals (such as *Journal of Business Research*, *Future Generations Computer Systems*, *Journal of Medical Systems*, *Knowledge Management*, *WSEAS Transactions on Business and Economics*, *Information Systems Frontiers*, and others) as well as peer-reviewed international conferences.

Furthermore, he holds a certification in data science and in agile coaching.

Bidan Pramanick

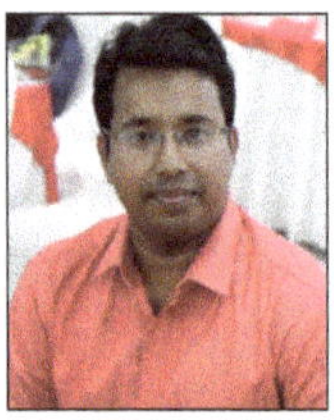

Dr Bidan Pramanick received BTech and MTech in electronics and communication engineering from Kalyani Government Engineering College, Kalyani, India, in 2005 and 2007, respectively, and obtained a PhD from the Indian Institute of Technology Kharagpur (IIT Kharagpur), India, in 2012. He has worked for more than two years as Assistant Professor in Indian Institute of Space Science and Technology, India and two years as Professor Postdoc in Tecnologico de Monterrey, Mexico in collaboration with University of California, Irvine, CA, USA. He is currently working at IIT Goa as an Assistant Professor. He has authored or co-authored more than 50 papers in international journals and conference proceedings, four book chapters and three books. His current research interests include MEMS-based drug delivery, carbon MEMS/NEMS devices, sensors, CD-based disease diagnostics and electrochemical biosensors. Dr Pramanick was a recipient of the CSIR SRF Fellowship (India) for his Doctoral Programme and Awarded with CONACYT Candidate level by Science and Technology department, Mexico (2016).

Mehedi Hasan Raju

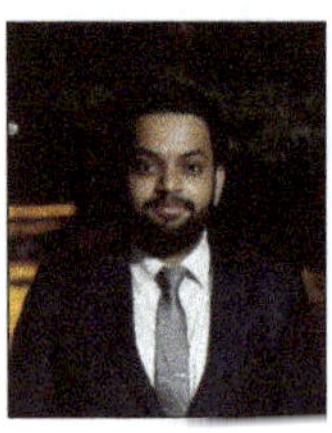

Mehedi Hasan Raju is a PhD student at Texas State University. He completed his BSc from Department of Information and Communication Technology, Bangladesh University of Professionals, Dhaka. His research interests include eye movements, biometrics, machine learning and signal processing.

Mridu Sahu

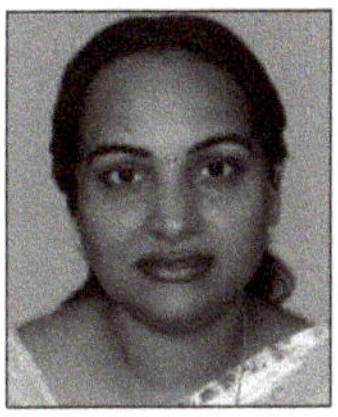

Dr Mridu Sahu received a degree in computer science and engineering from the Maulana Azad National Institute of Technology, Bhopal, in 2004, Master of technology in computer science and engineering from RIT Raipur, Raipur, India, in 2011, and PhD in computer science and engineering from the National Institute of Technology at Raipur, Raipur, in 2018. She has more than ten years' experience in teaching. She is working as an Assistant Professor with the Department of Information Technology, NIT Raipur. She has published more than 25 research articles in various journals and conferences and book chapters in the field of data mining, brain–computer interface, sensor devices, and visual mining techniques.

Hiba Shakeel

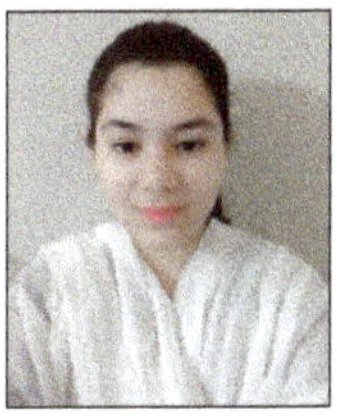

Hiba Shakeel received her bachelor's and master's degree in computer science and applications from Aligarh Muslim University, Aligarh, India, in 2017 and 2020, respectively. Her research interests include load balancing, cloud computing, fog computing, and IoT.

Palanivel Rajan Selvakumaran

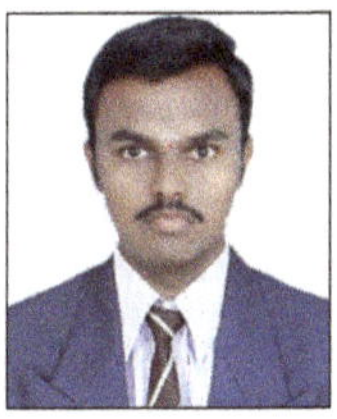

Dr Palanivel Rajan Selvakumaran is currently working as Professor and Head, Department of Electronics and Communication Engineering, M. Kumarasamy College of Engineering, Karur, Tamilnadu, India. He completed his PhD in Faculty of Information and Communication Engineering, Anna University Chennai, India, ME in communication systems, Thiagarajar College of Engineering, Madurai, Tamilnadu, India, BE in electronics and communication engineering, from Raja College of Engineering and Technology, Madurai, Tamilnadu, India. He is recognized as among the top 2% Scientists Worldwide Listed by Elsevier BV, Stanford University and also recognized as top Scientists Worldwide Listed by AD Scientific Index 2022. He is an Executive Editor, Editor-in-Chief, Editorial Board Member and also acts as reviewer in many SCI, SCIE and SCOPUS indexed journals. He has presented more than 55 technical papers in various international/national conferences. He has also published more than 45 research articles in various SCI, SCIE, SCOPUS and other refereed journals. In addition to his credit, he holds 12 patents (of which five were granted) based on his research work. He has received 'Best Article Reviewer Award' from a few SCOPUS journals. His individual 'Google Scholar H-Index is 22' and 'SCOPUS H-index is 12'. He is an authorized PhD Research Supervisor of Anna University Chennai, has guided three PhD scholars and is guiding eight PhD research scholars. His research interests include antennas, bio-signal processing, electrocardiography, telemedicine/telemetry, wireless networks and wireless communication. He is an active life member of ISTE, IE (I), IACSIT, ITE, IAAA, IAMI, TSI, BMESI, ISRD, IAENG and IETE.

Miss Hiral Rajivkumar Shah

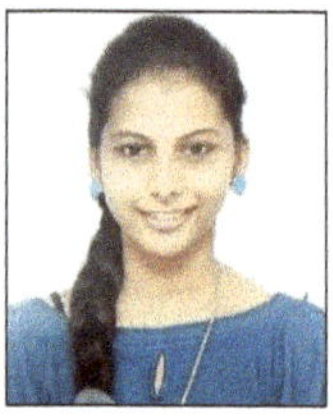

Miss Hiral Rajivkumar Shah, is currently a student pursuing her BTech in computer science and engineering from School of Engineering and Applied Sciences, Ahmedabad University, Ahmedabad and will complete her graduation in the year 2023. She completed her secondary (10th) and higher secondary education (12th) from St. Francis of Assisi Convent High School in 2017 and 2019, respectively.

Jash Shah

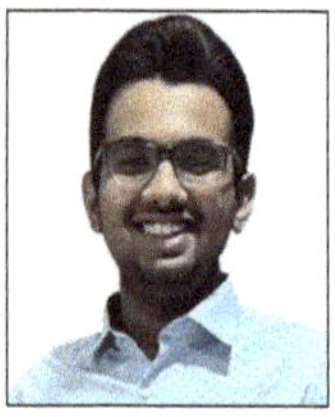

Mr Jash Shah, is currently a student pursuing his BTech in computer science and engineering from School of Engineering and Applied Sciences, Ahmedabad University, Ahmedabad and will complete his graduation in the year 2023. He completed his secondary (10th) from Bhulka Bhavan School and higher secondary education (12th) from Citizen School in 2017 and 2019, respectively.

Manan Shah

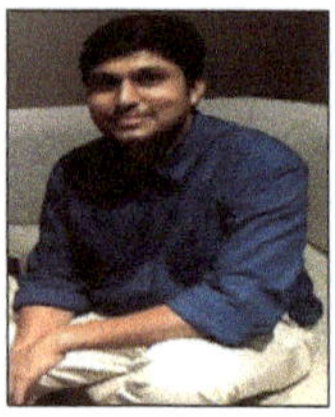

Dr Manan Shah studies a BE in chemical engineering from LD College of Engineering and MTech in Petroleum Engineering from School of Petroleum Technology, PDPU. He has completed his PhD in the area of exploration and exploitation of geothermal energy in the state of Gujarat. He is currently working as an assistant professor in Department of Chemical Engineering, School of Technology (SOT), PDPU, and he has published several articles in reputed international journals in the area of many sectors. He serves as an active reviewer for several reputable international journal publishers like Springer and Elsevier. Dr Shah is a young and dynamic academician and researcher in the various engineering fields. Dr Shah has received the best paper award for world's second best journal.

Manish Sharma

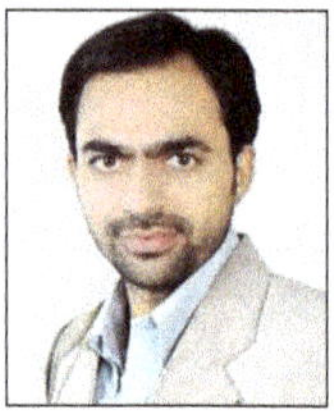

Dr Manish Sharma did a PhD at IIT, Bombay, in electrical engineering. He received the 'excellence in the PhD research work' (Best PhD thesis) award for his outstanding research contributions at IIT, Bombay, in 2015. He has been listed in the world's top 2% of scientists in a study carried out by Stanford University USA for two consecutive years (2019 and 2020). His research paper received the 'Honors Paper' award in recognition of outstanding work published in the SCI-indexed Elsevier journal *Computers in Biology* in 2018. He was a postdoctoral fellow at

IIT, Indore, during 2016–7. In June 2018, he was awarded the 'ERCIM' Alain Bensoussan Fellowship of the European Union for doing research work at the Norwegian University of Science and Technology (NTNU), Norway. He has been working as a faculty member in the Department of Electrical and Computer Science Engineering at IITRAM, Ahmedabad, India, An Autonomous University Established by the Government of Gujarat. He has more than 70 publications in reputed journals and conferences, of which 29 are h-indexed and 49 are i-10 indexed (Google Scholar, September 2022). His research includes machine learning, healthcare data analytics, signal processing, and the science of spirituality.

Priya Sharma

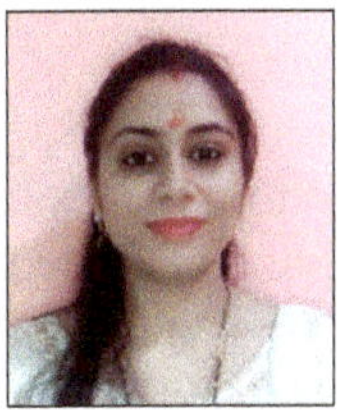

Priya Sharma is pursuing her PhD from the Gautam Buddha University Greater Noida. She obtained her MTech in CSE and BTech in computer science and engineering from the Galgotia University Greater Noida and Uttar Pradesh Technical University Lucknow, respectively. She is working as an Assistant Professor in the Department of Computer Science and Engineering of Delhi Technical Campus, UP, India. She has published various research papers in international journals and conferences. Her current research area is information security and IoT.

Rajeev Sharma

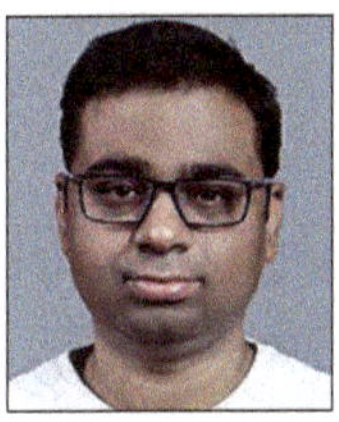

Dr Rajeev Sharma received his BE in electronics and communication engineering from RGPV Bhopal, India in 2009 and MTech from National Institute of Technology (NIT) Warangal, India in 2011. He received a PhD in the discipline of electrical engineering from Indian Institute of Technology (IIT) Indore, India in 2017. He is currently working as Sr Assistant Professor in the School of Electronics Engineering (SENSE) at VIT-AP University at Amaravati, AP India. His research interests include biomedical signal processing, image processing, speech processing, machine learning, and computer vision.

Arun Kumar Singh

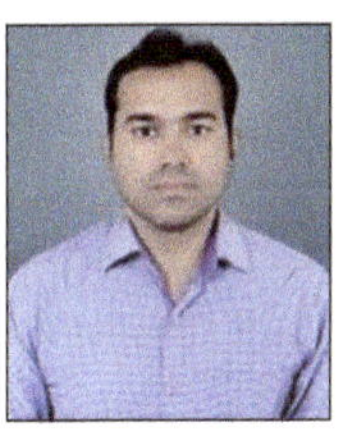

Dr Arun Kumar Singh, received his BTech from Uttar Pradesh Technical University Lucknow, Uttar Pradesh, Master's in information security from Indian Institute of Information Technology, Allahabad (IIITA), and PhD in computer science and engineering from Motilal Nehru National Institute of Technology Allahabad (MNNIT-Allahabad), Uttar Pradesh, India, in 2005, 2008 and 2015, respectively. His research interests are cyber security, cryptography, machine learning, Internet of Things (IoT), and computer forensics. Dr Arun has authored/co-authored many research papers and book chapters.

Uday Pratap Singh

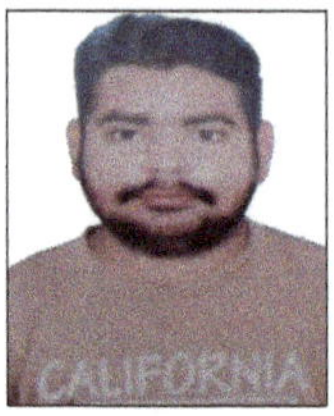

Mr Uday Pratap Singh is working toward a Master's in information technology, National Institute of Technology, Raipur, India. He earned his mastered scholarship position as a talented student. His research interests are network security like intrusion detection systems, malware detection system, Internet of Things, machine learning, deep learning, blockchain security architectures and privacy-preservation technique.

Abirami Tamilarasu

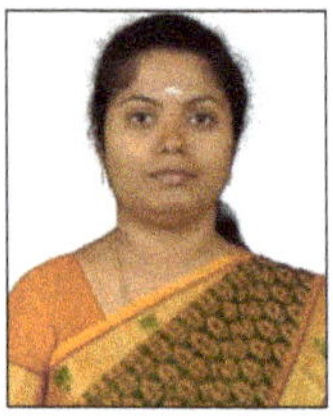

Abirami Tamilarasu is currently working as Assistant Professor, Department of Electronics and Communication Engineering, M. Kumarasamy College of Engineering, Karur, Tamilnadu, India. She is doing a PhD in Faculty of Information and Communication Engineering, Anna University Chennai, India. She has completed an ME in communication systems from M. Kumarasamy College of Engineering, Karur, Tamilnadu, India. She has completed a BE in electronics and communication engineering from Nandha Engineering College, Erode, Tamilnadu, India. She has presented 10 papers in various national/international conferences around Tamilnadu. She has published 12 research articles in Scopus and Web of Science indexed journals. Her research area includes biomedical, image processing, wireless communication, biotelemetry. She is an active member of IAENG and SWIDC.

Ashish Tripathi

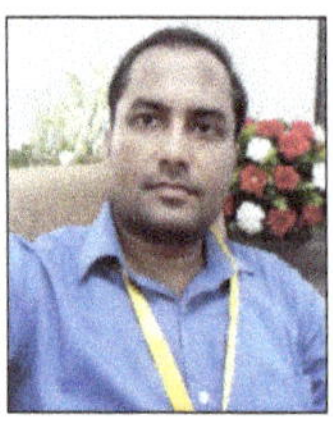

Dr Ashish Tripathi, PhD, received his MCA degree in computer applications from Sikkim Manipal University, East Sikkim, India, and MTech and PhD in computer science and engineering from Motilal Nehru National Institute of Technology Allahabad, Prayagraj, India. He has 12+ years of working experience in Industry and Academia. He has worked with many organizations. Since May 2018, he has been working as an Associate Professor in the Department of Information Technology. G L Bajaj Institute of Technology and Management, Greater Noida, affiliated to Dr A P J Abdul Kalam Technical University, Uttar Pradesh, India. His research interest includes optimization techniques, evolutionary computation, machine learning, deep learning, cloud computing, and software engineering. He has published more than 12 papers in high-impact factor and peer-reviewed journals (SCI/SCOPUS/WOS). He has written 14 book chapters and published 10 patents on different real-world problems. He has presented more than 40 papers in international and national conferences.

Chapter 1

IoT-based continuous cardiac monitoring system

Kapil Gupta, Varun Bajaj and Irshad Ahmad Ansari

As we saw in recent times, the deadly coronavirus has severely affected those who had been earlier diagnosed with cardiovascular diseases (CVDs). The fact is, if we look at the number of people who died due to coronavirus, the majority of them will be heart patients. The current death rate due to CVD is 5.6% in India and 32% worldwide. Research suggests that death can be avoided if proper detection is made in time. In the modern era, the Internet of Things (IoT) is shifting the technology infrastructure functions. Cardiac health monitoring is one of the prominent applications of IoT. This work proposes an IoT-based wearable cardiac healthcare system to prevent CVDs using continuous monitoring of electrocardiogram (ECG) signals and heart rate. An Arduino UNO, AD8232 sensor, an HC05 Bluetooth module, and Android mobile are used to design the proposed system. The key feature of the presented system is to provide timely intervention and 24 h improved monitoring for cardiac patients, thereby enhancing clinical services for such patients. In case of any fluctuation in the ECG pattern and heart rate of the patient, an alert message can be sent to the personal doctors or relatives about the patient's condition using the presented IoT-based system.

1.1 Introduction

The term 'cardiovascular diseases' (CVDs) refers to a wide range of blood vessel and heart disorders, that are the main root of mortality worldwide [1]. In 2019, 32% of all mortality was due to CVDs, causing the deaths of 17.9 million individuals. 85% of these fatalities were due to strokes and heart attacks. Almost 75% of CVD fatalities occur in middle and low-income nations [2]. The major cause of CVDs is a deposition of fatty plaques on the inner walls of arteries that supply the blood to the heart or brain [1]. Strokes and heart attacks are typically sudden events, that are caused by an obstruction that prohibits blood from flowing to the brain or heart. Blood bleeding or clotting from a blood vein in the cerebral region may be the cause of strokes [3]. Patients with cardiac disorders typically stay at home and seek medical

doi:10.1088/978-0-7503-5311-3ch1

assistance if they feel problems. The majority of the time, people do not begin to feel sick until the disease has severely affected the heart tissues, and the damage has already become irreparable. Furthermore, the majority of patients pass away before receiving any medical attention. Therefore, transforming the passive healthcare model into a widespread approach is crucial to improving heart disease healthcare performance and lowering the death rate. It follows that doctors should keep an eye on their patients' physical conditions and make decisions on when to provide healthcare based on the patient's actual situation. Real-time monitoring is an important feature of this pervasive healthcare approach. In the present era, when every physical thing can be connected to another to share information. IoT will be essential to this paradigm change in which things and systems become 'smart.' IoT-based systems allow for the monitoring of major human activities regardless of where they are or what they are doing. IoT is facilitating development of many complicated systems such as intelligent traffic control mechanisms, smart home appliances, intelligent office frameworks, smart environments, vehicles, and temperature control systems, among others, in very small spaces by providing effortless interaction between various modules [4]. IoT is currently a highly researched technology field. Nowadays, sensors are employed in practically every industry, from industrial monitoring systems to everyday products. IoT and sensor-based solutions for continuous monitoring of human health are the most extensively used [5]. The adoption of IoT-based e-health solutions has caused a notable revolution in the field of health management because they make it possible to monitor and collect patient data in real time and to improve clinical services, interventions, and treatments. IoT makes our lives easier, more effective, and more intelligent. Additionally, the recorded signals can be easily transmitted to distant doctors, assuring that these physicians are always and in real-time aware of the physical status of patients. Future cellular technologies will enable a wide range of applications and use instances that, among other things, will alter how devices connect in the health, energy, transportation, and environmental sectors. Due to the prevalence of mobile internet use nowadays, it is now relatively simple to combine mobile internet with an open-source Android health service system [6]. Continuous recording and monitoring of the electrocardiogram (ECG) signal of a CVD patient may help to provide timely treatment to save the life of an individual. Hybridization of IoT and ECG acquisition systems may provide easy access to the medical specialist to provide detailed analysis and proper treatment at the remote location. ECG has recently become a more prominent tool and easily accessible service to provide the diagnosis of various health problems. The functionality of the heart can be accurately determined by ECG signals. It is the combination of tiny electrical impulses produced by the cardiac muscle [7]. With the use of a smart device, medical professionals and patients may monitor the heart rate continually, gather crucial information, and take the necessary precautions to avoid severe harm. The number of beats in a minute is defined as the heart rate, and sometimes it's also denoted as the body pulse rate. A normal adult's pulse rate varies from 60 to 100 beats/minute. Males typically have a pulse rate of 70 beats/minute, whereas females typically have a pulse rate of 75 beats/minute. Heart rates in women above the age of 12 are higher than in men. Due to damage to the body, heart, and exercise, the rate alters throughout the disease. To assess one's health, heart rate is crucial. Hence, in this chapter, we present an IoT-based wearable system to prevent CVDs by continuous monitoring of cardiac health using ECG signals and the heart rate of a subject. This system continuously monitors, acquires, and transfers the ECG signals of a CVD patient to provide timely medical services. A sample prototype is also implemented to provide an overview of the system. This surveillance system meets the prerequisites for extensive healthcare for cardiovascular issues while also taking cost into account to ensure that the broad mode is as cost-effective as possible. Additionally, our developed technique is utilized in combination with real-time analysis tools to evaluate patients' health states and offer prior warnings of upcoming hazards, which can improve the intelligence of pervasive healthcare. The remainder of this chapter is arranged as follows. In section 1.2, related works will be described, and section 1.3 will provide three illustrations of the system, including its architecture, data acquisition, and data transmission components. The prototype implementation is provided in section 1.4. Conclusions and further research directions are presented in section 1.5.

1.2 Related works

Inadequacies in traditional healthcare services are becoming more obvious as the population of both older persons and patients with chronic diseases increases quickly. The most important one is that medical services are only provided in hospitals, which is difficult for old or disabled individuals, and unable to fulfill patient needs in an emergency. To overcome this obstacle and provide healthcare to everyone, everywhere, and always, the IoT-based healthcare concept is proposed. Numerous applications for IoT-based ubiquitous e-health systems have been developed in recent years. In [8], the authors presented an IoT-based system for the monitoring of CVD patients using the Hidden Markov Model (HMM) and ECG sensors. Various applications of IoT-based health monitoring systems have been reviewed by [9]. Krishnan *et al* [10] present an IoT-based system for the monitoring of individual health. They used heartbeat and temperature sensors to continually monitor the health of patients suffering from cardiac abnormalities. In [11], the authors proposed an IoT-based CVDs surveillance system for ubiquitous healthcare services. Their developed system sends physiological signals obtained from the patients to healthcare workers for providing service in real time. The authors of references [12, 13] used IoT to monitor ECG signals in real time and indicate the problems associated with real-time signal recording and transmission using the internet. ECG signals from a patient in an IoT environment—which could be non-clinical—transmit in real time to a particular hospital or clinic through the internet. The obtained signals were processed to appropriately portray the characteristics of the ECG signal before use and to extract certain necessary features (such as wavelet coefficients). The patient's location was, however, difficult to determine because of the persistence of signal acquisition. Authors of references [14–16] used an intelligent telemonitoring system that utilized wireless ECG data to diagnose CVD. To estimate user activity, position, and proxy server, as well as to make rules that are sent to the network router, the authors in [17] developed an optimized rule placement strategy to estimate the path of the user's location from the viewpoints of software-defined networking. Automatic classification of biomedical signals also plays a vital role to diagnose various diseases. Various deep learning networks are proposed in the literature to classify the signals and detect the types of abnormalities. In [18], the authors proposed a novel technique to detect sleep apnea using ECG signals. They used Gabor transform to convert ECG signals into 2D time–frequency (T–F) images and employed an S-G filter to smooth the obtained T–F images. They classified obtained smoothed images using three different convolutional neural networks (CNNs). Their developed architecture OSACN-Net attained a higher accuracy. Ballistocardiogram (BCG) signals have been classified to detect hypertension by Gupta *et al* [19]. They extracted the J-peaks of input BCG signals by employing the Pan–Tompkins algorithm and applied three different T–F toolboxes to evacuate 2D spectrograms. For the accurate detection of hypertension, the authors proposed a novel deep learning model namely, Hyp-Net. In [20], the author proposed an improved deep CNN framework for the detection of bundle-branch blocks using vector-cardiogram signals. These developed networks could be interfacing units to detect health abnormalities automatically over the internet. In summary, the monitoring system is an important component of the online healthcare service. Data accuracy in health applications is essential to overall performance and may even have a direct impact on patient lives. Therefore, this research provides a novel approach that enables monitoring of cardiac health while continuously communicating over widely available wireless network protocols and facilitating data-driven research for further enhancements.

The major contributions of this work are summarized as follows:

- Facilitate data-driven research and analysis like health history tracking, machine learning, and artificial intelligence for the prediction of cardiac arrest or health recommendations based on patterns found in big data collected over time.
- Lightweight and minimal hardware that can be easily embedded in apparel or wearables.
- Enablement of health data collection.
- Preventive/proactive approach against CVDs.

1.3 Proposed IoT-based system

The AD8232 sensor, which uses little power and reduces noise, is used to amplify the ECG signal once it is collected by placing electrodes on the body part. Arduino Uno receives the sensor's output signal on its analog pin and then transmits it over Bluetooth to an Android smartphone. With the help of the internet, recorded ECG signals are transmitted to the cloud server, where the signals are stored and a fixed heart rate threshold level is compared with the acquired signal. If any abnormalities are found, an alert message is sent to the patient, hospitals, and the patient's relatives. The proposed IoT-based system architecture is depicted in figure 1.1.

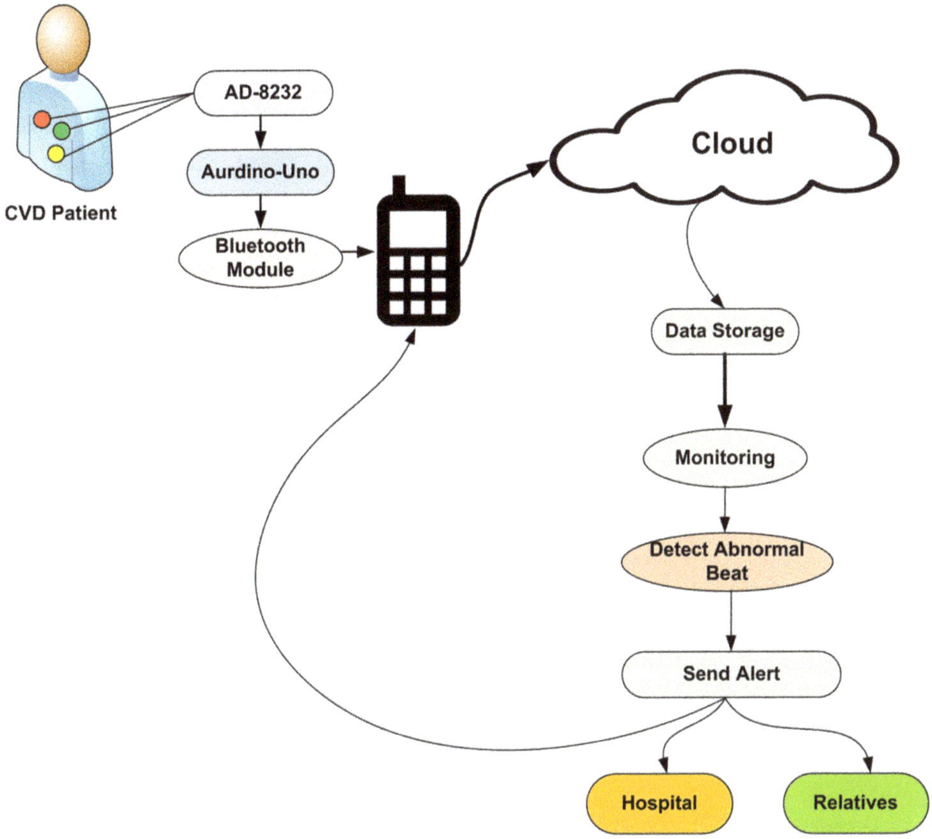

Figure 1.1. Proposed IoT-based system architecture.

1.3.1 ECG and its medical significance

The human body is continually producing bio-electrical impulses that include information about our health. This information can be measured and recorded using physiological instruments that measure various biomedical signals/data, such as an ECG. ECG represents a time and spatial summation of action potentials generated by millions of cardiac cells and defines different electrical stages of a cardiac cycle. It is a popular and crucial biomedical signal that contains vital information about the heart and aids in the diagnosis and prevention of various cardiac problems. The signals can be stored as digital data for further processing in various therapeutic applications [21]. ECG acquisition systems typically use 3, 6, or 12-lead or electrode-based sensors to record or monitor real-time signals. In this work, three-lead sensors are used to capture the data.

1.3.2 ECG electrodes

In the proposed system, to reduce the size and complexity, three-lead electrodes have been employed in place of 12-lead electrode systems and the bulk device. Disposable

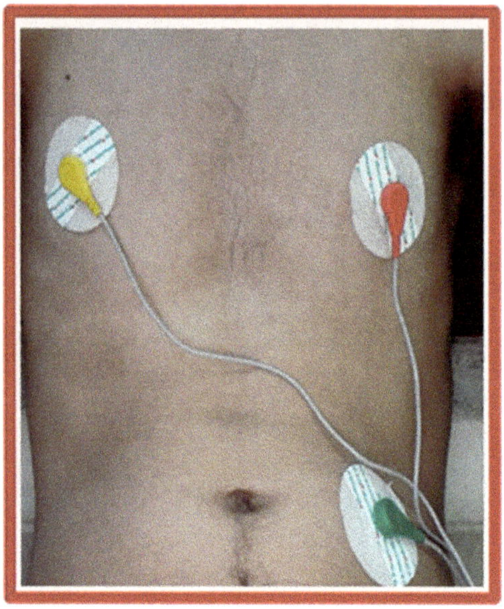

Figure 1.2. Schematic view of ECG electrode placement.

dry electrodes are used to design this presented system. These electrodes are the alternative to reusable or wet electrodes and offer more hygienic, fast, and easy recordings [22]. Figure 1.2 depicts the placement of electrodes on the right side of the heart (Y-Yellow), the left side of the heart (R-Red), and (G-Green) nearer to the stomach.

1.3.3 AD8232 ECG acquisition board

The AD8232 ECG sensor is a cost-effective, small, sensitive, professional board consisting of a right leg drive amplifier, an instrumentation amplifier, a mid-supply reference buffer, and an operational amplifier. The AD8232 also has circuitry for recognizing leads that have been disconnected, as well as an automatic fast reinstate circuit that quickly restores the signal. This board is used to record the tiny electrical impulses of the human heart. The result of this process is an analog reading, that can be plotted like an ECG signal. The AD8232 sensor functions similarly to an operational amplifier to help in acquiring a clear signal from the intervals quickly. In addition to other biopotential measurement applications, the AD8232 sensor is employed for signal conditioning in ECGs. The major function of this device is to amplify, retrieve, and filter biopotential signals that are weak in noisy environments, such as those created by replacing a remote electrode and moving an object [23]. It is built using a high-quality chip. It can be used to improve fitness, perform cardiac exercises, and monitor heart rate. It can be utilized as a handheld ECG or to monitor heart rate remotely. It is also useful to aid in the diagnosis of certain heart diseases. The board can be easily configured to any controller like Raspberry Pi, Arduino, and MSP430. Figure 1.3 represents the sensor module.

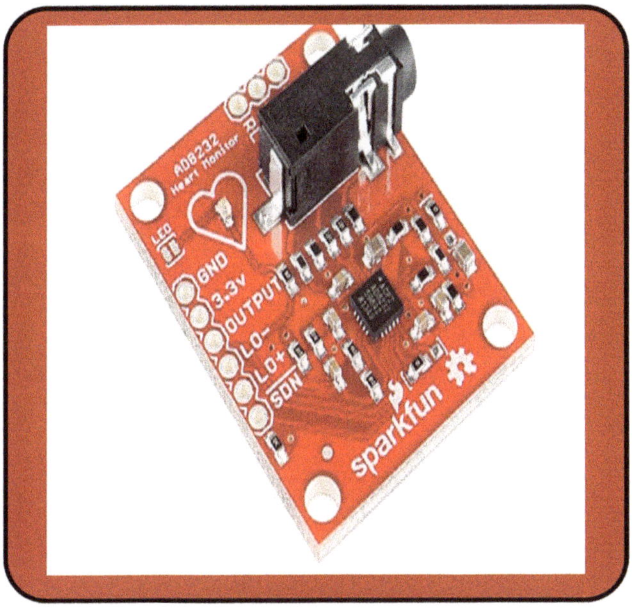

Figure 1.3. Schematic of AD8232 sensor.

1.3.4 Arduino UNO module

The module was designed by Arduino. cc and was initially released in 2010. It is an open-source microchip, that is based on the ATmega328P microcontroller. This board has six analog pins, 14 digital input/output pins, a 16 MHz ceramic resonator, a USB connection, a power jack, an ICSP header, and a reset button. Figure 1.4 represents the Arduino UNO module.

It comes with everything required to operate the microcontroller; to get started, simply attach a USB cable to connect it to a computer, or an AC-to-DC adapter or 9 sV battery to power it. It is programmed with open-source Arduino software. An embedded bootloader on the board's ATmega328 enables the upload of new code without the need for an external hardware programmer. This board operates at 5 V and can handle voltages ranging from 7 V to 20 V. It offers a max clock frequency of 20 MHz. Several sets of digital and analog input/output (I/O) pins are included on the board, allowing it to be interfaced with other circuits and expansion boards (shields).

1.3.5 HC-05 Bluetooth module

The HC-05 module is used in numerous applications, including wireless keyboards, mice, headsets, and game controllers. It has a range of up to 100 m, according to the source and destination, environment, and topographical and urban settings. It is a protocol established by IEEE 802.15.1 that can be used to establish a wireless Personal Area Network (PAN). It uses frequency-hopping spread spectrum radio to transmit data over the air. Serial communication is used to communicate with

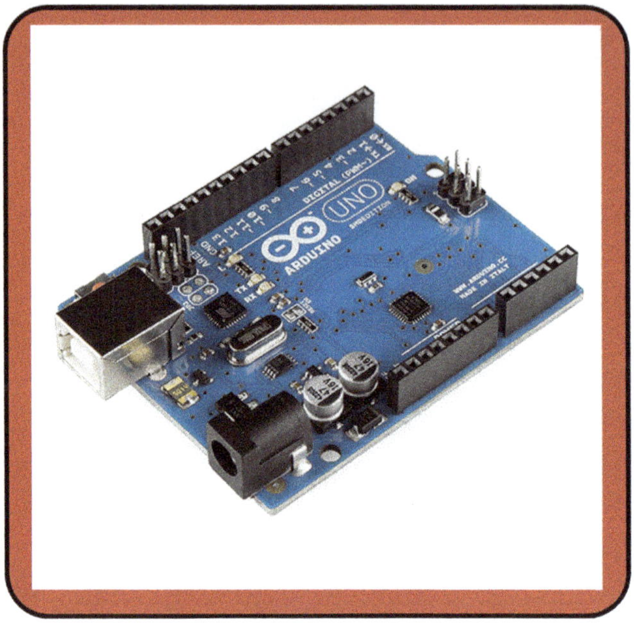

Figure 1.4. Arduino UNO module.

devices. It communicates with the microcontroller using the serial port. Both master and slave configurations of this module are possible. It uses 3.3 V and has six pins. There is a fixed 9600 baud rate for the slave. Bluetooth serial modules enable all serial-enabled devices to interact wirelessly with one another. Figure 1.5 represents the HC-05 Bluetooth module.

1.3.6 Android mobile

Adding the Android code to mobile requires modifying a configuration in developers. In this work, the Android mobile is used to receive the real-time data from the module and delivere it to the cloud server for continuous tracking and storing. If any alteration in the ECG pattern is detected at the server, an alert message is sent to the mobile by turning it on and displaying and showing the ECG heartbeat and its status.

1.4 Prototype implementation

Initially, an Arduino board is used to convert the cardiac electrical data from the AD8232 sensor into digital data. The monitor displays the voltage-converted serial data that was received over USB. The Bluetooth module is employed to transfer the data. To capture and monitor the characteristics of ECG signals, a variety of sophisticated commercial wireless sensors are used to implement the prototype of the proposed system. Due to the widespread use of smartphones and the openness of the Android platform, we chose an Android smartphone as the connecting device of the cloud server. A program on the smartphone was stored to adequately transfer the data on the device without disrupting the other essential mobile services.

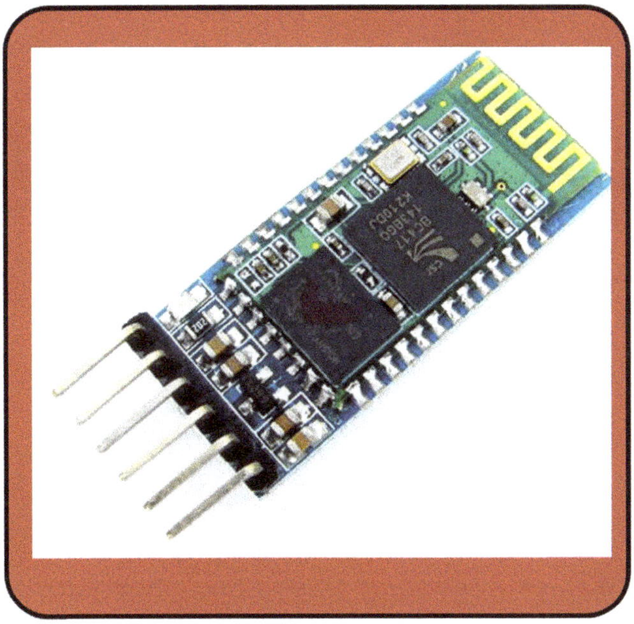

Figure 1.5. HC-05 Bluetooth module.

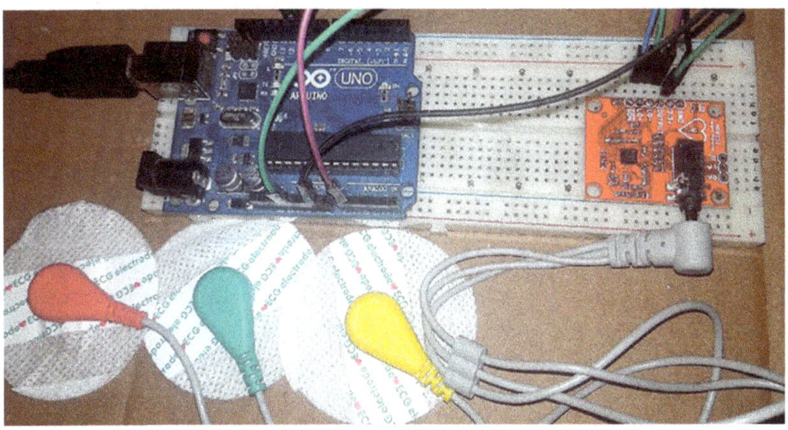

Figure 1.6. Developed monitoring system.

This program is in charge of receiving data through Bluetooth from the sensing devices, as well as transferring essential data following various operation modes. For the doctors to query the monitored data, a web-based application was developed on the cloud server. Figure 1.6 represents the developed monitoring system.

A program is written on the Arduino IDE to remove several artifacts from the recorded signals.

The serial plotter is utilized to plot the ECG signals on the system screen. Figure 1.7 depicts the recorded ECG signal at the baud rate of 9600 on the com3 port.

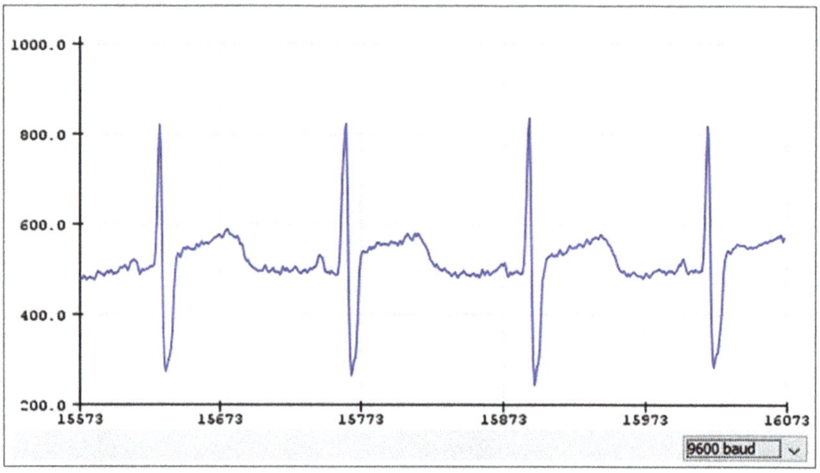

Figure 1.7. Recorded ECG signal.

1.5 Conclusion

Continuous monitoring of cardiac health, irregular heartbeat, alerts and notifications over widely-accepted wireless communication channels, and facilitation of data-driven research is the need of the hour. The proposed approach enables the continuous monitoring of cardiac health while continuously communicating over widely available wireless network protocols and facilitating data-driven research for CVD patients. To help with localization and prompt intervention for the treatment of CVD patients, this framework also shows patients' heartbeats tracked live data with time-stamps over the internet and alert management systems inside the clinics or hospitals. The real-time precision offered by three wearable monitoring electrodes is satisfactory. The Android mobile receives the filtered data and transmits it to the cloud server for storing and continuous monitoring of CVD patients. Additional research focuses on measuring the heart rate variability and enhancing the signal's accuracy level to assess various cardiac issues by employing a cloud-based monitor system. In the future, a suitable CNN will be interfaced on the cloud server to automatically diagnose various cardiac complications, such as hypertension, diabetes, sleep apnea, etc.

References

[1] Zhou S-s, Jin J-p, Wang J-q, Zhang Z-g, Freedman J H, Zheng Y and Cai L 2018 Mirnas in cardiovascular diseases: potential biomarkers, therapeutic targets and challenges *Acta Pharmacol. Sin.* **39** 1073–84

[2] Nowbar A N, Gitto M, Howard J P, Francis D P and Al-Lamee R 2019 Mortality from ischemic heart disease: Analysis of data from the world health organization and coronary artery disease risk factors from ncd risk factor collaboration *Circ. Cardiovasc. Qual. Outcomes* **12** e005375

[3] Ramalingam V, Dandapath A and Raja M K 2018 Heart disease prediction using machine learning techniques: a survey *Int. J. Eng. Technol.* **7** 684–7

[4] Qadri Y A, Nauman A, Zikria Y B, Vasilakos A V and Kim S W 2020 The future of healthcare internet of things: a survey of emerging technologies *IEEE Commun. Surv. Tutor.* **22** 1121–67

[5] Javaid M and Khan I H 2021 Internet of things (IoT) enabled healthcare helps to take the challenges of COVID-19 pandemic *J. Oral Biol. Craniofac. Res.* **11** 209–14

[6] Dang L M, Piran M J, Han D, Min K and Moon H 2019 A survey on internet of things and cloud computing for healthcare *Electronics* **8** 768

[7] Gupta K, Khare S K, Bajaj V and Ansari I A 2021 *Automatic Detection of Hypertension by Flexible Analytic Wavelet Transform Using Electrocardiogram Signals* (Bristol: IOP Publishing) pp 1–18

[8] Neyja M *et al* 2017 An IoT-based e-health monitoring system using ECG signal *GLOBECOM 2017–2017 IEEE Global Communications Conf.* (Piscataway, NJ: IEEE) 1–6

[9] Rahaman A, Islam M M, Islam M R, Sadi M S and Nooruddin S 2019 Developing IoT based smart health monitoring systems: a review *Rev. Intell. Artif.* **33** 435–40

[10] Krishnan D S R, Gupta S C and Choudhury T 2018 An IoT based patient health monitoring system *2018 Int. Conf. on Advances in Computing and Communication Engineering (ICACCE)* (Piscataway, NJ: IEEE) pp 1–7

[11] Li C, Hu X and Zhang L 2017 The IoT-based heart disease monitoring system for pervasive healthcare service *Proc. Comput. Sci.* **112** 2328–34

[12] Hernandez A I, Mora F, Villegas M, Passariello G and Carrault G 2001 Realtime ECG transmission via internet for nonclinical applications *IEEE Trans. Inf. Technol. Biomed.* **5** 253–7

[13] Azariadi D, Tsoutsouras V, Xydis S and Soudris D 2016 ECG signal analysis and arrhythmia detection on IoT wearable medical devices *2016 5th Int. Conf. on Modern Circuits and Systems Technologies (MOCAST)* (Piscataway, NJ: IEEE) pp 1–4

[14] Lin C-T *et al* 2010 An intelligent telecardiology system using a wearable and wireless ECG to detect atrial fibrillation *IEEE Trans. Inf. Technol. Biomed.* **14** 726–33

[15] Kumar R and Rajasekaran M P 2016 An IoT based patient monitoring system using Raspberry Pi *2016 Int. Conf. on Computing Technologies and Intelligent Data Engineering (ICCTIDE'16)* (Piscataway, NJ: IEEE) pp 1–4

[16] Masud M M, Serhani M A and Navaz A N 2016 Resource-aware mobile-based health monitoring *IEEE J. Biomed. Health Inf.* **21** 349–60

[17] Li H, Li P and Guo S 2014 MoRule: optimized rule placement for mobile users in SDN-enabled access networks *2014 IEEE Global Communications Conf.* (Piscataway, NJ: IEEE) pp 4953–8

[18] Gupta K, Bajaj V and Ansari I A 2022 Osacn-net: automated classification of sleep apnea using deep learning model and smoothed gabor spectrograms of ECG signal *IEEE Trans. Instrum. Meas.* **71** 1–9

[19] Gupta K, Bajaj V, Ansari I A and Acharya U R 2022 Hyp-Net: automated detection of hypertension using deep convolutional neural network and gabor transform techniques with ballistocardiogram signals *Biocybern. Biomed. Eng.* **42** 784–96

[20] Gupta K, Bajaj V and Ansari I A 2022 An improved deep learning model for automated detection of BBB using ST spectrograms of smoothed VCG signal *IEEE Sens. J.* **22** 8830–7

[21] Smulyan H 2019 The computerized ECG: friend and foe *Am. J. Med.* **132** 153–60

[22] Cosoli G, Spinsante S, Scardulla F, D'Acquisto L and Scalise L 2021 Wireless ECG and cardiac monitoring systems: state of the art, available commercial devices and useful electronic components *Measurement* **177** 109243

[23] Bravo-Zanoguera M, Cuevas-Gonz´alez D, Garc´ıa-V´azquez J P, Avitia R L and Reyna M 2019 Portable ECG system design using the AD8232 microchip and open-source platform *Proceedings* **42** 49

IOP Publishing

Internet of Things in Biomedical Sciences
Challenges and applications
Varun Bajaj and Irshad Ahmad Ansari

Chapter 2

IoT architectures for biomedical devices

Abu Jaffor Morshedul Abedin, Adiba Tabassum Chowdhury, Ifti Akib Abir, Mehedi Hasan Raju and Mosabber Uddin Ahmed

Significant technological advancements have been made in academia, industry, and healthcare facilities over the last decade. The healthcare sector is still struggling to deliver high-quality treatments though globalization continues. Complex analysis and diagnosis remain a major challenge for researchers who can assist physicians and humankind. The Internet of Things (IoT) has been incorporated into biomedical devices to make the healthcare system more dynamic, robust, trustworthy, and patient-centered. IoT allows healthcare practitioners to aid patients by utilizing smart biomedical devices and cutting-edge software thus improving treatment facilities and making the system more dynamic. In the IoT, artificial intelligence and machine learning (ML) are utilized to make crucial judgments on the basis of the information gathered, analyzed, and managed in real time and transmitted using cloud technologies in the IoT. This chapter presents an overview of the state-of-the-art of IoT, architectures in healthcare, and their applications in biomedical devices. Moreover, IoT architectures and frameworks in this sector, as well as a few specific areas of use for the IoT technology are mentioned. Finally, the chapter is concluded by pointing out the challenges that have been experienced, potential solutions, and aspects that will help to improve patient care in the future.

2.1 Introduction

The Internet of Things has lately created a new global viewpoint on data analysis in order to create a powerful geographical distribution by combining a range of real and digital 'stuff' with the developing extendable detectors. IoT was first proposed to merge well-known items and associated technological representations in an internet framework using transmitter-identifying innovation approaches. To encompass all types of 'things,' the term, IoT eventually entered use in a variety of detectors, incorporating processors, navigation programs, and smartphones [1]. A variety of exploratory problems, ranging between foundation architecture and information

doi:10.1088/978-0-7503-5311-3ch2

analysis and applications, have been posed by the agile methodology of the World Wide Web generation and the necessary facilities for such sensing devices. IoT advancement has developed quickly in several vocational studies in a variety of intellectual as well as engineering systems, particularly in the field of health treatment [2]. Consequently, the influence of IoT innovation and ML growth in health systems is the movement of routine clinical testing and other wellbeing support services from hospitals to homes, and the facilitation of the use of surgical resources by individuals and clinicians. Patients' access to medical treatment would have been made smoother, notably during troubling periods. By transferring essential duties to secluded areas, healthcare institutions help reduce the burden. Saving money is among the main advantages because individuals can avoid incurring health fees whenever they consult a psychologist. Another barrier seems to be the present network structure's inability to support a real segment to target employing the IoT. As a result, cloud-based connectivity is anticipated to be an appropriate connection architecture for such activities [3–6]. A modern innovation in the wellness business must be implemented soon to produce cutting-edge health services and utilize them to conveniently follow sufferers from other locations. Patient monitoring requires describing the person's current fitness level and medical history [7]. With the usage of labeling, IoT, sensor technology, etc having expanded considerably, portable devices could be combined with IoT technology to deliver greater insights. Pharmaceutical packaging can improve the product's usability by implementing an android operating system. Any industry, but especially the healthcare industry, will undergo a considerable shift when digital developments such as IoT are used. IoT may raise people's standards of living. The use of software applications would result in various enhancements to controlled connectivity, computer operations, and online data advisory operations [8–10]. There are several smart technologies and biomedicine which must be put into practice [11]. In this chapter, the scope of IoT and ML has been briefly discussed to discover the key components of individualized medical services. In addition to citing some earlier research on IoT and ML for individualized medical services, this section also identifies associated issues and difficulties.

2.2 IoT in biomedical devices and applications

IoT has the potential to empower the creation of a broad range of applications. New applications could undoubtedly enhance the quality of our lives in a wide range of contexts and settings, including those at home, when traveling, when we're ill, at work, while jogging, and in the gym, to name a few. Physical objects and gadgets can see, hear, and think thanks to the IoT concept, which allows them to 'speak' to one another and share information to coordinate choices. Giving these things the ability to speak with one another and elaborate on the information they pick up from their environment necessitates having various contexts in which a highly diverse variety of applications can be used [12–14].

The biomedical field being one of the most significant fields of application, much research has been conducted and is still being conducted. Utilizing IoT-based systems with worldwide connections, it is possible to easily collect, manage, and share all healthcare-related information, including therapy, diagnosis, recovery, inventory, and prescription. Due to their wireless interfaces and internet connections, IoT-based healthcare services facilitate mobility [13]. Numerous architectures and frameworks having different approaches fused with different technologies have been devised in the past years, which have been applied in a variety of applications in healthcare and biomedical devices [15].

2.3 Approaches to IoT-based applications

Technology selection and approaches are important while developing IoT-based healthcare and biomedical devices. This is so that an IoT system's capabilities can be improved by the usage of certain approaches.

So, to amalgamate profuse healthcare IoT applications countless cutting-edge technologies and approaches have been adopted [16]. An overview of different approaches is shown in figure 2.1.

2.3.1 Sensor-based approach

Various stimuli are converted into electrical signals for analysis by sensors in electronics-based medical devices. Sensors allow for distant and bedside monitoring of vital signs and other health parameters, as well as an improvement in the intelligence of medical devices such as life-supporting implants. A growing and aging population is hastening the creation of novel and distinctive medical devices, including a range of sensors that are incorporated into both the devices and the bodies of patients [17]. This chapter has categorized the sensor-based approach into three types—(a) wearable, (b) environmental, and (c) smartphone-based sensors.

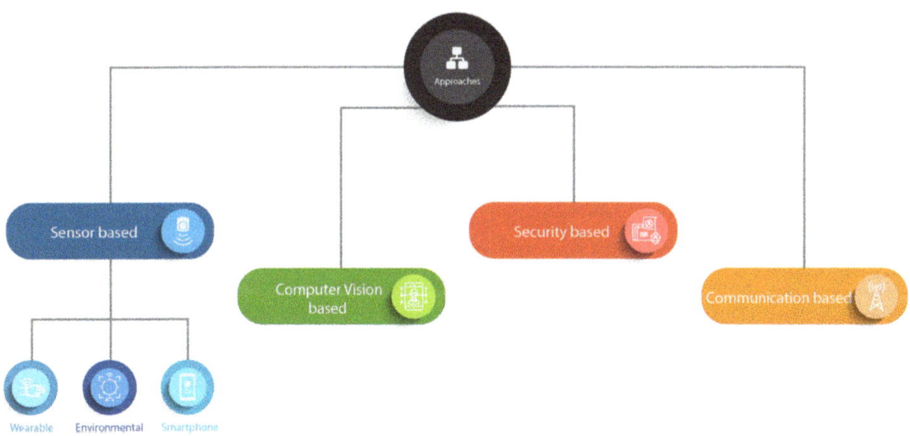

Figure 2.1. Different approaches to IoT-based biomedical devices.

2.3.1.1 Wearable sensors

All vital indicators in the body, including changes in skin conductance, heart rate, breathing rate, blood pressure, oxygen concentration, and blood glucose, may be monitored and interpreted using suitable sensors placed on clothing or directly on the body. Wearable sensors can be both in and out-of-body, depending on the application [18, 19].

Among the in-body sensors, the heart pacemaker, which is a small, battery-operated device, is used to monitor any irregularities in the heartbeat and deliver a signal to the heart to force it to beat at the proper rate after detecting anomalies in heartbeat. To monitor diabetes patients, blood glucose sensors are used to determine glucose concentration in the blood. Apart from the glucose sensor, there is another type of sensor that can be implanted under the skin [20]. When flexible endoscopy is unable to establish a diagnosis, CE (capsule endoscopy) is frequently used. It is made up of an imaging capsule, a data receiving, and storage device, a computer, and software. The actual capsule is made up of a transmission mechanism, a light source, a lens, and a battery [21].

A patient's heart is examined by ECG (electrocardiogram), and PPG (photoplethysmography), where ECG is used to measure and inspect heart rate, rhythm, and other information concerning the heart's condition, while PPG is used for determining blood flow rate controlled by the heart's pumping action. Body temperature is determined with the help of temperature sensors while the SpO2 sensor non-invasively measures blood's oxygen concentration [18].

The only item that changes over the course of a lifetime to fit our lifestyle is clothing. By incorporating intelligent devices into clothing, smart clothes can be produced. Smart cloth stands out as a promising contender to take the place of smartphones and other portable linked gadgets as the next point of contact between the physical and digital worlds. Additionally, shirts cover a bigger area of skin than wristbands or chest straps, making them more comfortable to wear and capable of tracking more biometric data. As a result, biometric tracking is made simpler because signals are captured exactly where they occur and can therefore be given as much meaning as feasible. Hence, patient monitoring can be done smoothly [22].

2.3.1.2 Environmental sensors

Environmental sensors include temperature sensors to measure environment temperature, surrounding air pressure sensors, humidity sensors for determining ambient humidity, PIR (passive infrared sensor) to detect movement, CO_2 sensors to measure carbon dioxide, and light sensors for measuring surrounding brightness. Environmental measurements are just one part of gauging the state of the environment. It may also consist of more intricate procedures involving people and environmental things. The environmental sensors embedded in devices are used for patient monitoring by detecting human activities. By analyzing the ambient sensor data along with other motion sensors, human activity recognition is performed by which patients, especially old people can be monitored thoroughly [23, 24].

2.3.1.3 Smartphone sensors

Smartphones and smartwatches are now equipped with a large number of sensors, making these devices multi-purpose devices, including biomedical devices. They have therefore become an important part of smart health solutions, essentially evolving into an ideal interface for actively receiving self-reported data from people, with the ability to collect active and passive data, which can be incorporated for detailed insight regarding patients' health. Built-in microphones and cameras of smartphones can capture behavioral cues such as gazes, facial expressions, and speech as well. Mobile devices also offer options for remote data transmission and temporary storage. These options can be used for further analysis or more complex evaluations by sending the data to the cloud [25].

2.3.2 Computer vision-based approach

Some of the tasks involved in computer vision include segmentation, object identification, and image classification. Medical image processing can greatly benefit from recent advancements in image categorization, and object recognition. Research has revealed good results in challenging medical diagnostics tasks covering pathology, radiology, and dermatology. Deep-learning systems may be able to assist doctors by offering additional viewpoints and emphasizing troublesome spots in photos. Medical picture analysis, disease diagnosis, patient rehabilitation, and other important tasks have become easier thanks to the use of computer vision in medical devices. Smart biomedical gadgets that support medical practitioners in making decisions at critical times by abstracting information have been produced by combining deep learning with computer vision algorithms, IoT, and cloud-based technology and incorporating cutting-edge cameras and sensors. Typically, a vision-based device works by capturing a digital image, and video then converting it into a usable format and analyzing it by applying proper algorithms [26, 27].

2.3.3 Security-based approach

Direct access to IoT devices is the predominant way of remote monitoring in modern IoT networks. Therefore, while in transit, biomedical data is open to multiple security breaches. The global risk report of The World Economic Forum published in 2019, declared cyber assaults and information leakage to be the fourth and fifth most intentional threats now confronting the world [28]. The healthcare industry, among others, has experienced an increase in cybersecurity breaches, which can be caused by a variety of circumstances. IoT formerly had a three-tier structure, with the perception layer, transport layer, and application layer being the key levels. However, the IoT reference model that CISCO established earlier contains seven layers, as shown in figure 2.2. Furthermore, levels 1–3 are referred to as the 'edge-side layer', levels 4–6 as the 'server/cloud-side layer' and finally, level 7 as the 'user-side layer' [29, 30]. These IoT components get attacked in several manners. Table 2.1 provides a comparative review of the cyber threats and potential countermeasures as proposed in the literature. In recent years, a lot of work has gone into addressing security concerns in the IoT paradigm. While some of these strategies aim to address

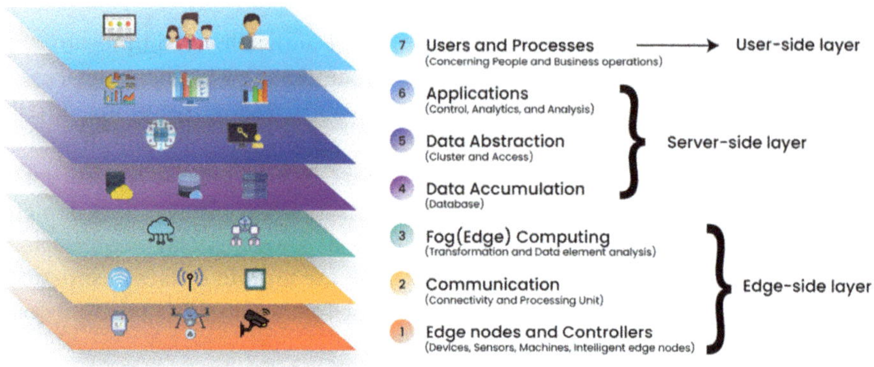

Figure 2.2. IoT reference model defined by CISCO.

Table 2.1. Summary of cyber attacks in IoT and countermeasures.

Security threat	Affected layer	Countermeasure
Sleep deprivation attack	Link layer	Cluster-based approach for intrusion identification [35]
Jamming	Physical layer	Channel surfing and spatial retreats [36], reckoning packet delivery ratio [37], anti-jamming tactics using cryptography [38]
Side channel attack	Edge node	Identification of Malicious Software [39], Willingly Noise Generation [40]
RFID tag	Edge node	Lightweight cryptographic protocol [41], personal RFID firewall [42]
Replay attack	Network layer	Timestamp introduced and enabled nonce options [43], content-chaining mechanism [44]
RPL routing attack	Network layer	Hashing and signature-based authentication, and monitoring end-to-end node behavior [45, 46]
Sybil attack	Network layer	Community detection algorithm, managing trusted/untrusted user list and user activity analysis [47–49]
Code Injection	Edge computing layer	IDS diglossia [50]
Virus, worms, spyware	Edge computing layer	Intrusion detection system, firewall, antivirus [51]

security concerns at a particular layer, others seek to offer end-to-end security for IoT. For delivering the quality of service (QoS) in an IoT-based healthcare system, security-based techniques basically focus on privacy, access control (authentication, authorization), confidentiality, and trust [31–33]. It is much more challenging to implement light and fast cryptographic methods while ensuring maximum security. However, in rare cases, a communication failure caused by a cybersecurity compromise may have fatal consequences for a patient. Therefore, an IoT-integrated health examining system impenetrable to attacks is an urgent necessity [34].

2.3.4 Communication-based approach

In the healthcare industry, biomedical devices collect data that includes both direct patient medical information from sensors like ECG, BPM, SpO2, temperature, and glucose sensors (on-the-body sensors) and indirect patient information from sensors like accelerometers, gyroscopes, ambient temperature, PIR, and other similar sensors. With the help of communication technologies and protocols, including wireless, wired, and M2M (machine-to-machine) ones, the vast amounts of data acquired from wearables, smartphones, and smartwatches are shared and exchanged. Wireless technologies are becoming more and more commonplace, even though all three of these technologies are employed for information sharing. The remarkable adoption of wireless and mobile technologies among the lowest populations demonstrates both the rise of this technology and its promise. The requirements for reliability, connectivity, data throughput, and latency may all be met by current communication technology. The end-to-end solution for emanating biomedical applications will, however, require a combination of technologies [52–54]. Table 2.2 presents a comparative overview of different communication technologies.

2.4 Implementation of IoT in healthcare and biomedical devices

With the growing need to make healthcare more personalized, pro-active, and affordable, the IoT can be seen and exploited as a noteworthy gadget in health management systems like patient monitoring, global pandemic (e.g., COVID-19), etc. The IoT allows health monitoring around the clock, anywhere with the use of WBAN technology. It is also able to handle emergencies, stop hospital infections, and deliver post-discharge care. The IoT has so completely changed how everything is done in the healthcare industry [56–58].

Table 2.2. A comparative overview of different communication technologies used to transfer biomedical data [53, 55].

Network technologies	Frequency	Data speed	Range
Zigbee	868.3 MHz, 902–928 MHz, 2.4 GHz	0.02–0.25 Mbps	100 m
Bluetooth (low energy)	2.4 GHz	1–2 Mbps	10 m
Wi-Fi	2.4 GHz, 5 GHz	11 Mbps–10 Gbps	<1 km (MSC10, 1 MHz)
SigFox	862–928 MHz	100–600 bps	10 km
LoRa	860–1020 MHz	290 bps–50 Kbps	15 km
5G	Lower bands	3.6 Gbps	10 km
	Higher bands	10 Gbps	<1 km

Additionally, because people are so busy today, appointments with doctors might take a long time because numerous diagnoses and tests are necessary. People frequently don't know how to maintain their physical health, so they only go to hospitals and clinics when a serious emergency arises. Also, this makes it difficult for doctors to monitor patients, provide rehabilitation, and discover diseases early and urgently. Because of this, a growing number of people are looking for an alternative, such as a wearable gadget, that can not only track their health in real time but also give them and their doctor fast information on a wide range of health parameters. Furthermore, using biomedical devices and IoT-based health systems, doctors and researchers can easily analyze a patient and corresponding medical information [59].

Numerous studies have been conducted to develop IoT-based health monitoring devices combined with biomedical devices. Since it is possible to keep track of patient data with IoT-based technology, doctors can easily monitor a patient by analyzing his/her health status. Also, there is a need for a cost-effective system in IoT-based health especially for developing countries to make it affordable. Keeping this in mind, Ahmed *et al* [60] designed a cost-effective and low-power consumption simple IoT-based architecture for patient health monitoring using wearable biomedical devices. The system consists of two sides, the patient side consisting of wearable sensors and a server side consisting of a database where a web application is used to connect the two sides. According to the paper, the designed system can reduce patient risk with its emergency alert system, additionally, the doctor can monitor patients' recorded data from anywhere via the internet. The block diagram of the proposed designed system has been illustrated in figure 2.3.

The remote health monitoring system for patients can now be measured and recorded in a comfortable atmosphere thanks to IoT technologies. IoT components including sensors, actuators, microcontrollers, and cloud-enabled systems help patients get care from home rather than having to frequently go to the hospital. Especially during a pandemic situation like COVID-19, an IoT-based health monitoring system plays a prominent role in patient monitoring. Wearable technology is able to track and forecast the occurrence of COVID-19 by deploying

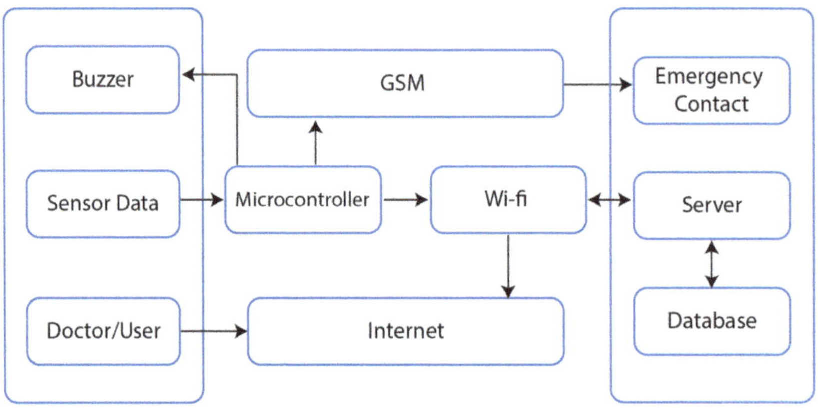

Figure 2.3. IoT-based block diagram for patient examining system.

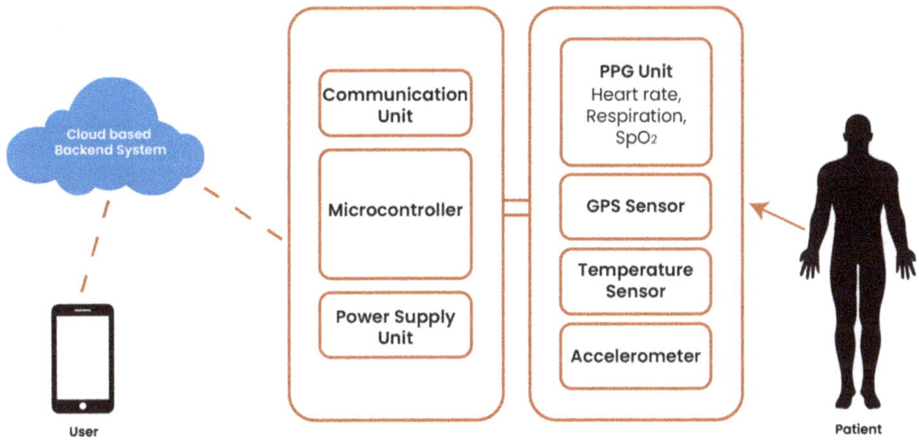

Figure 2.4. IoT-based framework for COVID-19 infected patient supervision.

sensors such as oxygen saturation, temperature, heart rate, and others as vaccines take time to develop and go on the market [61, 62]. To monitor, estimate vital signs, manage, and analyze COVID-19 infected patients by an IoT-based system, Al Bassam *et al* [63], proposed a system consisting of three-layered functionalities. The IoT sensor layer collects patients' data amassed in the cloud database in the cloud layer for taking instantaneous decisions and preventive measures. The cloud layer exchanges data with the Android web layer with Application Peripheral Interface (API), where the mobile application in the Android web layer can give alerts, and notifications when necessary. The proposed system is shown in figure 2.4. More literature that worked on IoT-based systems and biomedical devices for smart healthcare has been highlighted in table 2.3.

2.5 Implementation of cloud-based and fog-based technology in healthcare and biomedical devices

2.5.1 Cloud-based technology

2.5.1.1 Architectures and frameworks

Using servers online for data archiving, management, and processing is referred to as cloud computing. Virtual servers, databases, and collaboration tools offer potential customers several advantages. Information storage and consistency are among the flexible services offered by cloud-based architecture. Cloud architecture, which is useful in gathering resources at one location, is created by extending grid and cluster-based computing. Researchers from various fields have proposed unique emergent cloud computing service models [74, 75].

With the help of digital wearables, it is now possible for patients to self-analyze issues well before they develop into urgent situations that require attention. Self-diagnosis, on the other hand, can be dangerous, thus it is recommended to have a diagnosis made by professionals based on remote sensor data and observation before going to the hospital or being admitted. Hence, an IoT fused with

Table 2.3. Overview of IoT-based applications in healthcare proposed in literature.

Authors and Year	Major components	Application
Seshadri *et al* [61], 2020	ECG, PPG, accelerometer, temperature sensor, SpO2, heart rate, respiration rate, smartphone as receiving device	Remote patient monitoring and virtual assessment for COVID-19 patients
Turner *et al* [64], 2017	Heart rate sensor, Bluetooth, microcontroller, electrode pads, and smartphone	Heart rate monitoring using a smartphone
Asri *et al* [65], 2019	Activity sensor, pulse sensor, temperature sensor, Raspberry Pi, heart rate sensor	Miscarriage prediction system
Kolhar *et al* [66], 2020	Camera, cloud-based database and application server, face detection benchmark dataset (like WIDER FACE, FDDB), CNN architecture for face detection (MTCNN)	IoT-based face detection for cities under lockdown.
Hameed *et al* [67], 2020	Pulse rate, heartbeat rate, body temperature sensors, Arduino Uno, cloud server, and Android app	IoT-based healthcare system using a fuzzy network
Chianese *et al* [68], 2019	Smart medical cart (FIDRUN), smart medical cabinet (FIDROK), smart pocket dispenser (FIDRAY), and web-based application (FIDCARE)	IoT-based cost control and healthcare risk management
Muthu *et al* [69], 2020	Wearable sensor, generalize approximate reasoning base intelligence control (GARIC) architecture, Boltzmann belief network, regularization genome-wide association study (GWAS)	Disease prognosis and symptom analysis
Gupta *et al* [70], 2021	Sensors (camera, temperature, GPS tracker, etc), body area network (BAN), small base station (SBS), D2D link, SBS transmission, macro base station transmission (MBS)	The prospect of a 5G-based IoT structure
Wong *et al* [71], 2020	Body wearable sensors, camera, SBS, MBS, home care server, authentication and authorization server	Three-factor fast-authentication for multi-server e-health system in a 5G-based wireless sensor network in IoT
Hu *et al* [72], 2020	MySignal HW complete kit containing body sensors, Arduino UNO, ESP8266, and micro SD card (SD card reader SPI interface)	IoT-based sleep body position monitoring system
Chowdhury *et al* [73], 2020	Optical camera, software-defined networking (SDN), sensors, actuators	5G-based e-health architecture using optical camera communication

cloud-based architecture has been redefined in Lakshmi *et al* [76] which collects data from interconnected devices and sensors and analyzes data after aggregation for significant decision-making by professionals. Communication technologies like Wi-Fi and Bluetooth were used powered by Raspberry pi while Arduino nano was used to gather and send data to Raspberry pi through the serial port which displays results on a screen and transfers data to the cloud server. A smart software manager receives data from the cloud server and by proper analysis sends a warning to doctors. The proposed architecture is shown in figure 2.5. One area of healthcare that needs a lot of attention is the diagnosis and treatment of skin conditions that are still in their early stages. Skin conditions are occasionally disregarded and aren't always thought to be life-threatening. Negative or potentially fatal outcomes might arise from misdiagnosis, delayed diagnosis, or diagnostic incapacity. Irritation, side effects, significant skin deformity, and frequent skin cancer result from untreated skin conditions. For intelligent, efficient, real-time, and low-cost skin monitoring, Juyal *et al* [77] proposed an AI-enabled cloud-based IoT skin monitoring system.

The proposed architecture contains four phases such as data collection from environmental sensors, data acquisition from skin sensors (moisture level, image sensors, pH level, etc), disease classification and intelligent diagnosis, and research analysis and service. In the architecture SkinCare Van contains essential sensors that capture proper data and images from the patients, after which the collected individual health records are transmitted to the cloud. There, data is properly analyzed, and to improve the analysis an AI-enabled component is used. Notably, in the proposed model of architecture, a CNN-based model was used for two-level

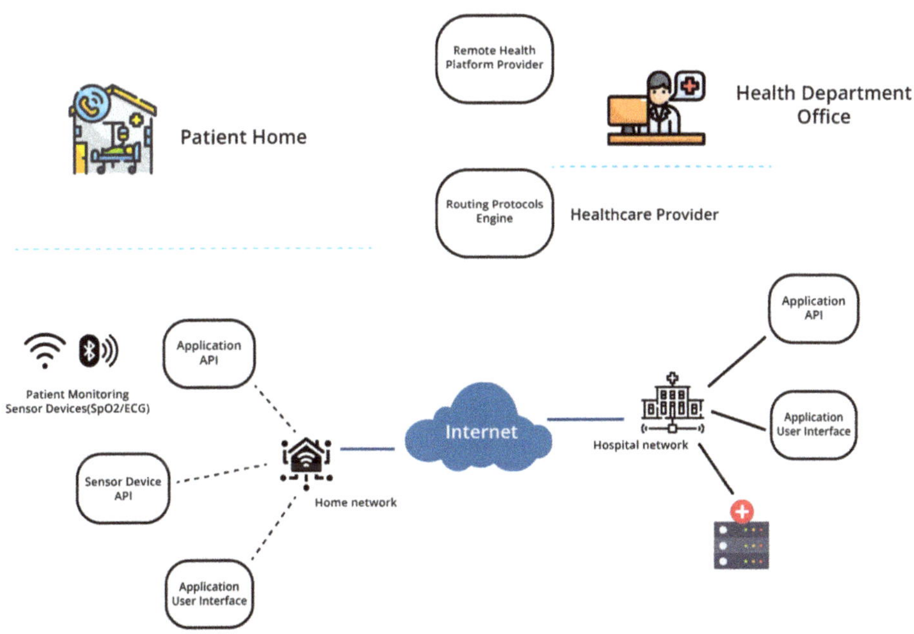

Figure 2.5. Cloud-based remote health monitoring platform.

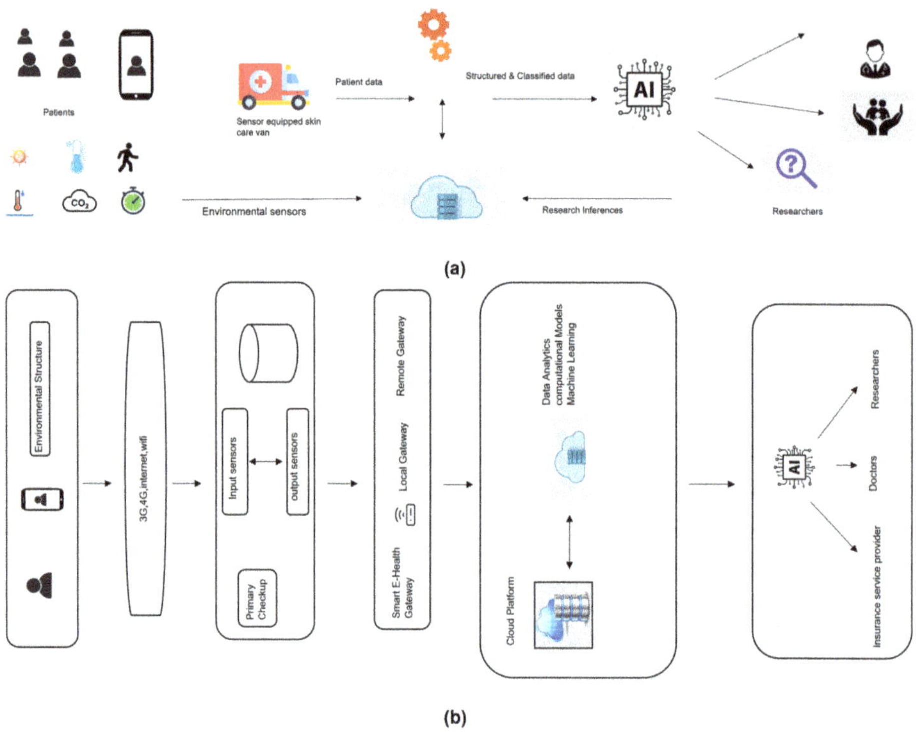

Figure 2.6. (a) Scenario of the AI-enabled cloud IoT-based skin care system. (b) The proposed model.

classification where the first level includes skin disease detection while in the second level classification the detected disease is classified into different levels of severity like regular, moderate, and bad, extreme. Figure 2.6 illustrates (a) a scenario of the recommended method, and (b) the introduced model. More studies on cloud-based applications are highlighted in table 2.4.

2.5.1.2 Challenges in cloud-based applications

Cloud-based technology is widely being applied for its flexibility and interoperability. Integrating cloud-based technology with IoT, cloud-based solutions have become more vigorous and user-centric [86]. Despite all the advantages of cloud integration, challenges still prevail.

However, cloud-based solutions are still constrained by geographical and multi-hop distance from the source. As a result of these restrictions, real-time interactions between users and the platform are frequently disrupted, with potentially fatal results. We may have a viable answer for this problem in fog-based systems [86]. A cloud server used in the smart medical system facilitates unsecured interaction between the doctor and patient. That the cloud is not completely secure is a huge worry. Numerous security concerns exist for this system, including those relating to data confidentiality, integrity, and other concerns, as well as issues with the doctor and patient anonymity and unlikability [31]. For ensuring a secured cloud-based

Table 2.4. Overview of a few cloud-based applications in healthcare.

Reference	Description	Application
Kumari *et al* [78], 2020	Cloud-based security framework using the elliptic curve cryptography (ECC)	Cloud-based security
Sharma *et al* [79], 2018	Cloud-based architecture and textile-based wearable system technology to improve the healthcare industry and ensure an efficient and comfortable patient monitoring system	Health monitoring and management
Kil *et al* [80], 2021	In this research for fully automated point of care molecular diagnostic devices, a cloud-based software architecture was brought to light	Fully automated point of care molecular diagnostic devices
Akhbarifar *et al* [81], 2020	For corroborating security for the massive medical data, distant health supervising cloud-based model applying a lightweight block encryption method was introduced	Early disease diagnosis
Stradolini *et al* [82], 2018	For online anesthesia supervision, a cloud-based IoT network was introduced. The introduced architecture assists anesthesiologist to remain connected to the sedated patients by an Android app, and data can be accessed by a web application	Online monitoring of anesthetized patients
Doukas and Maglogiannis [83], 2012	The paper proposed a platform for pervasive healthcare based on cloud-based technology and management of mobile and wearable sensors	Cloud computing toward pervasive healthcare
Chen *et al* [84], 2016	Healthcare system that uses the adaptability of cloud-based technology to protect the privacy and prevent interference from medical data exchange	Privacy protection of medical data sharing
Zhang *et al* [85], 2016	For patient-oriented applications, a cyber-physical system was put forward here, on the basis of big data analytics and the cloud	Healthcare cyber-physical system

system in the healthcare system, the literature has tried to propose models, frameworks, and architectures. For ensuring a secure authentication system and fighting against security attacks, Kumari *et al* [78] proposed a secured framework employing the elliptic curve cryptography method. To get most of the benefits of cloud computing, while inhibiting the lack of security, a model based on chain ontology was introduced by Al-Sharhan *et al* [87]. As the patient medical data is highly sensitive, transferring it over wireless media faces security issues like eavesdropping and alteration. Therefore, a lightweight secure access scheme to prevent unauthorized users from accessing and modifying patient data was proposed by Masud *et al* [88].

Cloud IoT health has a huge challenge due to the broad-ranging platforms, operating systems, appliances, and services available for unhackneyed and enhanced applications. Users who adopt multi-cloud solutions, or services that rely on many providers, run the danger of exacerbating this situation. A probable solution might be cloud brokering which third parties or cloud providers can effectuate [89].

Modern cloud IoT health applications regularly transmit data from sensors to the cloud, which in turn may employ smartphones as gateways, depleting the batteries on the objects and the gateway, curbing ceaseless operation to 24 h or fewer. Data processing and transmission energy efficiency is a major unsolved problem, according to relevant research. Energy-based tradeoffs must be balanced depending on offloading choice criteria, such as low energy reaction time or energy usage. To deal with this energy efficiency problem, Wu *et al* [90] brought forward a Lyapunov optimization-based energy-efficient algorithm. The proposed algorithm mitigates energy exhaustion of mobile devices while forwarding data to cloud infrastructure for execution remotely though slight response time is sacrificed. Applications are frequently hosted on virtual machines (VMs) to boost energy efficiency and to address one issue with this, namely QoS (Quality of Service). A QoS-aware VM scheduling approach (QVMS) for cloud-integrated systems for energy saving was developed by Qi *et al* [91].

2.5.2 Fog-based technology

2.5.2.1 Architectures and framework

As a result of its enormous storage capacity, flexibility, and processing power, cloud-based architecture is well-known as a productive method of handling data. The present cloud models, however, cannot be the ideal answer for important applications and addressing IoT difficulties due to various drawbacks such as unpredictable response times, high bandwidth limitations, and network infrastructure dependency [92–94]. Therefore, to address the issues faced by cloud computing, Cisco offered a new computing technology known as fog computing which can offer relevant amenities at the network's edge. Users can benefit from fog computing by reducing the strain on data centers, improving reaction times, using less energy, and conserving network bandwidth [95, 96].

Fog computing is built on the premise that fog nodes exist between the Earth and the cloud data centers where end users' devices are physically located. Edge devices are those owned by end users, and the duties associated with them, are referred to as 'edge computing' in this context [97]. Modern cloud-based models are said to be improved by the use of a new paradigm termed fog computing. In contrast to standard cloud computing, fog computing takes care of processing, storage, and communication at the network's edge. This allows computations requiring a delay while consuming less energy and reducing traffic. Based on its capacity, a fog node decides whether to execute a processing request received from end devices locally or send them to cloud servers. By lowering energy usage, minimizing delay, and saving bandwidth, fog computing improves performance and resource efficiency [98, 99].

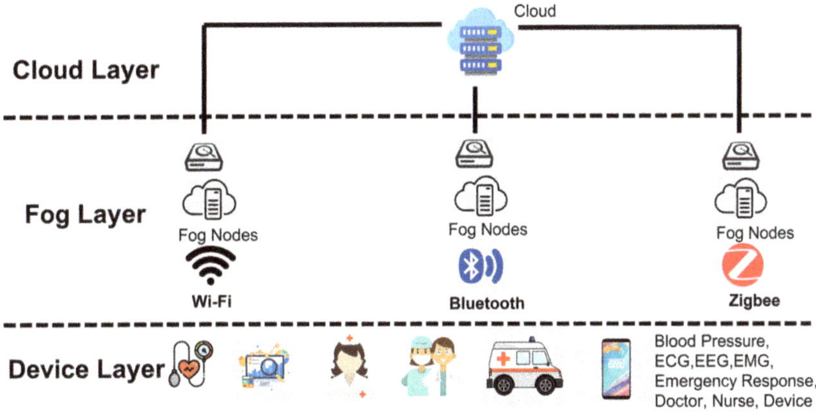

Figure 2.7. Fog computing three-level structure for health applications.

Fog computing architecture's reference model is an important research field. Countless concepts concerning fog computing have been offered in current history. Generally, they are gleaned from a three-layer structure. Cloud services are stretched by fog computing to the network edge by placing an additional layer of fog between end gadgets and the cloud [92]. A hierarchical three-layered fog architecture was mentioned in Ahmadi *et al* [100] which is shown in figure 2.7.

Among the three layers in the highlighted architecture are the bottommost layer (device layer), the middle layer (fog layer), and the top layer (the cloud layer), which is made up of data centers and robust servers for processing and analyzing enormous amounts of data. Bottom-positioned fog nodes are the foundational element of fog construction. They are either physical or virtual parts physically attached to smart appliances supplying them with processing power. The network links sensors with the upper tiers of the hierarchy and the cloud while offering the low latency and QoS necessary for providing time-critical statistics. The fog system's interconnection options include cable and wireless. Wireless networking offers greater flexibility and boosts productivity. Many different techniques, standards, and protocols are used in wireless interfaces. The degree of flexibility, mobility, and power consumption are all factors that affect the quality of connectivity [101, 102]. A few more applications of Fog technology have been highlighted in table 2.5.

2.5.2.2 Challenges in fog-based applications

While IoT-Fog-based applications have overcome the challenges faced by stand-alone cloud-based architectures, Fog itself has its limitations. With the advancement of IoT-based biomedical pieces of equipment and their usage, a colossal volume of medical data is being generated quotidianly. Furthermore, this immense data is being exchanged with servers and accessed for diagnosis and other medical purposes. Hence, with the increasing usage, users, access, and transfer of data, Fog-integrated IoT systems in healthcare are facing challenges [110].

Offloading is a key concept in resource management referring to the transfer of work from one unit to another or the act of a fog node shifting the load to another

Table 2.5. Overview of a few fog-based applications in healthcare.

Reference	Description	Application
Mahmoud *et al* [88], 2018	A proper simulation was performed, which showed 2.72% and 1.6% more energy savings compared to default fog and cloud-only	Energy-aware fog-based healthcare
Debauche *et al* [103], 2019	A fog IoT cloud-based health monitoring system was proposed in the paper. The proposed system monitors the health state and behavioral changes, rehabilitation, and recovery processes of elderly and lonely people	Patient and elderly monitoring
Tuli *et al* [104], 2019	A framework based on deep learning for heart disease diagnosis in integrated IoT and fog environments was proposed named as HealthFog	Heart disease diagnosis
Vijayakumar *et al* [105], 2018	A Fog-based intelligent system to discern and avert mosquito-borne diseases was proposed in the paper. A fuzzy K-nearest neighbor approach was used for the classification of the infected/uninfected class. Social network analysis in the cloud for representing the epidemic and location-based awareness to avert outbreaks can be provided by computing the PDO (probability of disease outbreak)	Detecting and preventing mosquito-borne diseases
Guo *et al* [106], 2020	A fog-based communication architecture along with an improved symmetric homomorphic cryptosystem was proposed to support time-sensitive monitoring and ensure secure analysis of medical data	Privacy assured data aggregation in e-healthcare systems
Lakhan *et al* [107], 2021	The research introduced a cost-effective, secure framework based on blockchain that enables fog technology, which aims to decrease the cost of healthcare applications	Cost-effective and secure mechanism based on fog-cloud network and blockchain
Ahmad *et al* [108], 2016	The study introduced a Health Fog framework which brings down the extra communication cost. Additionally, to amplify security and privacy cloud access security broker (CASB) was integrated	Health and wellness application
Gia *et al* [109], 2017	The research proposed a cost-effective monitoring system to monitor ECG along with analysis. The presented system contained a combination of energy-efficient sensor nodes and a fog layer	Energy efficient health system

node that is under less load. Offloading is necessary to maintain the low latency aspect of fog computing. Offloading presents a barrier for Fog computing since it requires decision-making. To maintain the QoS provided by Fog, decisions on when and how to offload tasks to other fog nodes must be made with the least amount of latency. When done improperly, offloading could have a negative impact on healthcare systems. The real-time monitoring of a patient's symptoms may be affected if the tasks' offloading adds more delay. If there is a delay, it could injure the patients or even result in death [111, 112]. For activities related to sophisticated applications and to deal with the offloading challenge, Aljanabi and Chalechale [113] suggested a hybrid offloading architecture between cloud and fog. The IoT node in this study will take the decision of offloading jobs to fog or cloud servers for load balancing and more effective task execution based on the task requirements.

In addition to heterogeneity, fog computing may run into issues with interoperability. For data to be transmitted to another device for processing or analysis, heterogeneity must exist. Heterogeneity in IoT end devices raises challenges with data collection, structure, and processing all at once. Computing and communication resources can be found in the fog layer, which is a logical step above it. When it comes to the design of architecture, heterogeneity plays an important role, especially when it comes to allowing various supervising machines to connect the patient as well as assessing medical data like blood pressure and heart rate [114, 115]. Because of this, an effective and dependable solution for managing fog servers in a heterogeneous environment is required. For such a challenge, Yang *et al* [116] introduced a maximal energy-saving scheduling algorithm. The algorithm was proposed based on multiple neighboring helper nodes under reasonable modulation schemes which share their computational resources.

Resource management in fog computing can be a challenging task when operating without the cloud. This is because there are fewer processing and storage resources in the fog than there are in the cloud. The data being exchanged and processed between IoT items and communication with the fog layer must have a purpose to avoid sharing redundant data and wasting precious resources. Management of these resources becomes increasingly crucial when numerous users or different system components are using the same resources to delay the devices being used as little as possible [112]. A novel resource management approach for the fog environment was presented by Wadhwa and Aron [117]. In the proposed technique for resource allocation and management (TRAM), to utilize resources at the fog layer, the expectation maximization (EM) algorithm is used to trace the level of intensity of an existing task and find out the present status of a task. Moreover, for the resource grading process, a scheduling algorithm was also proposed in the paper. To address the limitations of traditional methods for allocating computing resources in fog radio access network architectures (F-RAN), Khumalo *et al* [118] gave a proposal. In the study, the proposed algorithm based on Q-learning is provided as a solution for autonomous and dynamic resource allocation using reinforcement learning (RL). In resource allocation issues, RL offers several advantages, and simulations suggest that it works better than reactive approaches.

Because of where security fits in the network, fog computing security might be considered a research challenge. Recent research has brought attention to the necessity for security on fog servers because of the possible dangers of shared server resources and public network environments [119, 120]. Healthcare systems might be undermined by an assault on a gateway between a fog node and a sensor that analyzes and processes patient information. The patient's health may be jeopardized when the data being analyzed is remolded [91]. If privacy and security fail to be guaranteed, the full-fledged benefit of the application of biomedical devices in IoT-based healthcare will be obscured. Saha *et al* [121] proposed a secured framework for dealing with privacy issues of fog-based IoT applications in healthcare systems. The proposed framework enables accessing medical data with genuine access control without compromising privacy. Authentication is another major concern of privacy and security of fog computing. To develop an improved and robust authentication framework, Wu *et al* [122], proposed an improved authenticated key agreement scheme. The man-in-the-middle attack is a matter of great concern in software-defined networking (SDN) that uses OpenFlow channels when deployed in IoT-Fog networks. All controller commands being sent through the channel can be brought under complete control by the attacker when the channel is compromised. To deal with such potential threats Li *et al* [123] introduced a securing mechanism. The paper proposed a lightweight countermeasure using Bloom filters, after finding out the dreadful consequences of attacks when they used a feasible attack model and implemented the attack demonstrations.

2.6 Discussion and future direction

One of the core advantages of the technology revolution is the process of widespread IoT implementation. IoT is becoming more common in the modern healthcare sector. By facilitating connection with smart devices, the IoT can expand this field and realize the concept of 'anytime, anywhere, any media, anything' communications. Using communication technologies, cloud computing, and smart sensors, IoT has changed the medical sector. Many researchers have suggested IoT-based architectures to guarantee high service quality in the healthcare industry, some of which have been covered in this chapter. The structures combined several items of biomedical equipment with a few contemporary technologies like cloud-based, and fog-based technology along with deep learning algorithms and models. The architectures, frameworks, or suggested systems facilitated automation along with secure data collection, optimization of medical personnel, real-time transfer of massive amounts of medical data, improved disease diagnosis, effective prediction, analysis, and finally, patient monitoring, particularly for elderly patients, during pandemics like COVID-19, and rehabilitation.

Though IoT integration has revolutionized the healthcare system, it still has a long way to go as it faces new challenges and hurdles every day. Implementation of all the recent technologies discussed in this chapter has indeed ensured some dynamicity, interoperability, flexibility, and reliability in the medical sector. Yet, these technologies pose discrete challenges like power consumption of devices, scalability, cost, connectivity, and finally security and privacy issues, like the possibility of invasion while constantly monitoring a patient with devices attached to the body along with accessing the servers for analyzing patient data. All these problems thus need to be addressed.

Therefore, further research is required to develop systems that are safer, energy efficient, dependable, and versatile. Additionally, more research should be conducted to enhance the functionality of cloud- and fog-based technology in the healthcare system as well as to develop systems and devices with cost-effectiveness, seamless, uninterrupted communication, and high accuracy and precision.

In addition to addressing the technical problems described previously, the future potential of IoT-based technologies in healthcare can also be considered from an economic perspective. IoT-based healthcare will operate primarily in the medical sector and connect patients and doctors from across the world, as well as treat patients in less time and at a lower cost, despite its limitations and obstacles. According to Rayan *et al* [124], healthcare being one of the most propitious areas consuming enormous data, scientists believe that IoT combined with new technologies like cloud, fog computing, 5G, etc will shepherd an uprising in medicine in the coming years, and they predicted that by the next decade biomedical gadgets connected will escalate tenfold. Furthermore, according to Fortune Business Insights, the market value of IoT in healthcare will quickly increase from $57.62 billion in 2019 to $352.88 billion in 2027 [125]. Therefore, as IoT-based technology is the technology of the future, more advanced methods, and processes should be created to guarantee an effective and trustworthy IoT-based system.

2.7 Conclusion

One of several sectors of the economic industry that is growing the fastest right now is medical care, which has become increasingly expensive since more individuals need care. Government expenditure on healthcare has increased to a record level, yet it is now clear that stronger patient–physician relationships are crucial. Cognitive computing and big data are two examples of innovations that possess the capacity to provide physicians and nurses with adequate services at more affordable costs. Many companies and agencies have already made the initial move in this area. It encouraged the shift to healthcare services and scientific proof treatment. We would only have to figure out ways to display the information that is there. Additionally, unsupervised, or supervised learning relies greatly on the type and techniques available to classify inputs into specific groups. Humans make poor judgments, and occasionally we humans depend on the truth while making conclusions. People typically choose based on feelings, while machinery doesn't. Humans could make decisions based on their identification, moral standards, knowledge of the world, and governmental and religious beliefs. Several elements will be included in the information gathering used to intend learning for judgment calls. These elements might find difficulty in making the information gathering utilized for learning as liberated as it can be from mechanical biases. The goal of this chapter is to describe the broader viewpoint on IoT as it has been used in the public health system, the implementation utilized for customized medical services, and several other related publications and their perspectives on their findings in this domain, as well as the key limitations that were confronted by the digital healthcare system for the prospects of these concerns.

References

[1] Qi J, Yang P, Min G, Amft O, Dong F and Xu L 2017 Advanced Internet of Things for personalised healthcare systems: a survey *Pervasive Mob. Comput.* **41** 132–49

[2] Yadav S S and Jadhav S M 2019 Machine learning algorithms for disease prediction using IoT environment *Int. J. Eng. Adv. Technol.* **8** 4303–7

[3] Shavan A 2017 SDN-based load balancing scheme for fat-tree data center networks *Al-Nahrain J. Eng. Sci.* **20** 1047–56

[4] Askar S 2016 Adaptive load balancing scheme for data center networks using software defined network *Sci. J. Univ. Zakho* **4** 275–86

[5] Fizi F S and Askar S 2016 A novel load balancing algorithm for software defined network based datacenters *2016 Int. Conf. on Broadband Communications for Next Generation Networks and Multimedia Applications (CoBCom) (Graz, Austria, September 2016)* 1–6

[6] Keti F and Askar S 2015 Emulation of software defined networks using Mininet in different simulation environments *2015 6th Int. Conf. on Intelligent Systems, Modelling and Simulation (Kuala Lumpur, Malaysia, February 2015)* 205–10

[7] Reena J K and Parameswari R 2019 A smart health care monitor system in IoT based human activities of daily living: a review *2019 Int. Conf. on Machine Learning, Big Data, Cloud and Parallel Computing (COMITCon) (Faridabad, India, February 2019)* 446–8

[8] Atiqur R, Liton A M and Wu G 2020 Content caching strategy at small base station in 5G networks with mobile edge computing *Int. J. Sci. Bus.* **4** 104–12

[9] Aziz M N and Islam A K M M 2020 Reviewing data mining as an enabling technology for BI *Int. J. Sci. Bus.* **4** 46–51

[10] Rakhmatulin I 2020 Review of EEG feature selection by neural networks *Int. J. Sci. Bus.* **4** 101–12

[11] Aghdam Z N, Rahmani A M and Hosseinzadeh M 2021 The role of the Internet of Things in healthcare: future trends and challenges *Comput. Methods Programs Biomed.* **199** 105903

[12] Al-Fuqaha A, Guizani M, Mohammadi M, Aledhari M and Ayyash M 2015 Internet of Things: a survey on enabling technologies, protocols, and applications *IEEE Commun. Surv. Tutorials* **17** 2347–76

[13] Aktas F, Ceken C and Erdemli Y E 2018 IoT-based healthcare framework for biomedical applications *J. Med. Biol. Eng.* **38** 966–79

[14] Atzori L, Iera A and Morabito G 2010 The Internet of Things: a survey *Comput. Netw.* **54** 2787–805

[15] Catarinucci L *et al* 2015 An IoT-aware architecture for smart healthcare systems *IEEE Internet Things J.* **2** 515–26

[16] Pradhan B, Bhattacharyya S and Pal K 2021 IoT-based applications in healthcare devices *J. Healthc. Eng.* **2021** 1–18

[17] Thusu D R 2011 Sensors facilitate health monitoring *Fierce Electronics (1 April 2011)* https://fierceelectronics.com/components/sensors-facilitate-health-monitoring (accessed 27 June 2022)

[18] Katzis K, Berbakov L, Gardašević G and Šveljo O 2022 Breaking barriers in emerging biomedical applications *Entropy* **24** 226

[19] Kumar S, Arora A K, Gupta P and Saini B S 2021 A review of applications, security and challenges of Internet of Medical Things *Cognitive Internet of Medical Things for Smart Healthcare* ed A E Hassanien, A Khamparia, D Gupta, K Shankar and A Slowik vol 311 (Cham: Springer International Publishing) pp 1–23

[20] Zhang J X J and Hoshino K 2019 Implantable and wearable sensors *Molecular Sensors and Nanodevices* (Amsterdam: Elsevier) pp 489–545
[21] Hale M F 2014 Capsule endoscopy: current practice and future directions *World J Gastroenterol.* **20** 7752
[22] Fernández-Caramés T and Fraga-Lamas P 2018 Towards the internet-of-smart-clothing: a review on IoT wearables and garments for creating intelligent connected e-textiles *Electronics* **7** 405
[23] Demrozi F, Pravadelli G, Bihorac A and Rashidi P 2020 Human activity recognition using inertial, physiological and environmental sensors: a comprehensive survey *IEEE Access* **8** 210816–36
[24] Pateraki M *et al* 2020 Biosensors and Internet of Things in smart healthcare applications: challenges and opportunities *Wearable and Implantable Medical Devices* (Amsterdam: Elsevier) pp 25–53
[25] Khan W Z, Xiang Y, Aalsalem M Y and Arshad Q 2013 Mobile phone sensing systems: a survey *IEEE Commun. Surv. Tutorials* **15** 402–27
[26] Esteva A *et al* 2021 Deep learning-enabled medical computer vision *npj Digit. Med.* **4** 5
[27] Top 10 applications of deep learning and computer vision in healthcare, viso.ai, 19 August 2021. https://viso.ai/applications/computer-vision-in-healthcare/ (accessed 30 June 2022)
[28] World Economic Forum The global risks report 2019 [Online] https://weforum.org/reports/the-global-risks-report-2019 (accessed 5 August 2022)
[29] IoT reference model CISCO © 2014 Cisco [Online] https://studocu.com/in/document/visvesvaraya-technological-university/iot-and-wsn/iot-reference-model-cisco-module-1-iot-and-wsn/23547483 (accessed 5 August 2022)
[30] CISCO, Model, Internet of Things [Online] https://learniot.com/cisco-model (accessed 5 August 2022)
[31] Kaur M, Singh D, Kumar V, Gupta B B and Abd El-Latif A A 2021 Secure and energy efficient-based e-health care framework for green Internet of Things *IEEE Trans. Green Commun. Netw.* **5** 1223–31
[32] Tabrez Quasim M, Algarni F, Abd Elhamid Radwan A and Alshmrani G M M 2020 A blockchain based secured healthcare framework *2020 Int. Conf. on Computational Performance Evaluation (ComPE) (Shillong, India, July 2020)* 386–91
[33] Haghi Kashani M, Madanipour M, Nikravan M, Asghari P and Mahdipour E 2021 A systematic review of IoT in healthcare: applications, techniques, and trends *J. Netw. Comput. Appl.* **192** 103164
[34] Cherian M and Chatterjee M 2019 Survey of security threats in IoT and emerging countermeasures *Security in Computing and Communications (Singapore)* 591–604
[35] Bhattasali T and Chaki R 2011 A survey of recent intrusion detection systems for wireless sensor network *Advances in Network Security and Applications* ed D C Wyld, M Wozniak, N Chaki, N Meghanathan and D Nagamalai vol 196 (Berlin: Springer) pp 268–80
[36] Xu W, Wood T, Trappe W and Zhang Y 2004 Channel surfing and spatial retreats: defenses against wireless denial of service *Proc. 2004 ACM Workshop on Wireless Security—WiSe04 (Philadelphia, PA, USA)* 80
[37] Xu W, Trappe W, Zhang Y and Wood T 2005 The feasibility of launching and detecting jamming attacks in wireless networks *Proc. 6th ACM Int. Symp. on Mobile Ad Hoc Networking and Computing—MobiHoc05 (Urbana-Champaign, IL, USA)* 46

[38] Noubir G and Lin G 2003 Low-power DoS attacks in data wireless LANs and countermeasures *SIGMOBILE Mob. Comput. Commun. Rev.* **7** 29–30

[39] Msgna M, Markantonakis K and Mayes K 2013 The B-Side of side channel leakage: control flow security in embedded systems *SecureComm 2013. LNICST* vol 127 (Cham: Springer) pp 288–304

[40] Zhang M and Jha N K 2011 FinFET-based power management for improved DPA resistance with low overhead *J. Emerg. Technol. Comput. Syst.* **7** 1–16

[41] Ma J, Jin H, Yang L T and Tsai J J-P (ed) 2006 *Ubiquitous Intelligence and Computing* vol 4159 (Berlin: Springer)

[42] Rieback M R, Crispo B and Tanenbaum A S 2005 RFID guardian: a battery-powered mobile device for RFID privacy management *Information Security and Privacy* ed C Boyd and J M González Nieto vol 3574 (Berlin: Springer) pp 184–94

[43] Kim H 2008 Protection against packet fragmentation attacks at 6LoWPAN adaptation layer *2008 Int. Conf. on Convergence and Hybrid Information Technology (Daejon, South Korea)* 796–801

[44] Hummen R, Hiller J, Wirtz H, Henze M, Shafagh H and Wehrle K 2013 6LoWPAN fragmentation attacks and mitigation mechanisms *Proc. 6th ACM Conf. on Security and Privacy in Wireless and Mobile Networks—WiSec13 (Budapest, Hungary)* 55

[45] Dvir A, Holczer T and Buttyan L 2011 VeRA—version number and rank authentication in RPL *2011 IEEE Eighth Int. Conf. on Mobile Ad-Hoc and Sensor Systems (Valencia, Spain, October 2011)* 709–14

[46] Le A, Loo J, Lasebae A, Vinel A, Chen Y and Chai M 2013 The impact of rank attack on network topology of routing protocol for low-power and lossy networks *IEEE Sens. J.* **13** 3685–92

[47] Alvisi L, Clement A, Epasto A, Lattanzi S and Panconesi A 2013 SoK: the evolution of Sybil defense via social networks *2013 IEEE Symp. on Security and Privacy (Berkeley, CA, May 2013)* 382–96

[48] Zhang K, Liang X, Lu R and Shen X 2014 Sybil attacks and their defenses in the Internet of Things *IEEE Internet Things J.* **1** 372–83

[49] Mohaisen A, Hopper N and Kim Y 2011 Keep your friends close: incorporating trust into social network-based Sybil defenses *2011 Proc. IEEE INFOCOM (Shanghai, China, April 2011)* 1943–51

[50] Son S, McKinley K S and Shmatikov V 2013 Diglossia: detecting code injection attacks with precision and efficiency *Proc. 2013 ACM SIGSAC Conf. on Computer & Communications Security—CCS13 (Berlin, Germany)* 1181–92

[51] Deogirikar J and Vidhate A 2017 Security attacks in IoT: a survey *2017 Int. Conf. on I-SMAC (IoT in Social, Mobile, Analytics and Cloud) (I-SMAC) (Palladam, Tamilnadu, India, February 2017)* 32–7

[52] Alam M M, Malik H, Khan M I, Pardy T, Kuusik A and Le Moullec Y 2018 A survey on the roles of communication technologies in IoT-based personalized healthcare applications *IEEE Access* **6** 36611–31

[53] Ahad A, Tahir M and Yau K-L A 2019 5G-based smart healthcare network: architecture, taxonomy, challenges and future research directions *IEEE Access* **7** 100747–62

[54] Aceto G, Persico V and Pescapé A 2018 The role of information and communication technologies in healthcare: taxonomies, perspectives, and challenges *J. Netw. Comput. Appl.* **107** 125–54

[55] Misran N, Islam M S, Beng G K, Amin N and Islam M T 2019 IoT based health monitoring system with LoRa communication technology *2019 Int. Conf. on Electrical Engineering and Informatics (ICEEI) (Bandung, Indonesia, July 2019)* 514–7

[56] Garg L, Chukwu E, Nasser N, Chakraborty C and Garg G 2020 Anonymity preserving IoT-based COVID-19 and other infectious disease contact tracing model *IEEE Access* **8** 159402–14

[57] Gatouillat A, Badr Y, Massot B and Sejdic E 2018 Internet of Medical Things: a review of recent contributions dealing with cyber-physical systems in medicine *IEEE Internet Things J.* **5** 3810–22

[58] Habibzadeh H, Dinesh K, Rajabi Shishvan O, Boggio-Dandry A, Sharma G and Soyata T 2020 A survey of healthcare Internet of Things (HIoT): a clinical perspective *IEEE Internet Things J.* **7** 53–71

[59] Haghi M, Thurow K and Stoll R 2017 Wearable devices in medical Internet of Things: scientific research and commercially available devices *Healthc. Inform. Res.* **23** 4

[60] Ahmed Z U, Mortuza M G, Uddin M J, Kabir M H, Kabir M H, Mahiuddin Md and Hoque Md J 2018 Internet of Things based patient health monitoring system using wearable biomedical device *2018 Int. Conf. on Innovation in Engineering and Technology (ICIET) (Dhaka, Bangladesh, December 2018)* 1–5

[61] Seshadri D R *et al* 2020 Wearable sensors for COVID-19: a call to action to harness our digital infrastructure for remote patient monitoring and virtual assessments *Front. Digit. Health* **2** 8

[62] El-Rashidy N, El-Sappagh S, Islam S M R, El-Bakry H M and Abdelrazek S 2020 End-to-end deep learning framework for coronavirus (COVID-19) detection and monitoring *Electronics* **9** 1439

[63] Al Bassam N, Hussain S A, Al Qaraghuli A, Khan J, Sumesh E P and Lavanya V 2021 IoT based wearable device to monitor the signs of quarantined remote patients of COVID-19 *Inform. Med. Unlocked* **24** 100588

[64] Turner J, Zellner C, Khan T and Yelamarthi K 2017 Continuous heart rate monitoring using smartphone *2017 IEEE Int. Conf. on Electro Information Technology (EIT) (Lincoln, NE, May 2017)* 324–6

[65] Asri H, Mousannif H and Moatassime H A 2019 Reality mining and predictive analytics for building smart applications *J. Big Data* **6** 66

[66] Kolhar M, Al-Turjman F, Alameen A and Abualhaj M M 2020 A three layered decentralized IoT biometric architecture for city lockdown during COVID-19 outbreak *IEEE Access* **8** 163608–17

[67] Hameed K, Bajwa I S, Ramzan S, Anwar W and Khan A 2020 An intelligent IoT based healthcare system using fuzzy neural networks *Sci. Program.* **2020** 1–15

[68] Chianese R, Gargiulo F and Arciprete M 2019 An IoT-based HIS for healthcare risk management and cost control: a proposal *Proc. 2019 3rd Int. Symp. on Computer Science and Intelligent Control (Amsterdam Netherlands, September 2019)* 1–6

[69] Muthu B *et al* 2020 IoT based wearable sensor for diseases prediction and symptom analysis in healthcare sector *Peer-to-Peer Netw. Appl.* **13** 2123–34

[70] Gupta N, Juneja P K, Sharma S and Garg U 2021 Future aspect of 5G-IoT architecture in smart healthcare system *2021 5th Int. Conf. on Intelligent Computing and Control Systems (ICICCS) (Madurai, India, May 2021)* 406–11

[71] Wong A M-K, Hsu C-L, Le T-V, Hsieh M-C and Lin T-W 2020 Three-factor fast authentication scheme with time bound and user anonymity for multi-server e-health systems in 5G-based wireless sensor networks *Sensors* **20** 2511

[72] Hu X, Abdulghani A M, Imran M and Abbasi Q H 2020 Internet of Things (IoT) for healthcare application: wearable sleep body position monitoring system using IoT platform *Proc. 2020 Int. Conf. on Computing, Networks and Internet of Things (Sanya China, April 2020)* 76–81

[73] Chowdhury M Z, Hossan M T, Shahjalal M, Hasan M K and Jang Y M 2020 A new 5G ehealth architecture based on optical camera communication: an overview, prospects, and applications *IEEE Consum. Electron. Mag.* **9** 23–33

[74] Bharati S, Podder P, Mondal M R H and Paul P K 2021 Applications and challenges of cloud integrated IoMT *Cognitive Internet of Medical Things for Smart Healthcare* ed A E Hassanien, A Khamparia, D Gupta, K Shankar and A Slowik vol 311 (Cham: Springer International Publishing) pp 67–85

[75] Rishabh and Gianey H 2020 Implementation of Internet of Things and protocol *Inventive Computation Technologies* ed S Smys, R Bestak and Á Rocha vol 98 (Cham: Springer International Publishing) pp 272–8

[76] Lakshmi G, Ghonge M and Obaid A 2018 Cloud based IoT smart healthcare system for remote patient monitoring *EAI Endorsed Trans. Pervasive Health Technol.* **21** e4

[77] Juyal S, Sharma S and Shankar Shukla A 2021 Smart skin health monitoring using AI-enabled cloud-based IoT *Mater. Today Proc.* **46** 10539–45

[78] Kumari A, Kumar V, Abbasi M Y, Kumari S, Chaudhary P and Chen C-M 2020 CSEF: cloud-based secure and efficient framework for smart medical system using ECC *IEEE Access* **8** 107838–52

[79] Sharma A, Choudhury T and Kumar P 2018 Health monitoring and management using IoT devices in a cloud based framework *2018 Int. Conf. on Advances in Computing and Communication Engineering (ICACCE) (Paris, France, June 2018)* 219–24

[80] Kil B-H, Park J-S, Ryu M-H, Park C-Y, Kim Y-S and Kim J-D 2021 Cloud-based software architecture for fully automated point-of-care molecular diagnostic device *Sensors* **21** 6980

[81] Akhbarifar S, Javadi H H S, Rahmani A M and Hosseinzadeh M 2020 A secure remote health monitoring model for early disease diagnosis in cloud-based IoT environment *Pers. Ubiquitous Comput.*

[82] Stradolini F, Tamburrano N, Modoux T, Tuoheti A, Demarchi D and Carrara S 2018 IoT for telemedicine practices enabled by an Android™ application with cloud system integration *2018 IEEE Int. Symp. on Circuits and Systems (ISCAS) (Florence)* 1–5

[83] Doukas C and Maglogiannis I 2012 Bringing IoT and cloud computing towards pervasive healthcare *2012 6th Int. Conf. on Innovative Mobile and Internet Services in Ubiquitous Computing (Palermo, July 2012)* 922–6

[84] Chen M, Qian Y, Chen J, Hwang K, Mao S and Hu L 2020 Privacy protection and intrusion avoidance for cloudlet-based medical data sharing *IEEE Trans. Cloud Comput.* **8** 1274–83

[85] Zhang Y, Qiu M, Tsai C-W, Hassan M M and Alamri A 2017 Health-CPS: healthcare cyber-physical system assisted by cloud and big data *IEEE Syst. J.* **11** 88–95

[86] Mahmud R, Koch F L and Buyya R 2018 Cloud-fog interoperability in IoT-enabled healthcare solutions *Proc. 19th Int. Conf. on Distributed Computing and Networking (Varanasi India)* 1–10

[87] Al-Sharhan S, Omran E and Lari K 2019 An integrated holistic model for an eHealth system: a national implementation approach and a new cloud-based security model *Int. J. Inf. Manage.* **47** 121–30
[88] Masud M, Gaba G S, Choudhary K, Alroobaea R and Hossain M S 2021 A robust and lightweight secure access scheme for cloud based E-healthcare services *Peer-to-Peer Netw. Appl.* **14** 3043–57
[89] Darwish A, Hassanien A E, Elhoseny M, Sangaiah A K and Muhammad K 2019 The impact of the hybrid platform of internet of things and cloud computing on healthcare systems: opportunities, challenges, and open problems *J. Ambient Intell. Humaniz. Comput.* **10** 4151–66
[90] Wu H, Sun Y and Wolter K 2020 Energy-efficient decision making for mobile cloud offloading *IEEE Trans. Cloud Comput.* **8** 570–84
[91] Qi L, Chen Y, Yuan Y, Fu S, Zhang X and Xu X 2020 A QoS-aware virtual machine scheduling method for energy conservation in cloud-based cyber-physical systems *World Wide Web* **23** 1275–97
[92] Hu P, Dhelim S, Ning H and Qiu T 2017 Survey on fog computing: architecture, key technologies, applications and open issues *J. Netw. Comput. Appl.* **98** 27–42
[93] Fernando N, Loke S W and Rahayu W 2013 Mobile cloud computing: a survey *Future Gener. Comput. Syst.* **29** 84–106
[94] Ni J, Zhang K, Lin X and Shen X 2018 Securing fog computing for Internet of Things applications: challenges and solutions *IEEE Commun. Surv. Tutorials* **20** 601–28
[95] Andriopoulou F, Dagiuklas T and Orphanoudakis T 2017 Integrating IoT and fog computing for healthcare service delivery *Components and Services for IoT Platforms* ed G Keramidas, N Voros and M Hübner (Cham: Springer International Publishing) pp 213–32
[96] Mahmoud M M E, Rodrigues J J P C, Saleem K, Al-Muhtadi J, Kumar N and Korotaev V 2018 Towards energy-aware fog-enabled cloud of things for healthcare *Comput. Electr. Eng.* **67** 58–69
[97] Nair A R and Tanwar S 2021 Fog computing architectures and frameworks for Healthcare 4.0 *Fog Computing for Healthcare 4.0 Environments* ed S Tanwar (Cham: Springer International Publishing), pp 55–78
[98] Songhorabadi M, Rahimi M, Farid A M M and Kashani M H 2020 Fog computing approaches in smart cities: a state-of-the-art review arXiv:2011.14732
[99] Kashani M H, Ahmadzadeh A and Mahdipour E 2020 Load balancing mechanisms in fog computing: a systematic review arXiv.2011.14706
[100] Ahmadi Z, Haghi Kashani M, Nikravan M and Mahdipour E 2021 Fog-based healthcare systems: a systematic review *Multimed. Tools Appl.* **80** 36361–400
[101] Iorga M, Feldman L, Barton R, Martin M J, Goren N and Mahmoudi C 2018 Fog computing conceptual model *NIST Special Publication 500-325. March 2018* National Institute of Standards and Technology, Gaithersburg, MD https://doi.org/10.6028/NIST.SP.500-325
[102] Shi Y, Ding G, Wang H, Roman H E and Lu S 2015 The fog computing service for healthcare *2015 2nd Int. Symp. on Future Information and Communication Technologies for Ubiquitous HealthCare (Ubi-HealthTech) (Beijing, China, May 2015)* 1–5
[103] Debauche O, Mahmoudi S, Manneback P and Assila A 2019 Fog IoT for health: a new architecture for patients and elderly monitoring *Procedia Comput. Sci.* **160** 289–97

[104] Tuli S *et al* 2020 HealthFog: an ensemble deep learning based smart healthcare system for automatic diagnosis of heart diseases in integrated IoT and fog computing environments *Future Gener. Comput. Syst.* **104** 187–200

[105] Vijayakumar V, Malathi D, Subramaniyaswamy V, Saravanan P and Logesh R 2019 Fog computing-based intelligent healthcare system for the detection and prevention of mosquito-borne diseases *Comput. Hum. Behav.* **100** 275–85

[106] Guo C, Tian P and Choo K-K R 2021 Enabling privacy-assured fog-based data aggregation in e-healthcare systems *IEEE Trans. Ind. Inf.* **17** 1948–57

[107] Lakhan A *et al* 2021 Smart-contract aware ethereum and client-fog-cloud healthcare system *Sensors* **21** 4093

[108] Ahmad M, Amin M B, Hussain S, Kang B H, Cheong T and Lee S 2016 Health fog: a novel framework for health and wellness applications *J. Supercomput.* **72** 3677–95

[109] Nguyen Gia T *et al* 2017 Low-cost fog-assisted health-care IoT system with energy-efficient sensor nodes *2017 13th Int. Wireless Communications and Mobile Computing Conf. (IWCMC) (Valencia, June 2017)* 1765–70

[110] Quy V K, Hau N V, Anh D V and Ngoc L A 2021 Smart healthcare IoT applications based on fog computing: architecture, applications and challenges *Complex Intell. Syst.* **8** 3805–15

[111] Yousefpour A, Ishigaki G, Gour R and Jue J P 2018 On reducing IoT service delay via fog offloading *IEEE Internet Things J.* **5** 998–1010

[112] Al-khafajiy M, Webster L, Baker T and Waraich A 2018 Towards fog driven IoT healthcare: challenges and framework of fog computing in healthcare *Proc. 2nd Int. Conf. on Future Networks and Distributed Systems (Amman, June 2018)* 1–7

[113] Aljanabi S and Chalechale A 2021 Improving IoT services using a hybrid fog-cloud offloading *IEEE Access* **9** 13775–88

[114] Yi S, Li C and Li Q 2015 A survey of fog computing: concepts, applications and issues *Proc. 2015 Workshop on Mobile Big Data (Hangzhou China, June 2015)* 37–42

[115] Mouradian C, Naboulsi D, Yangui S, Glitho R H, Morrow M J and Polakos P A 2018 A comprehensive survey on fog computing: state-of-the-art and research challenges *IEEE Commun. Surv. Tutorials* **20** 416–64

[116] Yang Y, Wang K, Zhang G, Chen X, Luo X and Zhou M-T 2018 MEETS: maximal energy efficient task scheduling in homogeneous fog networks *IEEE Internet Things J.* **5** 4076–87

[117] Wadhwa H and Aron R 2022 TRAM: technique for resource allocation and management in fog computing environment *J. Supercomput.* **78** 667–90

[118] Khumalo N N, Oyerinde O O and Mfupe L 2021 Reinforcement learning-based resource management model for fog radio access network architectures in 5G *IEEE Access* **9** 12706–16

[119] Stojmenovic I and Wen S 2014 The fog computing paradigm: scenarios and security issues *2014 Federated Conf. on Computer Science and Information Systems (Warsaw, September 2014)* 1–8

[120] Hassija V, Chamola V, Saxena V, Jain D, Goyal P and Sikdar B 2019 A survey on IoT security: application areas, security threats, and solution architectures *IEEE Access* **7** 82721–43

[121] Saha R, Kumar G, Rai M K, Thomas R and Lim S-J 2019 Privacy ensured e-healthcare for fog-enhanced IoT based applications *IEEE Access* **7** 44536–43

[122] Wu T-Y, Wang T, Lee Y-Q, Zheng W, Kumari S and Kumar S 2021 Improved authenticated key agreement scheme for fog-driven IoT healthcare system *Secur. Commun. Netw.* **2021** 1–16

[123] Li C, Qin Z, Novak E and Li Q 2017 Securing SDN infrastructure of IoT–fog networks from MitM attacks *IEEE Internet Things J.* **4** 1156–64

[124] Rayan R A, Tsagkaris C and Iryna R B 2021 The Internet of Things for healthcare: applications, selected cases and challenges *IoT in Healthcare and Ambient Assisted Living* ed G Marques, A K Bhoi, V H C de Albuquerque and K S Hareesha vol 933 (Singapore: Springer) pp 1–15

[125] IoT stats, facts and trends, 18 July 2019. https://appventurez.com/blog/iot-market-trends (accessed 5 August 2022)

IOP Publishing

Internet of Things in Biomedical Sciences
Challenges and applications
Varun Bajaj and Irshad Ahmad Ansari

Chapter 3

AI role in making IoT-based medical devices a success

S Palanivel Rajan and T Abirami

In a healthcare system, Internet of Things (IoT), artificial intelligence (AI) and machine learning (ML) join together to monitor the health condition of sick people. The whole concept of a healthcare system is fully automated with sensors and transducers. To become very specific, the number of devices used in the system is huge. A sensor provides the physical quantity of the patient's health measurements via IoT, the data from the sensors are transferred to the cloud. From the cloud the consultant takes the data for further treatment process for remote patient monitoring. IoT helps in remote patient monitoring (RPM) technology. AI-based medical devices should make analysis and processing leading to the conclusion of their treatment process. AI is especially designed for chronic disease to provide a better solution of treatment. If any medication is required for this disease, that can also be mentioned and conveyed to the patients. Smartwatches like a glucometer are worn by the patient on their wrist to know the condition of their glucose level. Along with devices, an ML algorithm is also combined and make rules and regulation for monitoring the patient in remote area networks. In addition to the system, if the decision is made by the system with reference to the past data, this mechanism is known as AI. After producing each and every result, the past data will be erased and will give new decisions for treatment. Locked and continuous models are available in artificial networks. ML AI is used in acclimatized authoritarian, standards and frameworks to make sure of the precaution measurements in smart devices.

This chapter starts with the fundamental concept of IoT, AI and ML in medical devices. Interoperability is the major fact of AI and IoT to maintain the tracking of events on the devices and to react according to it. It involves a transformation towards an active patient, that can be accustomed in real time and a more complicated data management strategy. Thus IoT, AI and ML play a major role in medical devices.

doi:10.1088/978-0-7503-5311-3ch3

3.1 Introduction

Nowadays, the concepts of IoT, ML and AI combine together working to analyze the various parameters in the medical field. Initially the small device which is used to measure each parameter has been invented [1]. The measured parameters are transferred to the cloud via IoT. After receiving the data from the cloud, the consultant will make a decision to give appropriate treatment via remote access. For decision making and analysis we may use ML algorithms. AI is a machine which will think and act on its own. In IoT, many types of sensor are used like pressure sensors, temperature sensors, ECG sensors, etc.

The block diagram of an IoT-based healthcare network is shown in figure 3.1. In this diagram sensors are a major component to sense the information from the patient's body [2]. The collected information will be transferred via a portable device. This device is called an IoT agent. From this the data is moved to the cloud for analysis purposes by the doctor or consultant. For analysis of the data, ML algorithms may be used. The ML algorithm plays a major role after data collection via the cloud. The architecture of an IoT network is shown in figure 3.2.

3.2 Benefits of an IoT network

The smart device is used by patients in remote areas with wireless mode of treatments. The wireless mode of treatment will give various advantages over in-person visits to hospital. The following parameters are considered as the benefits of an IoT network in healthcare monitoring systems.

- Accuracy: System
  accuracy is a very important parameter to be considered for medical treatment. If the accuracy is not to the desired value the device needs to be checked in periodical duration.

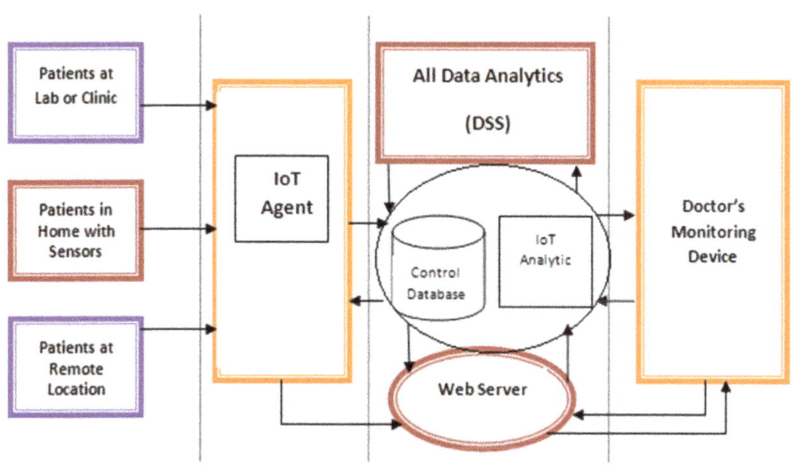

Figure 3.1. A model for IoT-based healthcare networks.

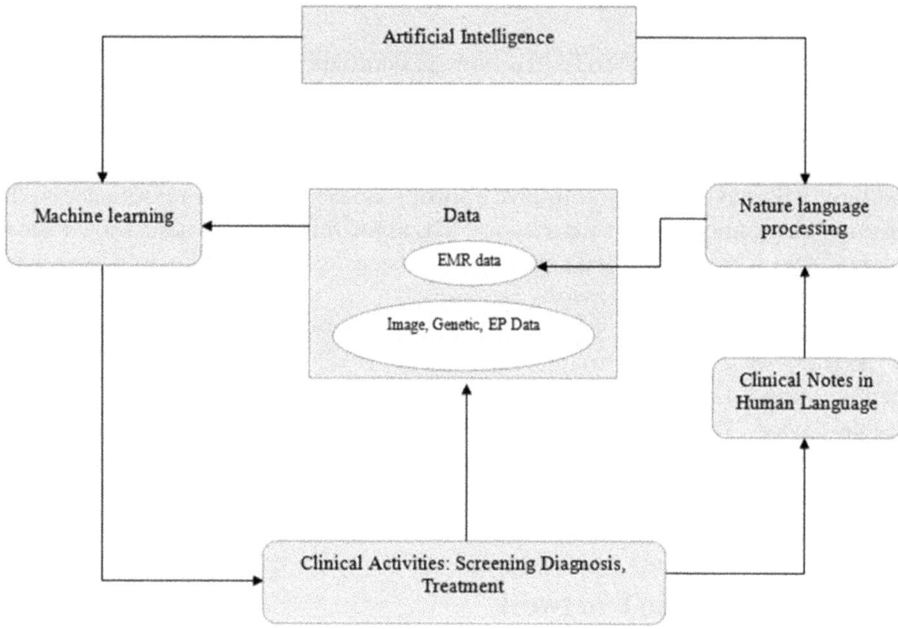

Figure 3.2. Architecture of IoT with ML and AI.

- Time consumption:
  For the patient to visit a hospital it will be a time-consuming process. A vehicle is required to take the patient to the hospital. The patient needs a care giver to stay in the hospital until the completion of treatment [3]. But an IoT system will not take much time to provide the treatment for patients. Time consumption of this process is very little.
- Less expensive:
  This system will provide the IoT kit for medical treatment. The cost of this treatment will be reduced.
- Data access and sharing:
  The device can support instant access to the entire data at any time. Here the cloud is used to store the data. Whenever the doctor needs to access the data it is possible. Data access should be in an effective manner.
- Updates in data:
  The data should be updated each and every second to allow convenient treatment for patients. Any delay in updates could lead to wrong direction of the treatment. This cannot be encouraged in healthcare monitoring via IoT.

3.2.1 Sensing elements for medical purpose

A sensor is a device which is used to predict the physical parameters from the patient or environment. Various sensors exist for finding parameters of medical usage. The measured values of the sensor are very accurate, easy to use for computations and reliable. Such a device can help patient monitoring for remote access. The various sensors are fixed on the human body as shown in figure 3.3. The sensor is also known as a transducer in that it can convert physical parameters into electrical signals.

- Electroencephalogram sensor:
  This sensor is available for measuring electrical movement of the brain. The brain is the heart of the body which will give the command to all other organs in the body.
- Blood pressure heart rate sensor:
  The pressure sensor is integrated with either microcontroller or microprocessor. It is mainly for diagnosis, pressure monitoring and infusion pumps. By means of pressure the heart rate can also be measured.
- Thermometer or thermister:
  The sensor measures the temperature of the human body. This device helps people to know the patient's condition because of rise and fall in the temperature. An increase shows that a patient is infected by disease.
- Implantable pacemaker:
  This is embedded with a controller that produces an electric stimulus to the heart for maintaining efficient cardiac tempo.
- Oximeter:
  Oximeter is a device to measure the ratio between oxygen saturated hemoglobin and total number of the hemoglobin.
- Glucometer:
  This device is a sensor which is worn to measure the glucose level in the blood.
- Electrocardiogram sensor:
  In short this is named ECG sensor. It will record the electric activity of the heart.

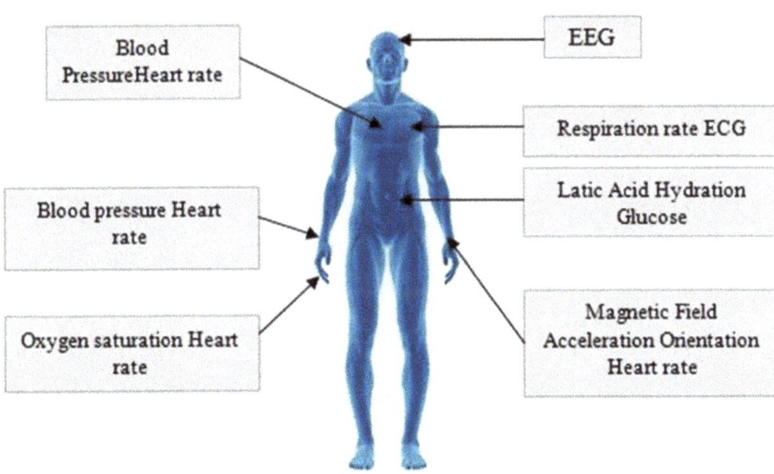

Figure 3.3. Various sensors in the human body.

- Sensor to measure heart rate:
  This sensor will give the heart beat per minute.
- Respiration rate sensor:
  It will produce a count of chest expansion per minute.

3.3 Machine learning

ML offers study tools for the researcher on the way to doing research in this domain. There will be comparison between traditional methods with ML algorithms [4]. In the traditional method, the data and predefined model should be the input, whereas in ML approach, data is only the input and the system will generate the model for it (figure 3.4).

It is divided into three types:

1. Supervised learning;
2. Unsupervised learning;
3. Reinforcement learning.

The methods of learning in ML will be in the following sections. First the concepts of supervised learning are given below.

3.3.1 Supervised learning

Here a labeled dataset is used. Labeled dataset means that the dataset has known outputs. It uses a number of training sets. When the input is received it automatically compares with the training set and it will produce an output. In supervised learning, the accuracy is high [5]. The algorithm may work under control of a supervisor. Therefore, it is called supervised learning. The pictorial diagram of supervised learning is shown in figure 3.5.

There are two classifications of a supervised learning algorithm. The algorithms are:

- Classification, and
- Regression.

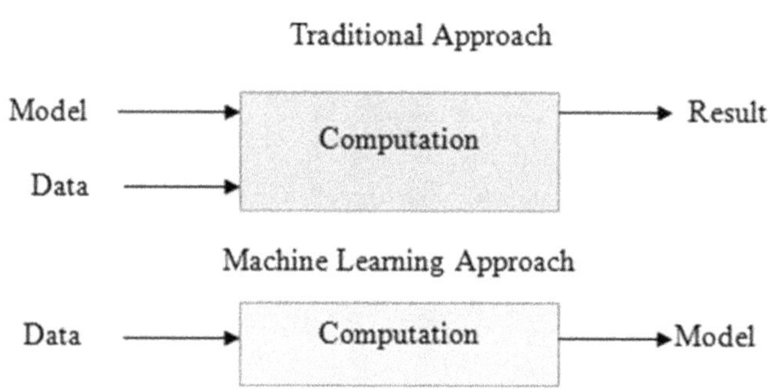

Figure 3.4. Comparisons between traditional approach and ML approach.

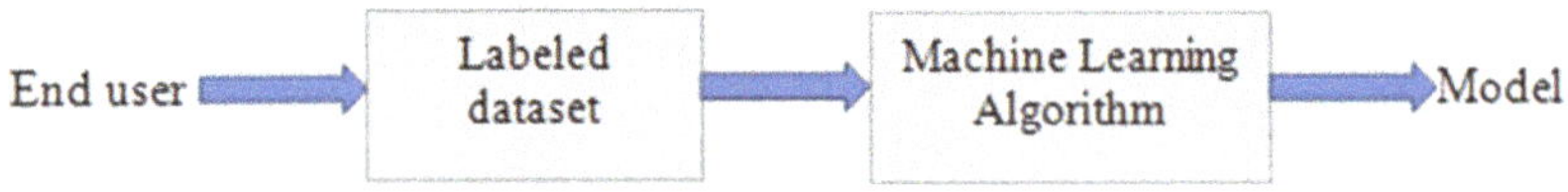

Figure 3.5. Example of supervised learning.

The classification type is used to classify the data. It may be called binary classification. There will be only two distinct outputs. In regression algorithm, it will predict the output for continuous incoming data.

- Classification:
  This is the process of finding an algorithm which helps in dividing the dataset into classes based on parameters. Suppose we have a model to predict gender, then this classification method is used for prediction and that will divide the dataset based on features and will give the results.
- Regression:
  Regression analysis is a fundamental concept which is trained with both the input and output labels. It is an algorithm which predicts the discrete value in the form of integer quantity.
  For an example, if we want to predict the experience of an employee in a company we need to know the age of the employee, and his salary and his date of joining in order to predict his experience. There are different algorithms used. A few algorithms are linear regression, K-nearest neighbor, decision trees, support vector machine and neural networks [6].
- Decision tree algorithm:
  This is widely used for finding the model and it is applicable for making decisions with the help of classification and regression algorithms. It is the concept of tree structure and it has root node, decisional node, branches, leaf and finally terminating node.
- K-nearest neighbor:
  This algorithm is a simpler algorithm than the other algorithms. This is under the category of supervised learning. Based on the similarities of the data, it classifies the new data. The other name of this algorithm is non-parametric algorithm, which is not based on the assumptions.
- Linear regression:
  Linear regressing is based on supervised learning and it performs regression tasks. In this we predict the target variable based on the independent variables. The relationship between the variables is linear.
- Support vector machine:
  This is used to create a new line or to create the boundary that segregates the dimensional space into different classes. It is good for reliable results when there is less data. Newly given data will measure future accuracy.
- Neural networks
  An artificial neural network is also called neural network or neural nets. It is based on the human nervous system. It is used to remember, recognize and correlate. It also makes us understand who we are, what we do and where we are.

3.3.2 Unsupervised learning

Here an unlabeled dataset is used. The unlabeled dataset means it doesn't know the output. This is why it is called an unlabeled dataset. The set of rules will be framed such that the input may be classified into a set of similar groups called a class [7]. Techniques used are clustering and associating the datasets. An example of unsupervised learning is shown in figure 3.6.

There are various types of unsupervised learning algorithms. The classifications are clustering algorithms, outlier detection, association rule mining and auto encoders.

- Clusters:

  This is an unsupervised learning technique. The method of dividing the objects into clusters is making two groups of objects with the help of similar and dissimilar objects. It has a finite number of data and clusters [8].

  For example, suppose a telecom company wants to segregate the customers based on their personalized calls and data plan, for this the cluster method is used.
- Association:

  Association is used for finding the relationship between variables in a large dataset. Discovering the probability of the association of the item is called collection.

  For example, when we are doing online shopping we will be searching for a product like TV and the other brands associated with that are displayed in the suggestion.

3.3.3 Reinforcement learning

Feedback and past experiences are major things to predict the values for the corresponding inputs. Each and every step there will be a feedback path so that it is also called trial and error method [9]. Q-Learning, deep adversarial networks, temporal difference are a few of the algorithms of reinforcement algorithms. A block diagram of reinforcement learning is shown in figure 3.7.

Reinforcement learning is used for decision making sequentially. Generally, the output will be dependent upon the current input and the next input will be the output of the previous input.

For example, when we are playing chess we will be moving a coin and that is considered as reward and punishment. If we make a right move then it will be reward and if we make a wrong move it will be considered as punishment.

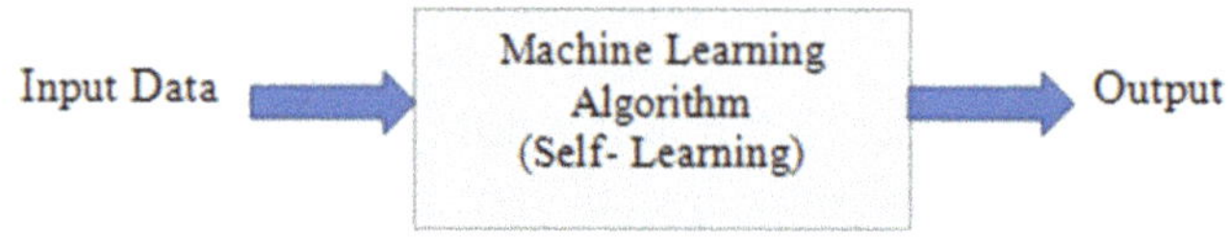

Figure 3.6. Example of unsupervised learning algorithms.

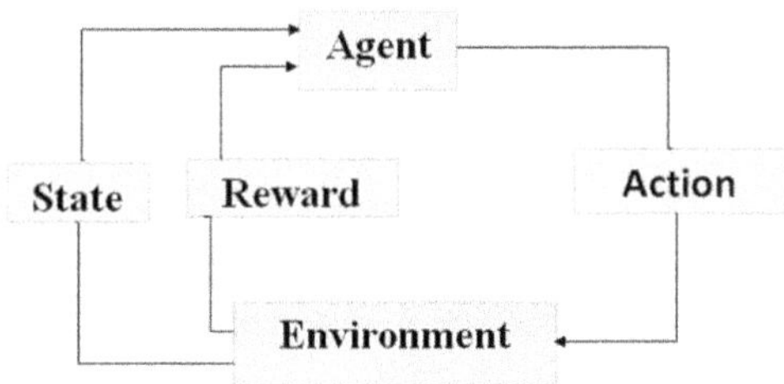

Figure 3.7. Example of reinforcement algorithms.

3.4 Machine learning and IoT

IoT is just internet of things, but if the IoT is used for healthcare means it is termed as H-IoT (healthcare-internet of things). There are different types of ML algorithm used for H-IoT applications. Various domains are mentioned for healthcare applications. The domains are monitoring, analyzing, prognosis, diagnosis, and logistics. In a healthcare application it is essential to produce accurate values. The accurate values will be produced by the various ML algorithms [10]. IoT with ML algorithms gives a number of advantages. ML-based systems use a large amount of data for training purposes. There are two different datasets: trained dataset and test dataset. The test datasets are taken from the device and given to the ML-based system for analysis.

3.4.1 H-IoT architecture

The architecture of H-IoT has three different layers in an end-to-end network. The three layers are collection layer of data, data storage layer and finally data processing layer. The data is collected by the various types of sensors and once collected can be stored and transferred through the internet. Finally, the data is processed by using different types of algorithms. Healthcare technologies combine different techniques to make an efficient architecture. An H-IoT technology diagram is shown in figure 3.8. RFID is used for identification technology. In this way, different communication modules can be combined that can work as an H-IoT network in healthcare applications.

There are various technologies in H-IoT.

i) Identification technology:

Initially, the identification technology accesses the data very securely. For accessing data, a unique identification is assigned for all data.

ii) Communication technology:

This can be short and long-distance communication. If the devices are very close it means using devices like Bluetooth, Zigbee, RFID. If long-distance communication is needed, the system requires the internet to transfer the data.

iii) Location technology:

GPS (global positioning system) is mainly used for tracking the location of H-IoT. In the case of poor connectivity, different location techniques may be used.

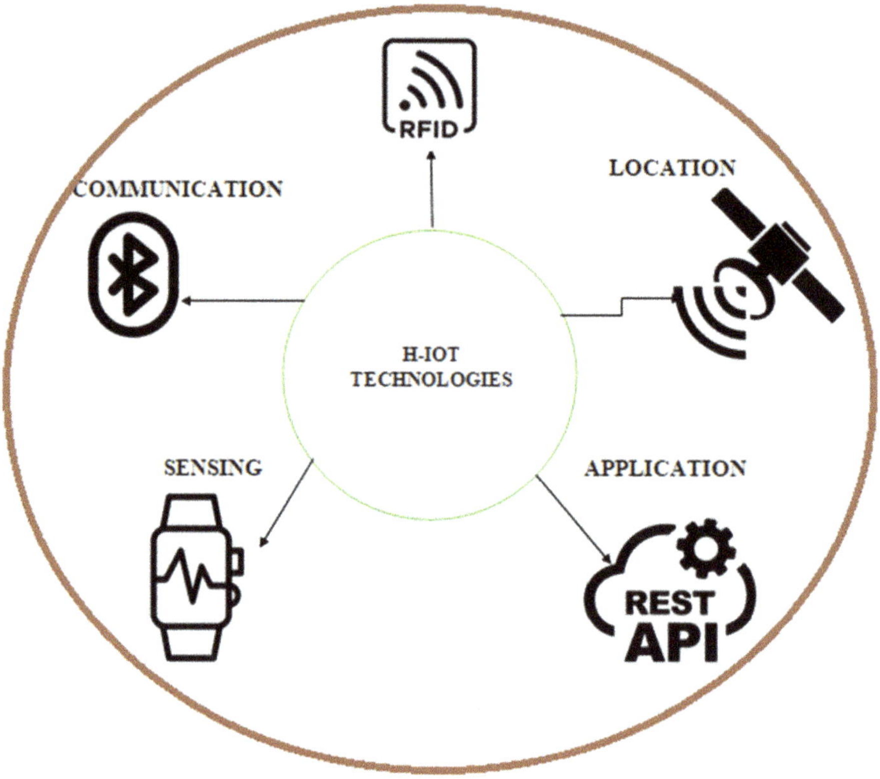

Figure 3.8. H-IoT technologies.

iv) Sensing technology:
This system is required for sensing physical changes in the human body. To capture data, various sensors are used as mentioned in the sensing elements topic.

v) Application level technology:
This technology uses service-based architecture.

3.4.2 H-IoT algorithms

Healthcare ML-based IoT systems will have different algorithms for classification, processing, and analyzing. There are two types of data in ML. ML mainly focuses on labeled datasets, whereas deep learning algorithms focus more on unlabeled data.

- K-nearest neighbors (KNN):
  This is one of the supervised learning algorithms. Data is classified into various categories based on similarity properties. Distance needs to be calculated. Distance is defined as the difference between the features of the object to the neighborhood features.

- K-means classifier:
  This algorithm mainly focuses on wireless sensor networks (WSNs). The algorithm gets the input data to compare with the trained dataset. It is going to predict the result as similar or dissimilar. It is used for continuous monitoring of ECG patients through wearable devices. Diagnosis can be done for the chikungunya disease among the possibilities. This algorithm may extend to test in the COVID-19 pandemic period also.
- Decision tree:
  This algorithm is like a tree that has nodes, branches and leaves, and is used to denote the features, decision making rules and finally the outcomes. This may also be helpful for tracking devices in a pandemic period. It may also be helpful for measuring heart rate.
- Random forest

A number of decision trees are combined to form a random forest algorithm to produce a single output. With the definition it is understood that it is very expensive. It can produce greater than 95% accuracy compared to all other algorithms to detect a virus-infected human body in a crowded area.

3.5 Artificial intelligence

AI is an intelligent machine which can perform actions on its own and make decisions automatically. This technology combines both hardware and software to support the vision of the system, understanding of machine languages, and finally for processing natural language [11]. AI makes use of conventional CMOS hardware and a few basic functions that drive the software. In future, the hardware may change to work with various machines.

The ideal quality of the AI system is reasoning and making decisions like a human being. The ML algorithm is a subtopic of AI to make the computer to do the operation automatically and make it adapt for new data without human assistance. Moreover, deep learning algorithms allow the autonomous system to acheive the best results from inputs in any one of the formats of text, photo, data or video.

- Problem solving
  AI provides the solution for a problem statement. It is a systematic approach to provide the potential activities to obtain a predetermined solution or goal for the given problem. The two different types of techniques of problem solving are specialized and universal. A special purpose of approach is created especially for a given problem statement. It takes the advantages of unique features of the context in which the crisis is well-established. This approach is used to solve many kinds of problems.
- How is AI used today?
  AI is widely used in different forms of applications. Very popular implementations include algorithms that recommend what you might like next and chat bots [12]. This can be found on websites or smartspeakers like Alexa or Siri. AI makes automatic production, reduces redundant cognitive

labor and offers weather forecasts. This technique is employed for a plethora of tasks, including different language processing, driving autonomous cars and online gaming.

3.5.1 The various types of AI

The types of AI are listed below. For making decisions reactive AI is used:
1. To store data, limited memory AI is used;
2. Theory of mind AI;
3. Self-aware AI in order to attain the objective.

An AI device is a machine that, like human beings, makes decisions and performs its own actions

- Reactive machine:
  This is a machine to carry out a fundamental mission. This level of AI is the common basic task. This kind of machine is used to provide some output in response to some input. Learning does not take place. Any AI starts off at this point. This machine accepts a human face as input and it will produce an output as a box of faces to recognize the face. Here learning is not happening and no data is stored [13]. The machines are models of static machines. They have unique architecture and are available in Github repositories. This type of model is able to download, make changes, share and upload for the developer's purpose.
- Limited memory:
  The important parameter of AI is storage capacity. The system stores the information and erases past data. The complication behind the ML algorithm is limited storage. Each and every model of the machine can be organized as a reactive model type even though it only needs a small amount of memory to be created. There are three prominent ML models that leverage restricted memory AI:

  - Reinforcement learning;
  - Long short term memory (LSTM);
  - Evolutionary generative adversarial networks (E-GANs).

3.5.2 AI and IoT

Today in modern trends, there are two ways to monitor the patient's health via remote access. The first is wearable devices like gadgets worn by the patient. AI and IoT play a major role in medical fields such as the patient's health monitoring, giving solutions for health problems through the gadgets. The second is developing the healthcare app to observe the patient's physical condition. Physical condition of the patient's health can be monitored and controlled continuously through AI and IoT.

In publications, 63% of people quote that this form of healthcare is giving very high value in such areas as radiology, pathology and generic pharmacy. From the researcher's point of view, 44% said that AI/ML is providing healthcare solutions in an effective way. This technology helps not only for the patient's health, but also advises individuals to adopt healthier habits either from the gadgets or through apps, by suggesting ways to live a healthy life. IoT is a comparatively innovative expertize that creates a connection of more smart gadgets without any flaws. Speed and accuracy are the required high effective parameters in IoT.

Why IoT needs AI?

IoT enables devices to talk to one another and act on these discoveries. These gadgets are only as useful as the information they offer. The data must be gathered, saved, processed, and analyzed in order to be valuable for decision making [14]. Organizations are faced with a dilemma as a result. Businesses are having trouble effectively processing the data and using it for practical decision making and insights as IoT use rises.

The cloud and data transit are to blame for these two issues. The bandwidth that is mandatory to move data from IoT to the cloud platform is constrained, and the cloud cannot scale proportionately to handle all the data that arrives from IoT devices. IoT device data collection generates latency and congestion regardless of the size and sophistication of the communications network.

Advantages of AI:

- It is possible to provide solutions to complex problems with low cost of service.
- AI devices provide full activity, without stopping and with no downtime experienced.
- People with disabilities can improve their capability.
- Across industries, AI may have large market potential.
- Decision making by the AI helps improving the process.

Disadvantages of AI:

- High cost.
- No creativity.
- Makes humans lazy.
- Emotionless.

Applications of AI:

- AI is used in law and order based services.
- AI provides services in manufacturing industries.
- AI is used in banking sectors.
- AI is applicable for transportation and makes high security.

3.5.3 Remote patient monitoring (RPM)

RPM is mostly used in the following chronic problems: diabetes, post-surgery patients, cardiac patients, pediatrics, prenatal care and hyper tension. Various devices can be used as remote patient monitoring devices, such as:

- For measuring oxygen level in blood, a pulse oximeter is used.
- For monitoring glucose level, a glucometer is used.
- ECG for heart patients.
- Movement tracking by a smart watch.

Devices are installed or ready to use by the patient, the values in the devices are recorded and directed to vendors for checking health conditions [15]. Based on the measured values, actions are taken by the consultant or doctors. In case of any abnormal conditions, the device has a risk alarm system to warn of a dangerous situation. This device provides real-time healthcare solutions for accuracy of a patient's health condition [16]. Because of this device the following benefits are achieved:

- Better outcome;
- Readmissions are reduced;
- Reduction in cost;
- High efficiency;
- Enabled self-care;
- Enlarge the patient meeting.

3.5.4 Diabetes disease

Kaiser Permanente has introduced the Bluetooth-enabled glucometer. It has been worn by two patients for monitoring glucose level. With the help of IoT, measured readings are sent to the healthcare team. The record says that 45 000 people used this device. This may help people in the period of COVID-19 pandemic. During the pandemic period, their care has improved. The number of users can be increased in future. The RPM device will grow rapidly with its adoption. It can be expected to be used by about 30 million US patients by the year 2024.

Diabetes is a metabolic disease that may increase or decrease. If the sugar level of the human is decreased it is called low sugar. Insulin is required to increase the glucose level. If it is increased it is called as high sugar. Rise in sugar can be reduced by means of regular food habits. Patients are advised to take twice the glucose level in the device. Before eating they need to take a sugar level test and again after. The normal range of glucose level is 80–130 mg dl^{-1} for the human being.

3.5.5 Cardiovascular disease (CVD)

CVD affects the blood vessels or heart. It is connected with the deposit of unwanted fat inside arteries and it causes clots in blood. Blood clots will damage the other organs such as kidneys, brain and eyes [17]. Finally, it causes either disability in the body or death. There are various types of CVD. The categories are:

1. Coronary heart disease:

   This heart disease occurs with a rise in the oxygen level of blood to block the function of the heart. It will increase strain in the heart. The different types of coronary heart disease are angina, heart attack, heart failure.
2. Strokes and transient ischemic attacks:

   The supply of blood to the brain is suddenly stopped causeing brain damage or death [18]. The symptoms of stroke are in any part of the body such as face, arms, restricted speech.

3. Peripheral arterial disease:
   This happens in the legs because of blockage in the arteries. Moreover, the legs are affected with various causes like hair loss in legs, weakness of the leg, etc.
4. Aortic disease:
   This mainly affects the number of vessels. The vessels are used to supply the blood from the heart to the rest of the body and from the rest of the body to the brain.

3.5.6 Wearable device using IoT

Sensor technology plays a major role in wearable devices. The sensor is used to sense or detect physical parameters and in that device next to the block is a transducer which is used to transfer physical parameters into an electrical signal [19]. The eyeglass was the first wearable device, introduced in 1286. The eyeglass is a wearable device that overcomes problems of eyesight. Today, eyeglasses can be replaced by laser treatment of the retina. Abacus rings and roulette shoes were developed in 1600 and 1601, respectively. The abacus ring is for doing mathematical calculations. For a long period inventions of wearable devices have been improving and modification in inventions has continued.

Some devices are used for medical purposes and others are for attaining fitness of the body. The wearable device is classified into two types:

i) Medical wearable device.
ii) Fitness wearable device.

- Medical wearable device:
  This device is essential for medical purposes. The device is used to collect information about the patient and it is used for analysis of the patient's health condition. The glucose meter is a good example.
- Fitness wearable device:
  This device is used for maintaining proper condition of health. It is only for detecting wellness. FDA approval is not required before usage. The best examples of the device are fitness bands and smart watches. It is used for tracking various vessels including for temperature, stress levels, heart rate, oxygen level etc; all the data are collected from the wrist.
- Implantable device:
  This non-removable device can be fixed inside the body and is used to obtain health-related data. With the help of the device, the information of the entire change in the body will be monitored by the consultant and it will help to give proper and appropriate treatment. There are many implanted devices, of which a few can be mentioned here. Glucose monitoring: this device has multiple layers of sensors placed in the abdominal skin cells to do the treatment effectively [20]. The data is received from the device with time duration of 5 min and it will monitor the glucose level. One more implanted device is neural stimulator: this device monitors neural activity to give the proper direction of the brain. With the help of the device, pressure level in the structure of the brain can be reduced.

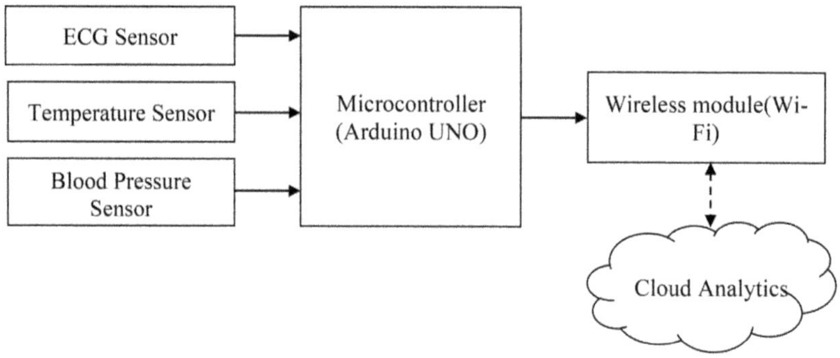

Figure 3.9. Block diagram of health monitoring devices.

3.6 Real-time applications of health monitoring devices

- **Arduino UNO:**

  Arduino UNO is the heart of our projects, which operates multiple sensors together depending upon the given input to the Arduino board. Arduino UNO is a type of microcontroller consisting of ATmega328P which is an IC that controls the operations (figure 3.9).

  Arduino UNO has 14 pins of digital input and outputs. Out of 14 pins, 6 are used as pulse width modulation (PWM) outputs, 6 pins are analog inputs, 16 MHz ceramic resonator, a USB (A to B Type) with connector and power jack. Basically, Arduino is the device which converts programming language into machine language and controls the sensor through the given code.
- **ECG sensor:**

  This is a device which measures the heart's rhythm and electrical movement. These sensors are fixed in the body in order to sense the electrical signal and produce the measured value for further processing.

  ECG sensor has a number of electrodes to trace electrical signal of ECG. Some models are attached to the skin on the chest using sticky patches. Here it connects the ECG sensor to the Arduino UNO to measure the heart rate. Finally, the data is uploaded to the cloud with the help of a Wi-Fi module.
- **Temperature sensor:**

  This is a device used to measure the surrounding room temperature and the body temperature etc. Here we use the temperature sensor to find the temperature of the human body. There are many types of temperature sensors such as thermocouple, RTDS thermister, and semiconductor-based integrated circuits.

  The temperature sensor is connected to the Arduino board and measured temperature of the body data is uploaded to the cloud.
- **Blood pressure sensor:**

  This is a device used to determine blood pressure. The blood pressure sensor works on the principle of blood flowing through an artery between systolic and diastolic pressure. It causes vibrations in the arterial well which can be sensed and the transducer converts into electrical signals.

Measuring your blood pressure is the only way to know whether the blood pressure is high or not. High blood pressure has no caution signs. Then we connect the blood pressure sensor to the Arduino board and all sensor data are uploaded to the cloud with the help of a Wi-Fi unit.

- **Wi-Fi module:**

  This is a device in which the function is used to convert from the serial port or TTL level into an embedded module. Wi-Fi module connects the wireless network communication standard, with the wireless network protocol. Wi-Fi module ESP32 will help to upload the data of all sensors to the cloud.

  WSP32 is a Wi-Fi module that can operate as a whole standalone system or as a slave device in order to reduce the communication stack on the main application processor. The ESP32 Wi-Fi module interfaces with other systems to provide the functions of Wi-Fi and also Bluetooth functionality through the SPI/SDIO or I2C/VART connectors.

- **Cloud analysis:**

  ThingSpeak is an IoT analytics platform. It provides the service that allows aggregating, visualizing and analyzing live data streams to cloud. The data can be sent to the ThingSpeak from devices, creating instant visualizations of live data, and sending alerts using web services. ThingSpeak module and MATLAB tool are combined to execute the MATLAB code to perform pre-processing, visualizations, and analyses. ThingSpeak enables the prototype to build IoT systems without setting up servers or developing web software.

  To write the data to channel:

  REST and MQTT APIs are used to update channels with software or devices.

  To read data from channel:

  REST and MQTT APIs are needed to read channels using software or devices.

  To prepare and analyze data:

  Filtering the data, to transform, and give a response to data in MATLAB tool.

  To visualize data:

  Transformation and visualization of data in MATLAB tool.

  To act on data:

  ThingSpeak app is required to trigger an action or transform and visualize the data.

  Specialized analysis with MATLAB toolbox:

  ThingSpeak is the best example that demonstrates the usage of the advanced tools available in add-on toolboxes.

  API Reference:

  REST and MQTT APIs are needed to update the ThingSpeak channels and to chart numeric data stored in the channels.

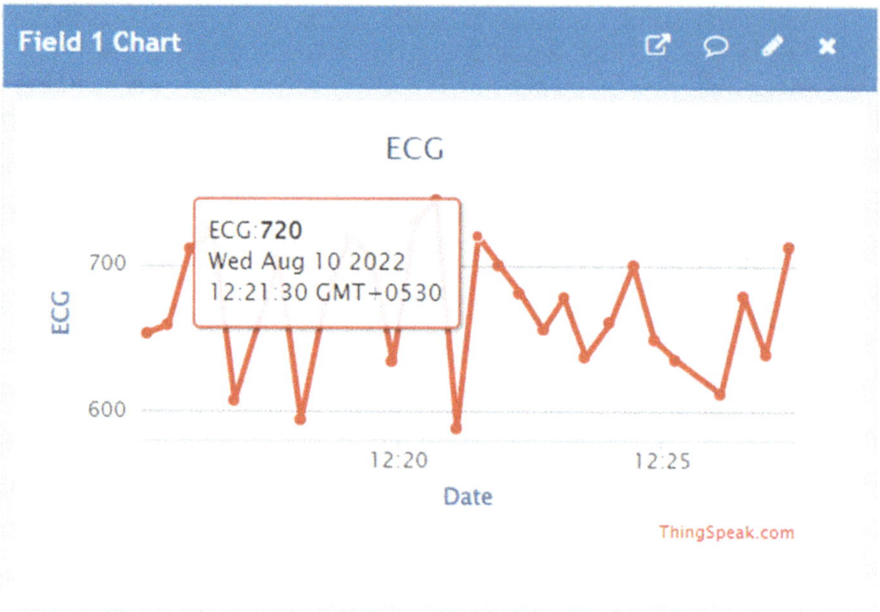

Figure 3.10. ECG output waveform.

- **ECG output wave form:**

  The ordinary range of the ECG signal has different values for males and females. For men, the normal range of the heart is 49–100 bpm (figure 3.10). For women, the ordinary range of the heart is 55–108 bpm. P wave has duration from 81 to 130 ms versus 84–130 ms and the PR interval differs from 119 to 210 ms versus 120–202 ms. Finally the QRS duration is about 74–110 ms.
- **Temperature output wave form:**

  Normal body temperature is generally accepted as an average of 98.6 °F (37 °C). There is a wide range of temperature from 97 °F (36.1 °C) to 99 °F (37.2°C). If temperature is above 100.4 °F (38 °C), this most often means they have a fever caused by a virus or disease (figure 3.11).
- **Systolic blood pressure output in waveform:**

  The pressure on the walls of the arteries in the heart every time it beats is called systolic blood pressure (figure 3.12). Briefly, systolic blood pressure means the blood pressure when the heart increases in its beats. The normal systolic blood pressure range is less than 120 mm Hg. The systolic blood pressure abnormal range is 120–139 mm Hg.
- **Diastolic blood pressure output in wave form**

  Diastolic pressure is the pressure in the arteries when the heart is resting between its beats. The resting between the beats is the time to fill the blood and get the oxygen needed (figure 3.13). Briefly, diastolic pressure means pressure of blood in the heart resting time between beats. Diastolic pressure has a value between 60 and 80 mm Hg. The abnormal diastolic pressure range is above 80 mm Hg.

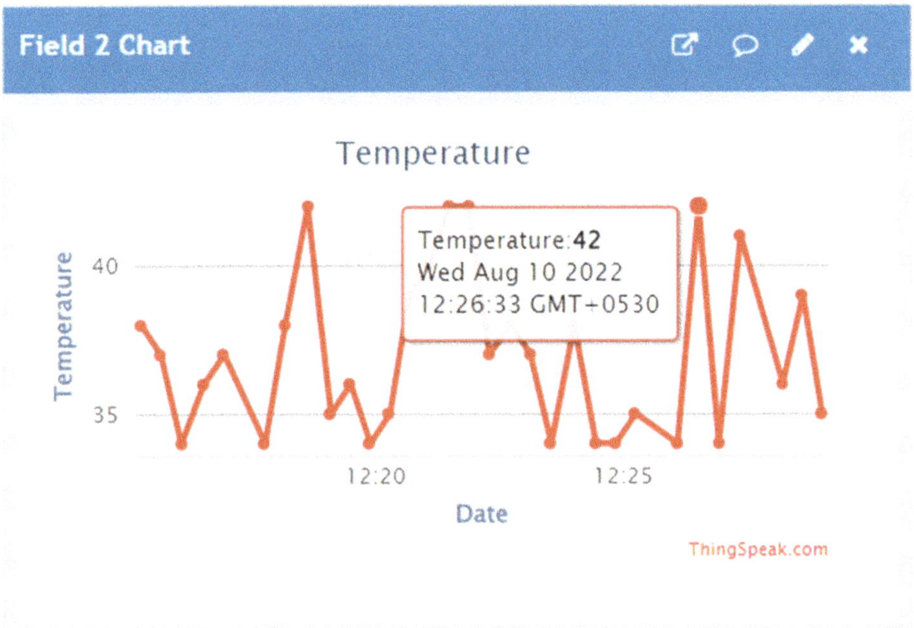

Figure 3.11. Temperature output waveform.

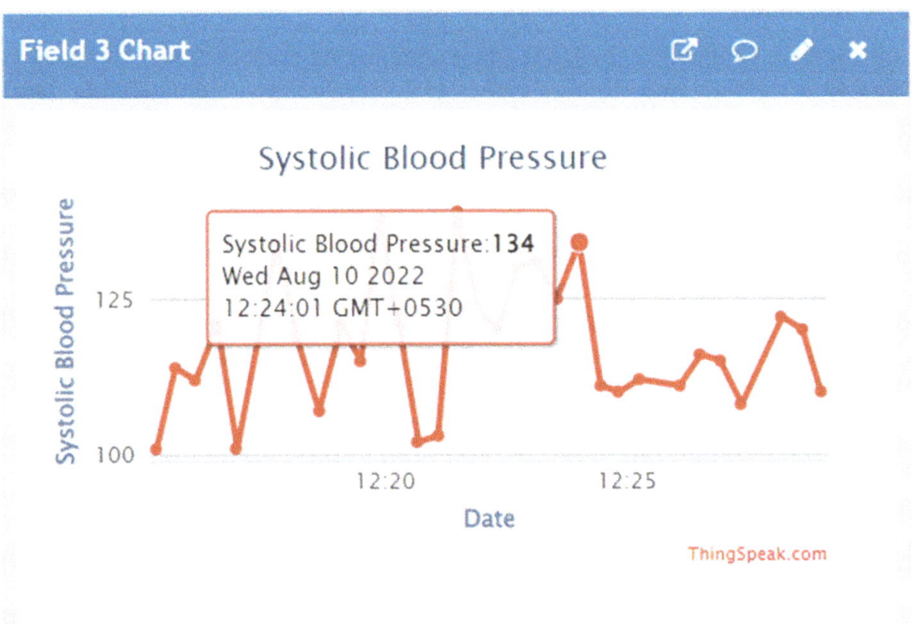

Figure 3.12. Systolic blood pressure output waveform.

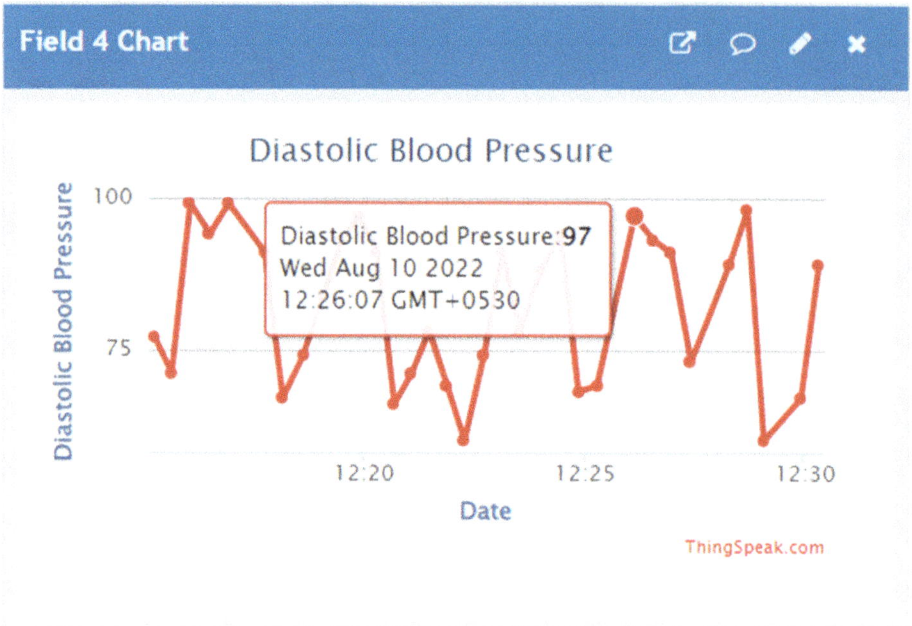

Figure 3.13. Diastolic blood pressure output waveform.

3.7 Conclusion

In a healthcare application, IoT, ML algorithm and AI are joined together to help in predicting disease and classifying diseases in an appropriate manner. The patient is not in a position to move to hospital for checking his/her health condition. During the pandemic period this technology played a major contribution to detect disease. This technology has helped with remote access health monitoring. This technique has produced very accurate data with no fault analysis of this mechanism found. With this conclusion these three areas work together more efficiently to predict disease in an accurate manner. In particular, it has helped older people who are less able to come to hospital for regular checkup. For these people this technique has been invented, and now doctors and consultants may virtually visit the patient's home frequently to provide healthcare.

References

[1] https://rfwireless-world.com/Articles/Medical-sensor-basics-and-medical-sensor-types.htm

[2] Yin Y, Zeng Y, Chen X and Fan Y 2016 The Internet of Things in healthcare: an overview *J. Ind. Inf. Integr.* **1** 3–13

[3] Ahmed F 2017 An Internet of Things (IoT) application for predicting the quantity of future heart attack patients *Int. J. Comput. Appl.* **164** 36–40

[4] Ganesan M and Sivakumar N 2019 IoT based heart disease prediction and diagnosis model for healthcare using machine learning models *Proc. IEEE Int. Conf. on System, Computation, Automation and Networking (ICSCAN) (March 2019)* 1–5

[5] Panda S and Panda G 2020 Intelligent classification of IoT traffic in health-care using machine learning techniques *Proc. 6th Int. Conf. on Control, Automation and Robotics (ICCAR) (April 2020)* 581–5

[6] Wiens J and Shenoy E S 2018 Machine learning for healthcare: on the verge of a major shift in healthcare epidemiology *Clin. Infect. Dis.* **66** 149–53

[7] https://softwaretestinghelp.com/types-of-machine-learning-supervised-unsupervised/

[8] Qayyum A, Qadir J, Bilal M and Al-Fuqaha A 2021 Secure and robust machine learning for healthcare: a survey *IEEE Rev. Biomed. Eng.* **14** 156–80

[9] Chnar M M and Askar S 2021 Machine learning for IoT healthcare applications: a review *Int. J. Sci. Bus.* **5** 42–51

[10] Bharadwaj H K, Agarwal A, Chamola V, Lakkaniga N R, Hassija V, Guizani M and Sikdar B 2021 A review on the role of machine learning in enabling IoT based healthcare applications *IEEE Access* **9** 38859–90

[11] What is Artificial Intelligence (AI)?—definition from Techopedia n.d. from https://techopedia.com/definition/190/artificial-intelligence-ai (accessed 1 June 2019)

[12] Rong G, Mendez A, Assi E B, Zhao B and Sawan M 2020 Artificial intelligence in healthcare: review and prediction case studies *Engineering* **6** 291–301

[13] https://ai4.io/blog/2021/08/26/how-ai-and-iot-play-an-important-role-in-healthcare-today/

[14] Bagula A, Lubamba C, Mandava M, Bagula H, Zennaro M and Pietrosemoli E 2016 Cloud based patient prioritization as service in public health care *Proc. ITU Kaleidoscope, ICTs Sustain. World (ITU WT) (November 2016)* 1–8

[15] https://apexon.com/blog/how-iot-is-advancing-remote-patient-monitoring/

[16] Park K, Park J and Lee J 2017 An IoT system for remote monitoring of patients at home *Appl. Sci.* **7** 260

[17] Azariadi D, Tsoutsouras V, Xydis S and Soudris D 2016 ECG signal analysis and arrhythmia detection on IoT wearable medical devices *Proc. 5th Int. Conf. Modern Circuits and Systems Technologies (MOCAST) (May 2016)*

[18] Kakria P, Tripathi N K and Kitipawang P 2015 A real-time health monitoring system for remote cardiac patients using smartphone and wearable sensors *Int. J. Telemed. Appl.* **2015** 373474

[19] Sood S K and Mahajan I 2017 Wearable IoT sensor based health-care system for identifying and controlling chikungunya virus *Comput. Ind.* **91** 33–44

[20] Ani R, Krishna S, Anju N, Aslam M S and Deepa O S 2017 IoT based patient monitoring and diagnostic prediction tool using ensemble classifier *Proc. Int. Conf. on Advances in Computing, Communications and Informatics (ICACCI) (September 2017)* 1588–93

IOP Publishing

Internet of Things in Biomedical Sciences
Challenges and applications
Varun Bajaj and Irshad Ahmad Ansari

Chapter 4

IoT-enabled biosensors for cancer and disease detection

Bidhan Pramanick and Anto Manuel

IoT-enabled biosensors have tremendous potential for openly acknowledging and analyzing various anomalies related to the human body, particularly diseases like cancer. Lung cancer (LC) rates as a significant cause of mortality and a major obstacle to raising life expectancy in every nation since it is the principal factor in cancer-related death internationally. The death rate may be decreased to some extent by earlier detection as most LC patients are diagnosed at the advanced stages when curative therapy is no longer an option. A better comprehension of the disease's molecular origins and evolution can help in the treatment and prevention of cells that start to grow out of control. LC can be treated using a variety of techniques that are used to screen for cancer based on tumor size. The available techniques are expensive and not suitable for widespread screening as they are time-consuming and have a high rate of false-positive results. Therefore, it is required to design a simple, cost-effective, early detection platform to improve clinical prognosis and survival rates. Biomarker-based cancer treatment aims to achieve the indicated parameters at an appropriate level by using molecular biomarkers (BM). For the goal of detecting illnesses, non-invasive exhaled breath analysis helps to discover and analyze volatile organic compounds (VOCs). Acetone, pentane, ethanol, and isoprene are the four carbonyl VOCs associated with LC, and depending on the kind of cancer, different concentration ranges exist. In contrast to healthy people, LC patients must have distinct metabolic pathways that lead to VOC production or metabolism. The ideal system may include a number of VOC sensors, electronic signal conditioning circuits for signal extraction from the sensor, a data-transferring unit for instituting with IoT, a server for data collection, and software for data analysis and better prediction of lung cancer with high accuracy. In this chapter, various biosensors for LC detection will be discussed followed by the reported works on IoT-enabled biosensor systems.

4.1 Introduction

The major cause of mortality in every nation on earth is cancer, and it is a major barrier to raising life expectancy [1]. Data from the World Health Organization (WHO) indicate that until the age of 70, cancer is the second most frequent reason for death. When compared to cancer mortality rates, stroke and coronary heart disease mortality rates have significantly improved in many countries, which has contributed to the growth of the main cause of mortality being cancer [2]. The alarming rise in LC mortality and its disproportionately high occurrence in Nature has prompted the implementation of several cancer control studies and early diagnosis initiatives [3]. According to statistics released by the WHO, figure 4.1 shows the percentage of lung cancer deaths to all other cancer deaths in 2021.

Most LC patients are diagnosed only after the disease has progressed to the point where curative treatment is no longer an option. LC has a higher fatality rate than other common cancers such as prostate, breast, and skin cancers all around the world [1]. Its mortality rate can be lowered to some extent if it is detected sooner. It's also crucial to understand the various sorts of detection [4].

4.2 Lung cancer and its detections

4.2.1 Lung cancer

Cancer is a condition in which the body's cells proliferate unchecked. In LC, lungs are where cancer first appears. Three procedures are involved: diagnosis, staging, and treatment. The process of diagnosing LC varies from person to person; the medical team selects tests based on a variety of considerations. Finding out whether and how far LC has spread is referred to as staging. A treatment strategy is influenced by the tumor's stage [2].

The majority of LC patients only receive a diagnosis when the disease has progressed to the point that curative therapy is no longer an option [3]. Compared to other common cancers including prostate, breast, and skin worldwide, LC has a

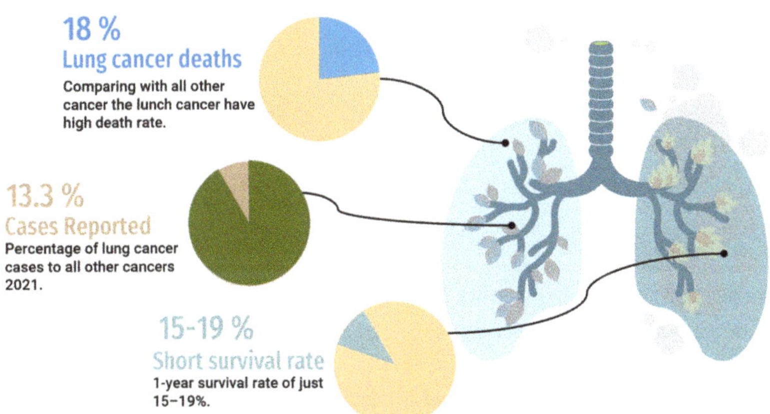

Figure 4.1. Percentage of LC deaths to all other cancer deaths 2021 (derived from the references [1, 2]).

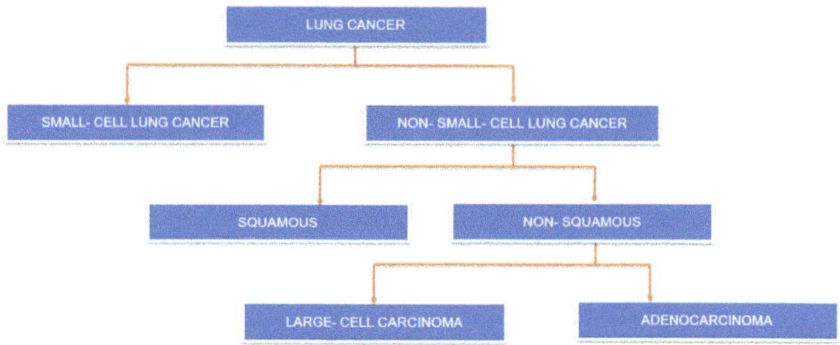

Figure 4.2. Classification of lung cancer (derived from reference [6]).

higher mortality rate. Early identification can help to some extent in lowering its fatality rate. Knowing the various forms of detection is also crucial [2].

The two predominant forms of LC are small-cell (SC) and non-small-cell (NSC) LC, as shown in figure 4.2. Despite advancements in early detection and conventional therapy, NSCLC generally has a dismal prognosis and is discovered at an advanced stage. Major unmet needs in the treatment and prevention of LC can likely be fulfilled better by understanding the molecular causes and progression of the condition [5].

In a healthy organism, normal cells develop, reach adulthood, and expire, ultimately being replaced by other healthy cells. In the body, abnormal cells can develop and proliferate at any time. Similar to how white blood cells combat pathogens, the body's specified systems may work to eliminate the aberrant cells if it detects these cells as 'abnormal.' Because your body doesn't fight these abnormal cells when you have cancer because it identifies them as a part of you, the cells grow out of control [7]. Despite advancements for detection in advanced and conventional therapy, LC is typically identified at an advanced stage [6].

4.2.2 LC symptoms

LC is the development of malignant cells that begin in the lungs. Typically, early-stage LC has no symptoms. The most notable signs of LC appear in its advanced stages. A persistent cough that becomes worse over time and persists, headache, a persistent feeble feeling, ongoing discomfort in the chest, hoarseness, breathing problems, blood in the sputum, body and joint discomfort, and weight loss, are all typical signs of LC [8].

4.2.3 Treatment options

The location, size, metastases, and DNA of the tumor will all affect the therapy options. The selections will also depend on general health and shape. Most likely, the course of treatment will involve a mix of prescription medications, such as immunotherapy or targeted therapy. The decision to perform surgery on a patient with LC entirely depends on the cancer's stage and their ability to survive the procedure. Patients who receive an early diagnosis are the only ones who undergo surgery. Depending on the severity of the infection, the surgeon may decide the right option [3–8].

4.2.3.1 Radiation-based therapy

Strong beams produced by x-ray and proton emission are used in radiation therapy to destroy cancer cells. The patient rests on a table as the damaged region is exposed to radiation from a moving machine during the procedure. Radiation may be administered following surgery, in the early stages of NSCLC, or to uncomfortable areas to relieve symptoms [3–8].

4.2.3.2 Chemotherapy

Drugs are used as part of the treatment to kill cancer cells. These medications can be administered intravenously or orally. A series of treatments lasting a few weeks or months is provided by the combination of the medications. In order to eliminate any cancer cells that may have survived the surgery, chemotherapy is typically administered. Stage III cancer is treated with chemotherapy in addition to radiation therapy, and stage IV cancer is typically solely treatable with chemotherapy [3–8].

4.2.3.3 Targeted drug therapy

Targeted medication therapy is advised for patients with stage IV LC caused by a particular type of cancer cell mutation (EGFR, ALK, ROS, MET, etc). Drugs used to eliminate cancer cells disrupt the abnormality in the cell. These medications have significantly increased the survival rate of advanced-stage cancer due to advancements in cancer research and clinical science [3–8].

4.2.3.4 Immunotherapy

A new weapon in the repertoire against LC is immunotherapy. These medications are injected into the patient. By removing the immune system's protective proteins, it paves the way so that cancer cells can be combated by the patient's immune system. Currently, only patients with advanced LC are advised to use immunotherapy drugs [3–8].

4.2.4 Factors determining LC stage

The size, position, and involvement of the local lymph nodes are characteristics that are utilized to identify the stage of LC. All around the body, lymph nodes are tiny, ball-shaped immunological organs [3]. It is crucial to determine if the lymph nodes around the lung have been affected by the LC. The metastatic status (M) denotes the organs to which the cancer has metastasized. A combination of all of these factors determines the stage of LC (TNM) [9].

4.3 Detection methods and their disadvantages in LC

4.3.1 Early detection methods of LC

LC cures are typically dependent on early detection of the disease, and suitable diagnostic methods lead to lower LC incidence rates. LC is being treated using seven different procedures—chest radiography (CXRs), cytology sputum, computed tomography (CT) breath studies, positron emission tomography (PET) functional imaging technique, and magnetic resonance imaging (MRI). Molecular level detection can be a possible way of identifying cancer in earlier stages [10].

4.3.2 Disadvantages of the traditional methods over breath biopsy

The sensitivity of some of the most popular imaging methods used today to detect cancer is largely dependent on tumor size. The procedures are expensive and time-inefficient, making them unsuitable for mass screening [7].

Figure 4.3 shows the disadvantages of the traditional methods of testing. The US Preventive Services Task Force estimates that low-dose CT has an overall sensitivity and specificity of 80%–100% for LC detection. However, false-positive findings and the dangers associated with radiation exposure are relatively high. With the aid of this technique, it is possible to increase clinical prognosis and survival rates. Compared to traditional testing procedures, breath analysis provides benefits that early detection is straightforward and affordable, and testing methods range from invasive to non-invasive [12]. Since early-stage LC is frequently asymptomatic, the majority of cases are discovered when therapy is no longer curative [13].

4.4 Biomarkers

4.4.1 What are biomarkers?

A feature that is assessed as a sign of typical biological activities, pathogenic processes, or responses to exposure or treatment, involving both is referred to as a biomarker (BM) [14]. Human exhalation contains several BMs that may be used to diagnose various disorders. The different components in exhaled breath are depicted in figure 4.4.

BMs might be molecular, histologic, radiographic, or have physiological properties. Many types of BM include pharmacodynamic/response/susceptibility BM, diagnostic BM, safety BM monitoring BM, predictive BM, and prognostic BM [15].

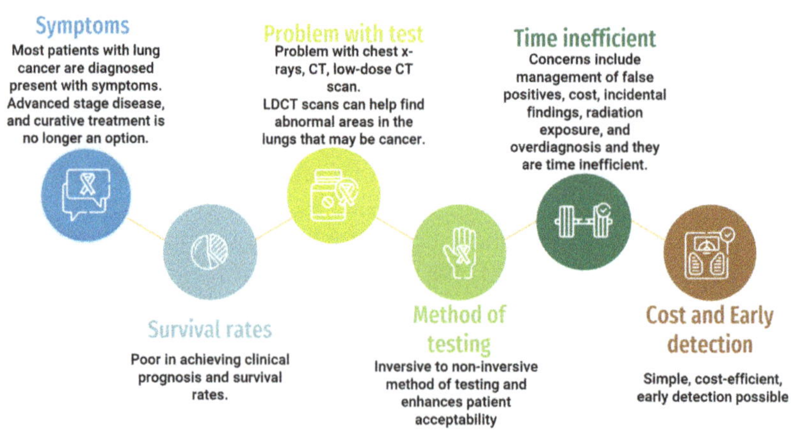

Figure 4.3. Disadvantages of the traditional methods as against new systems (derived from references [6–11]).

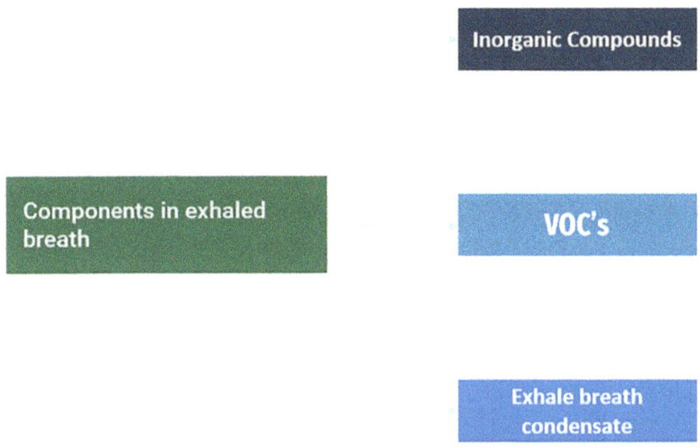

Figure 4.4. Exhaled breath components.

In addition to N, O_2, and CO_2, human exhaled breath also contains 100–3000 other organic and inorganic VOCs, which are created by both external and internal sources [16]. Because the different levels of VOCs in the exhaled gas of normal healthy persons and a person with specific disorders differ, these volatile organic molecules (VOMs) serve as disease-specific indicators [17].

4.4.2 VOCs as biomarkers

There are around 3000 VOCs that have been discovered in human breath at least once, with most breath samples including more than 200 VOCs [18]. There are a few VOCs in exhaled breath with quite high quantities (values in brackets) [19], acetone (450–504 ppb) [20], ammonia (800–866 ppb) [20], isoprene (90–122 ppb), etc [21]. Most VOCs in the exhaled human breath with concentration ranges of less than 1.00 ppb. When compared to healthy participants, unwell individuals' exhaled VOC concentrations are often not higher [22]. The body produces VOCs, which then circulate throughout the body via circulation before crossing the alveolar barrier to appear in exhaled breath. Parts-per-million by volume (ppmv) and parts-per-billion by volume (ppbv) or lower traces of these VOCs may be found [23]. Though they might not always enter the circulation, the trace chemicals produced in the mouth seem to be exhaled. By accurately analyzing levels of VOCs in breath, it is possible to establish whether a person is in a healthy or ill state. The ability to differentiate between healthy and unhealthy conditions may be determined by analyzing the parts of VOCs in breath with adequate accuracy. As a result, these methods can diagnose illnesses in their early stages, painlessly and non-invasively [24].

4.4.3 Choice of appropriate VOCs as biomarkers

Exhaled gas is considered exclusively relevant for physical parameters or gas-phase constituents. The only absorption rate of oxygen, carbon dioxide elimination, and rate of respiration are measured during exercise physiology examinations [25, 26].

The different VOCs of patients with LC in exhaled breath are depicted in figure 4.5. The quantities of acetone, phenol, isoprene, propenal, nitric oxide, nonanal, carbon oxides, and pentane in the exhaled breath are examined in more thorough breath tests as indicators of many medical disorders, such as diabetes, metabolic efficiency, lipid peroxidation, and so on [27–30]. Two study groups led by H J O'Neil and Michael Phillips were among the first to discover LC BMs in 1988 and 1992, respectively. The primary breath indicators related to LC are listed in figure 4.5 for cancer diagnosis. It is now possible to identify and test VOCs in exhaled gas more precisely. Linus Pauling, a two-time Nobel laureate, announced in 1971 that gas chromatography (GC) had been used to quantify 250 volatiles in a breath sample [11].

Any molecule containing carbon that is sufficiently volatile to be discernible in the gas phase at room temperature is considered a VOC. Patients with LC have been shown to exhale a large number of VOCs, certain benzene derivatives, and alkanes [11]. For people with LC to have a distinct pattern of breath VOCs, the biochemical pathways that contribute to their synthesis or metabolism must differ from those who do not have LC [35]. The primary carbonyl VOCs associated with LC are shown in table 4.1 along with their ranges for both healthy individuals and those who have the disease. Around 42 VOCs are used as LC BMs, with the following VOCs being the most important [36].

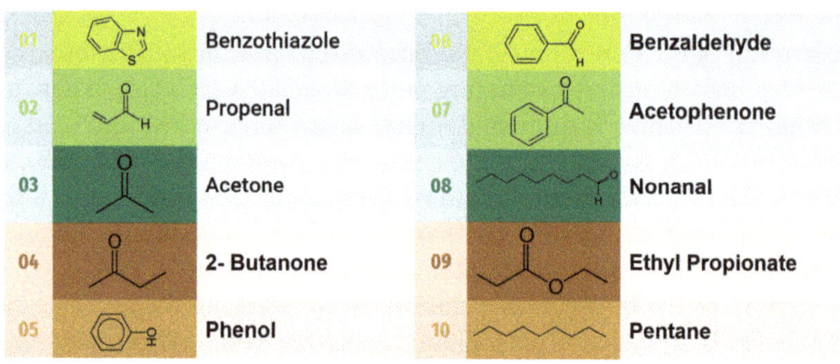

Figure 4.5. VOCs of patients with LC.

Table 4.1. VOC concentration range healthy, cancer (derived from references [14, 31–34]).

	Minimum concentration (ppb) (μg m^{-3})		Maximum concentration (ppb) (μg m^{-3})		Minimum mass (μg) (μg m^{-3})		Maximum mass (μg m^{-3})	
VOC	Healthy	Cancer	Healthy	Cancer	Healthy	Cancer	Healthy	Cancer
Acetone	240	1250	970	1690	12	624	485	845
Ethanol	37	170	130	207	18	85	65	103
Isoprene	70	450	340	580	35	225	170	300
Pentane	2	>14	14	>27	1	>7	7	>13

4.4.4 Potential of VOCs in disease detection

Sensor-based electronic noses (e-nose) successfully detect VOCs and breathprints in respiratory disorders [37]. VOCs are utilized to diagnose cystic fibrosis and tuberculosis [38]. Non-respiratory illnesses, including Barrett's esophagus and inflammatory bowel disease, pneumonia [39] and diagnosing ketosis [40], and diabetes [41] can also be spotted using an e-nose [42].

VOCs from exhaled breath can help detect different diseases. The potential of VOCs in disease detection is depicted in figure 4.6 and exhaled breath includes VOCs that can be utilized to identify a number of disorders, as shown in figure 4.7. The nature of the content will vary depending on the metabolites involved in the production of the same and also depends on the portion of the human body that served as the platform for the analysts to develop.

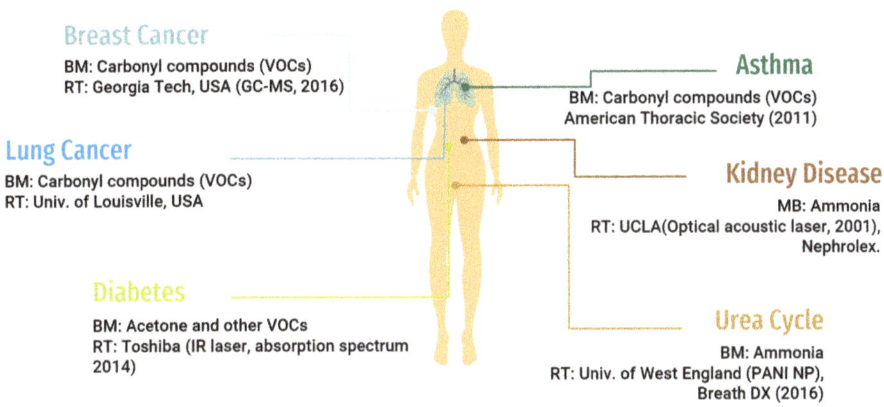

Figure 4.6. Breath analysis for biomedical applications overview (BM—biomarker) (RT—research team) (derived from references [43–47]).

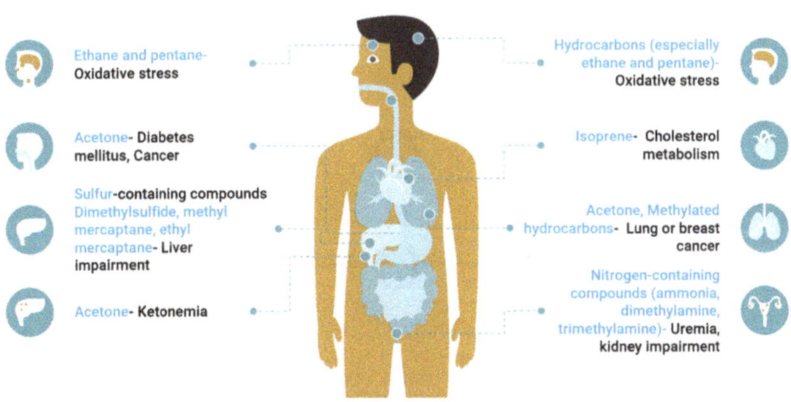

Figure 4.7. Breath analysis for biomedical applications overview (derived from references [22, 43, 48, 49]).

4.4.5 Acetone (C3H6O) as biomarker

Among the most typical VOCs in human exhaled breath is acetone. Different studies found that acetone has a high potential in detecting LC [10]. Acetone is implicated in the metabolism of dextrose and lipolysis [50]. Figure 4.8 depicts acetone structure.

Lipolysis or lipid peroxidation generates acetoacetate, which is then decarboxylated to develop acetone [51]. In ketonemic individuals, patients with prediabetes, and during famine, ketone bodies in the blood are elevated [52]. Ketones are created when the body uses fat as fuel rather than glucose. Due to the shortage of oxalacetate, which is involved in creating glucose in the gluconeogenesis pathway, acetyl-CoA cannot enter the Krebs cycle [53].

4.5 IoT-enabeled biosensor

Wi-Fi's point-to-point architecture, frequency range of 2.4–5 GHz, range of 10–100 m, and data throughput of 6.75 Gbps make it suitable for the implementation of an IoT system [55]. Security in health care is also a concern in the transmission of the data to a server which is described in different studies [54]. The sensor gadget has a cryptography algorithm built in so that the packets created with the patient's health data are encrypted there before being transferred. The system can establish two-way communication in the IoT owing to the data transmitting unit [56].

The evolution of wearable sensing technology, the first stage of IoT-enabled systems, is shown in figure 4.9. Technology for tracking health and well-being has been used more and more throughout time, and these systems are now present in smart homes, workplaces that are accessible to older workers, public locations, and other places. To support functional, physiological, and behavioral monitoring, address social interaction aspects of daily life, and either focus on specific health-related conditions or support the more general goal of comfort, quality of life, and well-being, they use a wide range of commercially available smart sensors and medical equipment. Figure 4.10 illustrates the technologies employed in IoT for establishing connectivity.

4.6 Typical block diagram

Typical block diagram of the IoT-enabled system is shown in figure 4.11. The exhaled breath will first be collected in a bag, with sensors in the bag providing an

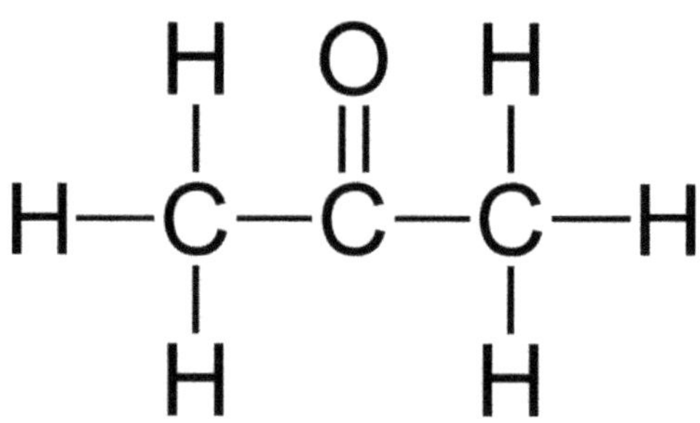

Figure 4.8. Structure of acetone VOC [22].

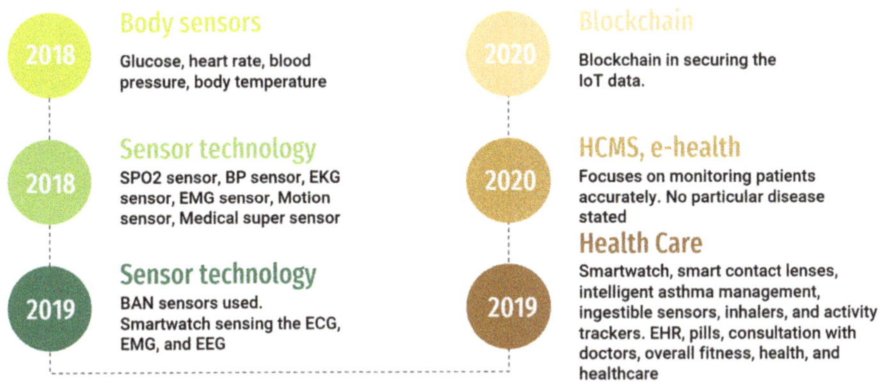

Figure 4.9. Wearable sensor technology milestones.

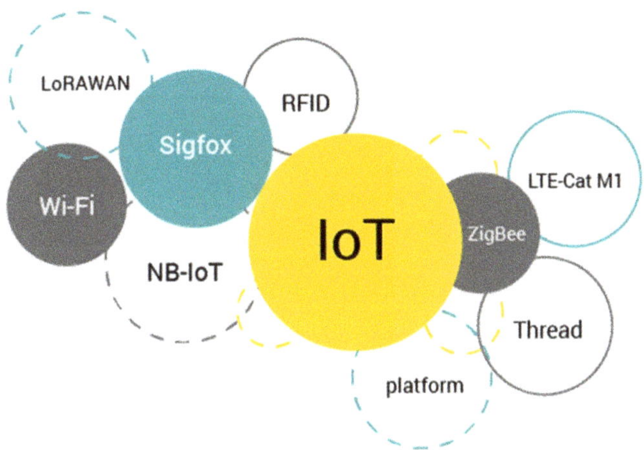

Figure 4.10. Technologies used in IoT (derived from reference [57]).

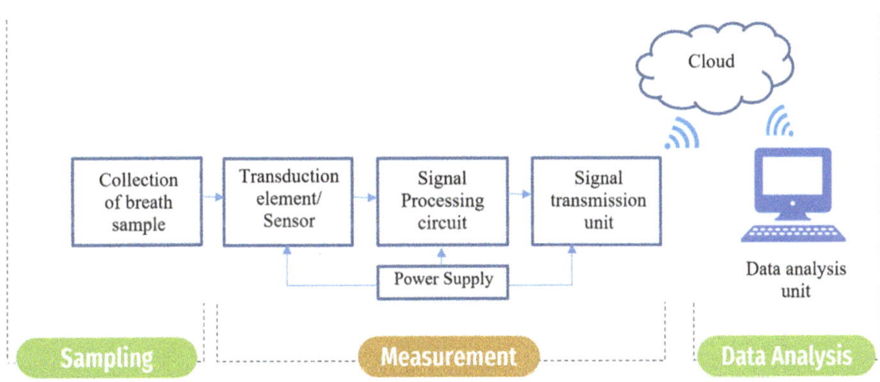

Figure 4.11. Typical block diagram of the system.

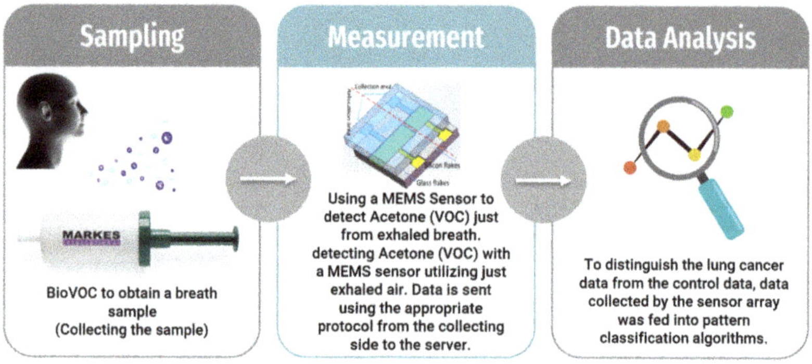

Figure 4.12. Process flow diagram (derived from references [58–60]). Image credit: Markes International Ltd.

electric signal based on the sample. The signal will be processed by the processing unit and sent into the transmission unit based on the electrical signal.

The data transmission unit is responsible for storing all real-time data in the server by a breath sample. This identifies the risk of cancer and other ailments using artificial intelligence and diverse sample data on the server. Figure 4.12 depicts the flow diagram of a typical system process.

4.6.1 Sampling-breath sample collection method

Many ways have been reported for collecting breath samples accurately without losing parameter features or all contaminated bodies remaining in the exhaled breath [61]. From all the collection processes documented in various research, a suitable method of breath collection was identified as commercially available equipment, Markes International Ltd, Rhondda Cynon Taff, UK, recommends a breath sampling protocol. Following a 60-min rest period, the individuals were instructed to inhale slowly through a Teflon-bulb-connected valve for one vital capacity (VC) breath, which collects the last of the exhaled gas 150 ml [62]. Figure 4.13 demonstrates how to collect a breath sample using BioVOC. More than 10 environmental samples were collected from the test subjects' rooms to compare the amounts of VOCs in their breath with the air outside [63].

4.6.2 Measurement—a sensor for acetone detection

4.6.2.1 Sensor for the detection of acetone: a review

There are many types of acetone gas sensors reported in various studies. However, the sensor report in several studies faces lots of lagging factors in the detection because of the selectivity and sensitivity of the acetone at the lower concentration. Figure 4.14 depicts the many sensors that may be used to detect acetone gas sensor categorization.

The dependable parameters related to the sensitivity and selectivity of acetone sensors are mainly seven: collection mechanism of the exhale breath; humidity in the collected sample; temperature of the collected sample; keeping a high requirement of temperature in the receiver session [66]; selectivity of the acetone from another

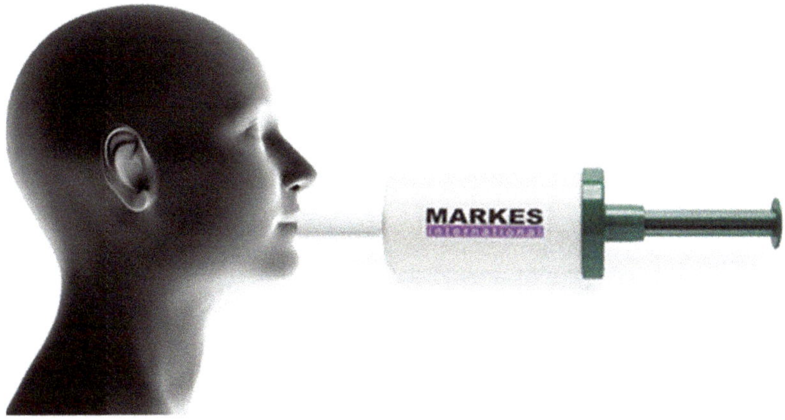

Figure 4.13. Using the BioVOC to obtain a breath sample is depicted in this illustration (derived from reference [64]). Image credit: Markes International Ltd.

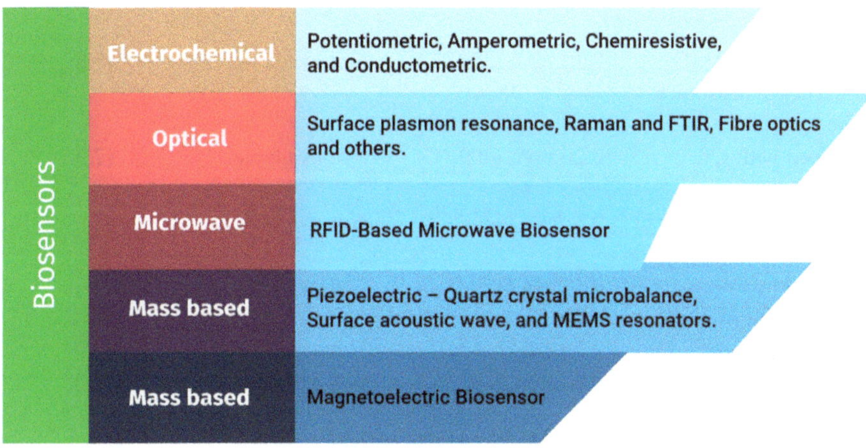

Figure 4.14. Transduction-based classification of breath acetone biosensors [65].

parameter of exhaling breath VOCs; sensitivity range of the acetone required for the detection. The graphic depicts the major approaches with details that can be considered for detection. The different types of sensors able to detect BMs with the specified rage are reviewed in table 4.2.

A significant shift in the microelectronics industry has been brought about by MEMS' low cost, small size, great integration capabilities, and high throughput capabilities [86]. Mechanical vibration, stress, humidity and temperature effect, and particle pollution are only a few of the causes of MEMS devices' lack of selectivity and sensitivity; these are all essential considerations while looking for an effective acetone detection sensor.

Internal and external factors are the two sorts of elements that influence the functioning of the gas sensor. Internal variables like shape, crystal lattice structure, intrinsic flaws, doping, depletion layer at heterojunctions, and surface chemistry all

Table 4.2. Acetone sensor a review.

Method for detection and material used	Acetone detection range (operating temperature)	Processing	Reference	Year
P-type (Metal oxide) NiO—(4 wt. % W)	0.1–1000 ppm (250 °C)	Annealing process (450 °C, 1 h), Hydrothermal (150 °C–160 °C, 12 h).	[67]	2015
Solid-state gas sensor metal oxides resistance change	0.0200 ppm (350 °C)	Not available	[68]	2019
SnO_2 nanotubes—functionalized with Pt and Au resistance change	0.100 ppm (350 °C)	Not available	[69]	2014
SnO_2—fibers catalyzed with Pt resistance change	0.120 ppm (300 °C)	Not available	[70]	2014
Pt-functionalized–WO_3 resistance change	0.120 ppm (300 °C)	Not available	[71]	2014
WO_3—nanofibers, Rh_2O_3 nanoparticles, resistance change	0.10 ppm (350 °C)	Not available	[72]	2016
WO_3—doped with Cr, resistance change	0.20 ppm (400 °C)	Not available	[73]	2008
ZnO–Fe_3O_4 inverse—optical gas sensor	0.1 ppm (485 °C)	Not available	[74]	2017
single-crystalline Fe_2O_3 mesoporous nanospheres	0.1 ppm (170 °C)	Not available	[75]	2017
Monolayer graphene	0.1 ppm (NA)	Not available	[76]	2017
Synthesis of In_2O_3 hollow nanofiber	0.02 ppm (300 °C)	Not available	[77]	2017
Pt@In_2O_3 nanowires	0.02 ppm (320 °C)	Not available	[78]	2018
Hierarchical porous ZnO:Ni	0.116 ppm (340 °C)	Not available	[79]	2017
WO_3 nanofibers	0.1 ppm (270 °C)	Not available	[80]	2016
Yb ferrites-nanocrystalline powders	0.1 ppm (230 °C)	Not available	[81]	2017
SmO_3 loaded-mulberry-shaped tin oxide	0.1 ppm (250 °C)	Not available	[82]	2018
Pt-functionalized SnO_2 hemipill network	0.0036 ppm (300 °C)	Not available	[83]	2018
WO_3—C-doped carbon spheres hollow spheres	0.2 ppm (300 °C)	Not available	[84]	2017
Optical gas sensor NiO-doping with rGO Acetone	0–500 ppm (27 °C)	Not available	[85]	2021
FAIMS	0–500 ppm (27 °C)	Not available	[85]	2021

impact the sensing processes. The exhaled breath collection technique, the humidity of the collected sample, foreign entities' impact on the acquired sample, and the temperature of the collected sample are the external factors impacting acetone sensing mechanisms [96]. Figures 4.15 and 4.16 depict the major approaches with details that can be considered for detection.

Electrochemical sensors in the detection of VOCs, like metal oxide semiconductor (MOS) and organic and inorganic chemiresistive gas sensors, rely heavily on the sensing materials used, which include nano- and microparticles, metals, and conducting polymers [99]. These sensors feature a simple design and are less expensive to produce. Standard altering conditions of the environment, like temperature and humidity, have little effect on their sensing activity [100]. Because of the higher working temperature of MOS sensors, they waste a lot of energy during sensing, and organic chemiresistive sensors have low sensitivity [101]. The wavelength of the oscillating crystal changes with the mass on the quartz surface [102].

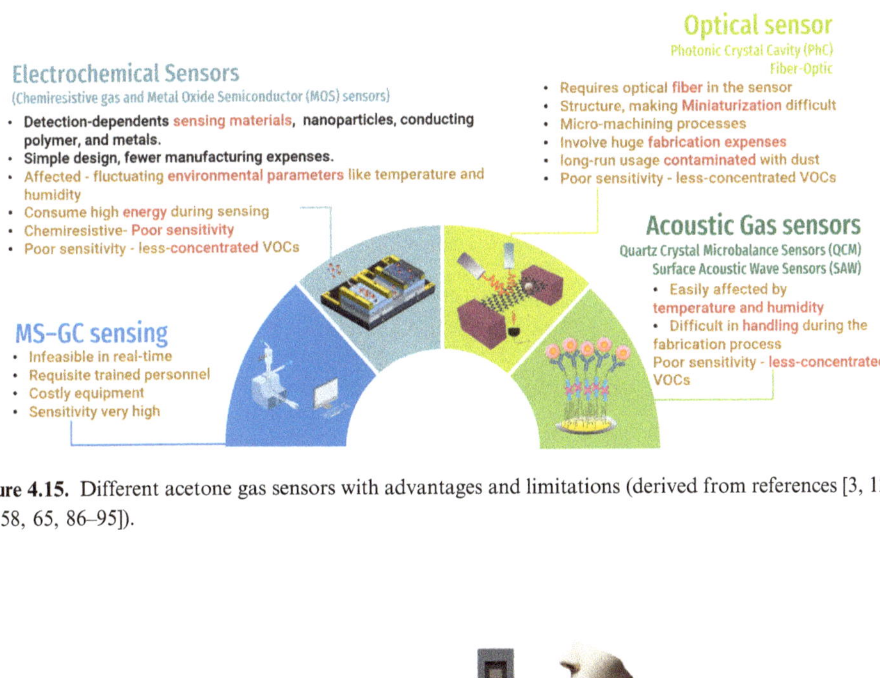

Figure 4.15. Different acetone gas sensors with advantages and limitations (derived from references [3, 12, 17, 33, 58, 65, 86–95]).

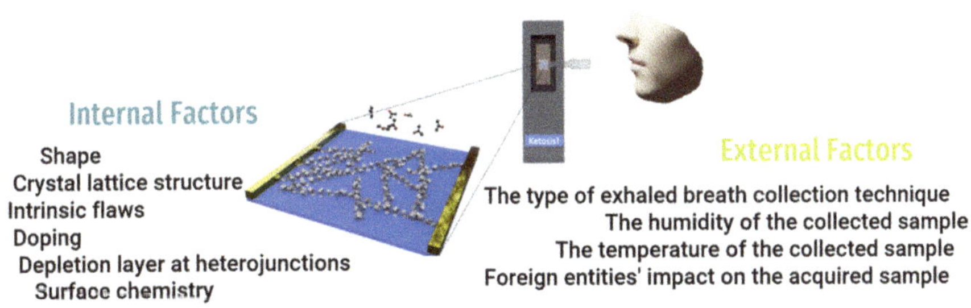

Figure 4.16. Factors impacting acetone sensing mechanisms are depicted in a diagram (derived from references [66, 96–98]).

4.6.2.2 Sensing mechanism of acetone

VOCs are nonreactive and very slightly adsorb to solid surfaces, so they are challenging to detect [103]. GC–MS (gas-based chromatography with mass-based spectrometry) remains the most effective and feasible approach for recognizing potential BM like acetone with high sensitivity and selectivity [104]. VOCs, as well as other key components including nitrogen, oxygen, carbon dioxide, and water, are present in small levels in an exhaled breath so it is necessary to identify a sensor with high selectivity and low dependability of mentioned compounds [105]. For more sensitive acetone detection at lower concentration levels, an ion mobility spectrometry (IMS) and MEMS sensor combination is preferable [106].

The system is said to have areas for gas ionizing, ion migration, and ion collection as shown in figure 4.17. The signal that the MEMS sensor (which collects ions) captures is sent to the next stage of processing from where it is then transmitted to the server. Figure 4.17 shows the setup for an IMS and MEMS sensor combo to detect acetone.

Before approaching the migration zone, the ions must be isolated from the gas molecules. The gas has to be identified as charged negatively due to ionization or

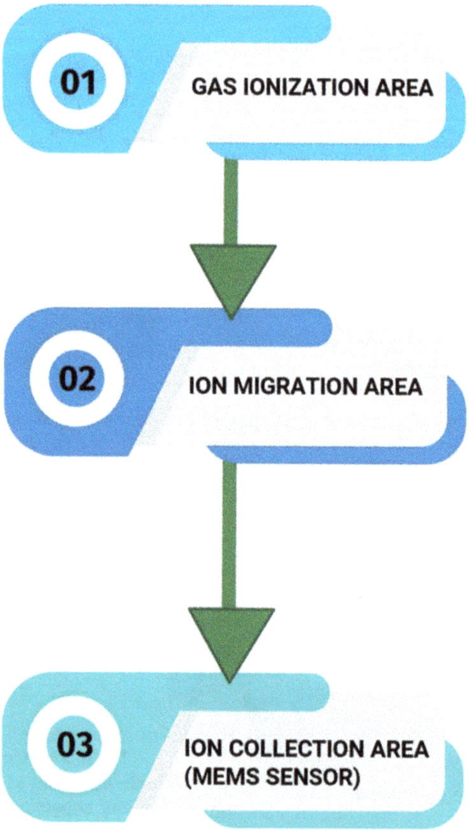

Figure 4.17. Setup for detection of acetone using a combination of IMS with MEMS sensor (derived from references [58, 105–108]).

charged positively due to ionization in the ionization zone. In the migration zone, the ions are then confronted with a high field (electrical) asymmetric (FA) voltage and a DC compensating voltage (DCCV). As acetone ions contact the electrode, the charged ions that need to be detected move from the migration zone into the collecting zone.

Voltage detection in the collecting zone is then taken to identify different gas mixtures. A MEMS-based FAIMS system is schematically depicted in figure 4.18. Acetone gas is ionized as it travels through this ionization lamp because the acetone gas molecule has an ionization energy of 9.43 eV [108].

The ions go to the area of detection and set up the required circuit for the identification of electrical signals. A micro-current detecting method is used in the detection area. In order to measure concentration, charged ions flow to the electrode plate of the detecting region and make a little current flow across the electrode pole plate. An external amplifier circuit then increases the voltage of this feeble current.

4.6.3 Signal processing circuit and signal transmission unit

Initially, the system is connected with an oscilloscope for the initial analysis then by generating the database as the next step develop a circuitry for the processing. IoT communication involves both physical connectivity options (such as cellular, satellite, and LAN) and particular protocols that are utilized in certain IoT contexts (ZigBee, Wi-Fi, Thread, Z-Wave, MQTT, LwM2M). Choosing the best communications solution is one of the most important steps in constructing any IoT system. The technology employed will have an impact on how data is sent to and received from the cloud, as well as how well devices are maintained and communicate with one another. Numerous studies have used a variety of methodologies; nevertheless, ZigBee, LoRaWAN, Wi-Fi, and Bluetooth are the most flexible and trustworthy ones [109, 110].

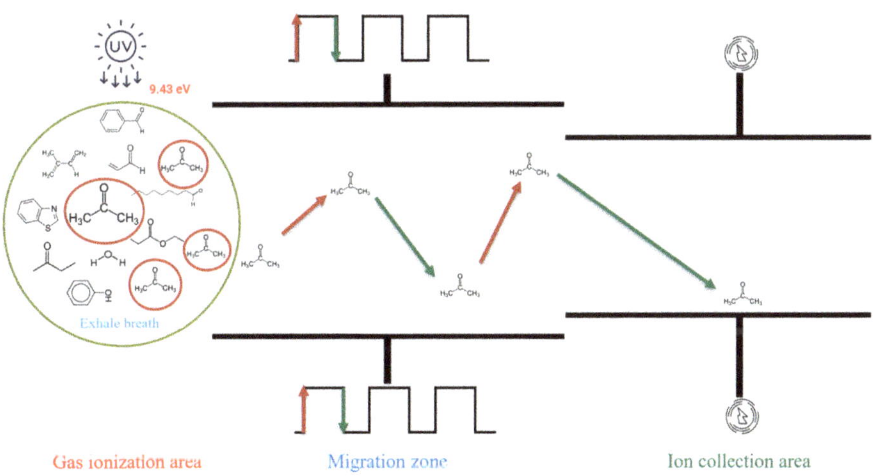

Figure 4.18. The FAIMS device assembly (derived from reference [107]).

4.6.4 Data analysis

To distinguish the data on LC from the control data, pattern classification algorithms were used for the multi-dimensional data collected with the aid of different sensors. SVM, 2-class SVM, 1-class LDA, and MLP were among the generic classification models that were taken into consideration in the search for the best classification model for this application [17]. By projecting the dimension onto the principle components, they had chosen using principle component analysis (PCA), researchers were able to compare the characteristics of LC data with healthy control data. PCA is also used to analyze the distribution of high-dimensional sensing data [111].

4.7 Conclusions

This chapter's major goal is to enlighten readers on the most recent advancements in IoT-enabled biosensor technology. The details of VOCs are also reported here, which are the essential elements for detecting lung cancer. Several biosensors with high sensitivity and selectivity for various biological applications with excellent repeatability using MEMS technology are also discussed. As technology develops, it should benefit people in many sectors, particularly in the biomedical industry, for illness detection and understanding. The VOC detection-based techniques make it simple and painless to do non-invasive analyses of the most prevalent and articulable diseases, such as cancer, kidney, lung, stomach, and brain-related ailments. Before the development of this device or system in the biomedical area, the non-invasive approach for detection and analysis was most commonly used. With the use of BM, breath analysis-based detection can do this. Most MEMS sensors in this region have several issues that have been noted as a result of internal and external factors, such as temperature, humidity, self-heating, and others, which also result in inaccurate results. The novel technique discussed here is very sensitive and stable for the detection of acetone, designated as a BM in the detection, to solve this issue. By combining MEMS sensor technology with ion mobility spectroscopy, this is made achievable.

Acknowledgments

The Indian Institute of Technology, Goa, India, and St. Joseph's College of Engineering and Technology, Palai, Kerala, India, have both supported the writers of this chapter, which they would like to acknowledge.

References

[1] WHO 2022 https://who.int/news-room/fact-sheets/detail/cancer *WHO* **59**

[2] Sung H, Ferlay J, Siegel R L, Laversanne M, Soerjomataram I, Jemal A and Bray F 2021 Global Cancer Statistics 2020: GLOBOCAN estimates of incidence and mortality worldwide for 36 cancers in 185 countries *CA: Cancer J. Clin.* **71** 209–49

[3] Binson V A and Subramoniam M 2018 Advances in early lung cancer detection: a systematic review *2018 Int. Conf. on Circuits and Systems Digital Enterprise Technology (ICCSDET 2018)* 1–5

[4] Mazzone P J *et al* 2017 Evaluating molecular BM for the early detection of lung cancer: when is a biomarker ready for clinical use? An official American Thoracic Society Policy Statement *Am. J. Respir. Crit. Care Med.* **196** e15–29

[5] Thakur S K, Singh D P and Choudhary J 2020 Lung cancer identification: a review on detection and classification *Cancer Metastasis Rev.* **39** 989–98

[6] Zamay T N, Zamay G S, Kolovskaya O S, Zukov R A, Petrova M M, Gargaun A, Berezovski M V and Kichkailo A S 2017 Current and prospective protein BM of lung cancer *Cancers (Basel)*. **9** 1–22

[7] Reckamp K L (ed) 2016 *Lung Cancer* (Cham: Springer International Publishing)

[8] Cares N H 2022 All you need to know about lung cancer *Narayana Health* 1–18 https://narayanahealth.org/lung-cancer

[9] Li W, Liu H, Xie D, He Z and Pi X 2017 Lung cancer screening based on type-different sensor arrays *Sci. Rep.* **7** 1–12

[10] Gashimova E, Temerdashev A, Porkhanov V, Polyakov I, Perunov D, Azaryan A and Dmitrieva E 2020 Investigation of different approaches for exhaled breath and tumor tissue analyses to identify lung cancer biomarkers *Heliyon* **6** e04224

[11] Pauling L, Robinson A B, Teranishi R and Cary P 1971 Quantitative analysis of urine vapor and breath by gas–liquid partition chromatography *Proc. Natl Acad. Sci. USA* **68** 2374–6

[12] Haick H, Hashoul D, Haick H and Hashoul D 2019 Expert review of respiratory medicine lung cancer breath tests *Expert Rev. Respir. Med.* **13** 597–9

[13] Jia Z, Zhang H, Ong C N, Patra A, Lu Y, Lim C T and Venkatesan T 2018 Detection of lung cancer: concomitant volatile organic compounds and metabolomic profiling of six cancer cell lines of different histological origins *ACS Omega* **3** 5131–40

[14] van Geffen W H, Lamote K, Costantini A, Hendriks L E L, Rahman N M, Blum T G and van Meerbeeck J 2019 The electronic nose: emerging BM in lung cancer diagnostics *Breathe* **15** e135–41

[15] McShane L M 2021 BEST (Biomarkers, EndpointS, and other Tools) Resource vol November 2

[16] Schnabel R, Fijten R, Smolinska A, Dallinga J, Boumans M L, Stobberingh E, Boots A, Roekaerts P, Bergmans D and Van Schooten F J 2015 Analysis of volatile organic compounds in exhaled breath to diagnose ventilator-associated pneumonia *Sci. Rep.* **5** 1–10

[17] Binson V A and Subramoniam M 2021 Artificial intelligence based breath analysis system for the diagnosis of lung cancer *J. Phys. Conf. Ser.* **1950** 012065

[18] Phillips M, Gleeson K, Hughes J M B, Greenberg J, Cataneo R N, Baker L and McVay W P 1999 Volatile organic compounds in breath as markers of lung cancer: a cross-sectional study *Lancet* **353** 1930–3

[19] Turner C, Španěl P and Smith D 2006 A longitudinal study of ammonia, acetone and propanol in the exhaled breath of 30 subjects using selected ion flow tube mass spectrometry, SIFT-MS *Physiol. Meas.* **27** 321–37

[20] Turner C, Španěl P and Smith D 2006 A longitudinal study of breath isoprene in healthy volunteers using selected ion flow tube mass spectrometry (SIFT-MS) *Physiol. Meas.* **27** 13–22

[21] Turner C, Španěl P and Smith D 2006 A longitudinal study of methanol in the exhaled breath of 30 healthy volunteers using selected ion flow tube mass spectrometry, SIFT-MS *Physiol. Meas.* **27** 637–48
[22] Boto R E F, Almeida P and Queiroz J A 2008 Human exhaled air analytics: BM of diseases *Biomed. Chromatogr.* **288** 278–88
[23] Smith D and Španěl P 2007 The challenge of breath analysis for clinical diagnosis and therapeutic monitoring *Analyst* **132** 390–6
[24] Lourenço C and Turner C 2014 Breath analysis in disease diagnosis: methodological considerations and applications *Metabolites* **4** 465–98
[25] Kharitonov S A and Barnes P J 2002 BM of some pulmonary diseases in exhaled breath *BM* **7** 1–32
[26] Harald S S S 2015 *Biomarker Validation Technological, Clinical and Commercial Aspects* (New York: Wiley)
[27] Miekisch W, Schubert J K and Noeldge-Schomburg G F E 2004 Diagnostic potential of breath analysis—focus on volatile organic compounds *Clin. Chim. Acta* **347** 25–39
[28] Salerno-Kennedy R and Cashman K D 2005 Potential applications of breath isoprene as a biomarker in modern medicine: a concise overview *Wien. Klin. Wochenschr.* **117** 180–6
[29] Schwarz K *et al* 2009 Breath acetone—aspects of normal physiology related to age and gender as determined in a PTR-MS study *J. Breath Res.* **3** 027003
[30] King J, Mochalski P, Kupferthaler A, Unterkofler K, Koc H, Filipiak W, Teschl S, Hinterhuber H and Amann A 2010 Dynamic profiles of volatile organic compounds in exhaled breath as determined by a coupled PTR-MS/GC–MS study *Physiol. Meas.* **31** 1169–84
[31] Kinoyama M, Nitta H, Watanabe A and Ueda H 2008 Acetone and isoprene concentrations in exhaled breath in healthy subjects *J. Heal. Sci.* **54** 471–7
[32] Machado R F *et al* 2005 Detection of lung cancer by sensor array analyses of exhaled breath *Am. J. Respir. Crit. Care Med.* **171** 1286–91
[33] Bhattacharya D, Rathore P K and Majumdar S 2018 Non-invasive piezoelectric sensor for detection of lung cancer *Proc. 3rd Int. Conf. on Communication and Electronics Systems (ICCES 2018)* 418–21
[34] Fenske J D and Paulson S E 1999 Human breath emissions of VOCs *J. Air Waste Manag. Assoc* **49** 594–8
[35] Mazzone P J 2008 Analysis of volatile organic compounds in the exhaled breath for the diagnosis of lung cancer *J. Thorac. Oncol.* **3** 774–80
[36] Fernandes M P, Venkatesh S and Sudarshan B G 2015 Early detection of lung cancer using nano-nose—a review *Open Biomed. Eng.* **9** 228–33
[37] De Vries R *et al* 2018 Clinical and inflammatory phenotyping by breathomics in chronic airway diseases irrespective of the diagnostic label *Eur. Respir. J.* **51** 1–10
[38] Saktiawati A M I, Stienstra Y, Subronto Y W, Rintiswati N, Sumardi, Gerritsen J W, Oord H, Akkerman O W and Van Der Werf T S 2019 Sensitivity and specificity of an electronic nose in diagnosing pulmonary tuberculosis among patients with suspected tuberculosis *PLoS One* **14** 1–18
[39] Huang J, Kumar S, Singanayagam A, George P M, Kon O M, Takata M and Hanna G B 2013 Exhaled breath acetone for therapeutic monitoring in pneumonia using selected ion flow tube mass spectrometry (SIFT-MS) *Anal. Methods* **5** 3807–10

[40] MUSA-VELOSO K 2002 Epilepsy and the ketogenic diet: assessment of ketosis in children using breath acetone *Pediatr. Res.* **52** 443–8

[41] Salehi S, Nikan E, Khodadadi A A and Mortazavi Y 2014 Highly sensitive carbon nanotubes–SnO_2 nanocomposite sensor for acetone detection in diabetes mellitus breath *Sens. Actuators* B **205** 261–7

[42] O' Neill H J, Gordon S M, O'Neill M H, Gibbons R D and Szidon J P 1988 A computerized classification technique for screening for the presence of breath biomarkers in lung cancer *Clin. Chem.* **34** 1613

[43] Amann A and Smith D 2004 *Breath Analysis for Clinical Diagnosis and Therapeutic Monitoring* (Singapore: World Scientific)

[44] Haick H and Hashoul D 2019 Lung cancer breath tests *Expert Rev. Respir. Med.* **13** 597–9

[45] Daniel D A P and Boss R S C 2012 A review of early detection of cancers using breath analysis *Int. Conf. on Pattern Recognition, Informatics and Medical Engineering (PRIME-2012) (Salem, India)* 433–8

[46] Broza Y Y and Haick H 2013 Nanomaterial-based sensors for detection of disease by volatile organic compounds *Rev. Nanomed.* **8** 785–806

[47] Buszewski B, Kesy M, Ligor T and Amann A 2007 Human exhaled air analytics: BM of diseases *Biomed. Chromatogr.* **21** 553–66

[48] Chen X, Xu F, Wang Y, Pan Y, Lu D, Wang P, Ying K, Chen E and Zhang W 2007 A study of the volatile organic compounds exhaled by lung cancer cells *in vitro* for breath diagnosis *Cancer* **110** 835–44

[49] Waves A and Applications D 2015 Application of saw gas chromatography in the early screening of lung cancer *2015 Symp. on Piezoelectricity, Acoustic Waves, and Device Applications (SPAWDA) (Jinan)* 22–5

[50] Miekisch W and Schubert J K 2006 From highly sophisticated analytical techniques to life-saving diagnostics: technical developments in breath analysis *TrAC Trends Anal. Chem.* **25** 665–73

[51] Ma W, Liu X and Pawliszyn J 2006 Analysis of human breath with micro extraction techniques and continuous monitoring of carbon dioxide concentration *Anal. Bioanal. Chem.* **385** 1398–408

[52] Deng C, Zhang X and Li N 2004 Investigation of volatile BM in lung cancer blood using solid-phase microextraction and capillary gas chromatography–mass spectrometry *J. Chromatogr.* B **808** 269–77

[53] Libardoni M, Stevens P T, Waite J H and Sacks R 2006 Analysis of human breath samples with a multi-bed sorption trap and comprehensive two-dimensional gas chromatography (GC × GC) *J. Chromatogr.* B **842** 13–21

[54] Besher K M, Subah Z and Ali M Z 2021 IoT sensor initiated healthcare data security *IEEE Sens. J.* **21** 11977–82

[55] Mamdiwar S D, Akshith R, Shakruwala Z, Chadha U, Srinivasan K and Chang C Y 2021 Recent advances on iot-assisted wearable sensor systems for healthcare monitoring *Biosensors* **11** 1–37

[56] Firouzi F, Chakrabarty K and Nassif S 2020 *Intelligent Internet of Things: From Device to Fog and Cloud* (Cham: Springer)

[57] 2019 https://avsystem.com/blog/iot-technology/ **8**

[58] Zhang J, Lei C, Liang T, Liu R, Zhao Z, Qi L, Ghaffar A and Xiong J 2021 Acetone sensor based on faims-mems *Micromachines* **12** 1–21

[59] Marzorati D, Mainardi L, Sedda G, Gasparri R, Spaggiari L and Cerveri P 2021 MOS sensors array for the discrimination of lung cancer and at-risk subjects with exhaled breath analysis *Chemosensors* **9** 1–19
[60] Nowshin N, Mazumder P, Soikot M A, Probal M and Qadir M U 2019 Designing and implementation of microcontroller based non-invasive health monitoring system *1st Int. Conf. on Robotics, Electrical and Signal Processing Technique (ICREST 2019)* 134–9
[61] Vicent-Claramunt A and Naujalis E 2021 Cheap and easy human breath collection system for trace volatile organic compounds screening using thermal desorption—gas chromatography mass spectrometry *MethodsX* **8** 101386
[62] Phillips M 1997 Method for the collection and assay of volatile organic compounds in breath *Anal. Biochem.* **247** 272–8
[63] Lawal O, Ahmed W M, Nijsen T M E, Goodacre R and Fowler S J 2017 Exhaled breath analysis: a review of 'breath-taking' methods for off-line analysis *Metabolomics* **13** 1–16
[64] Markes International Ltd 2022 https://selectscience.net/products/bio-voc-breath-sampler/?prodID=196978 (accessed 2–5 June 2022)
[65] Usman F, Dennis J O, Ahmed A Y, Meriaudeau F, Ayodele O B and Rabih A A S 2019 A review of biosensors for non-invasive diabetes monitoring and screening in human exhaled breath *IEEE Access* **7** 5963–74
[66] Kao K W, Hsu M C, Chang Y H, Gwo S and Andrew Yeh J 2012 A sub-ppm acetone gas sensor for diabetes detection using 10 nm thick ultrathin InN FETs *Sensors (Switzerland)* **12** 7157–68
[67] Wang C, Liu J, Yang Q, Sun P, Gao Y, Liu F, Zheng J and Lu G 2015 Ultrasensitive and low detection limit of acetone gas sensor based on W-doped NiO hierarchical nanostructure *Sens. Actuators* **220** 59–67
[68] Abdelghani R, Hassan H S, Morsi I and Kashyout A B 2019 Chemical nano-architecture of highly sensitive SnO_2-based gas sensors for acetone and ammonia using molecular imprinting technique *Sens. Actuators* B **297** 126668
[69] Righettoni M, Tricoli A, Gass S, Schmid A, Amann A and Pratsinis S E 2012 Breath acetone monitoring by portable Si:WO_3 gas sensors *Anal. Chim. Acta* **738** 69–75
[70] Jang J S, Kim S J, Choi S J, Kim N H, Hakim M, Rothschild A and Kim I D 2015 Thin-walled SnO_2 nanotubes functionalized with Pt and Au catalysts via the protein templating route and their selective detection of acetone and hydrogen sulfide molecules *Nanoscale* **7** 16417–26
[71] Choi S J, Lee I, Jang B H, Youn D Y, Ryu W H, Park C O and Kim I D 2013 Selective diagnosis of diabetes using Pt-functionalized WO_3 hemitube networks as a sensing layer of acetone in exhaled breath *Anal. Chem.* **85** 1792–6
[72] Kim N H, Choi S J, Kim S J, Cho H J, Jang J S, Koo W T, Kim M and Kim I D 2016 Highly sensitive and selective acetone sensing performance of WO_3 nanofibers functionalized by Rh_2O_3 nanoparticles *Sensors Actuators* B **224** 185–92
[73] Wang L, Teleki A, Pratsinis S E and Gouma P I 2008 Ferroelectric WO_3 nanoparticles for acetone selective detection *Chem. Mater.* **20** 4794–6
[74] Zhang L *et al* 2017 Three-dimensional ordered ZnO–Fe_3O_4 inverse opal gas sensor toward trace concentration acetone detection *Sens. Actuators* B **252** 367–74
[75] Wang P, Zhang X, Gao S, Cheng X, Sui L, Xu Y, Zhao X, Zhao H and Huo L 2017 Superior acetone sensor based on single-crystalline α-Fe_2O_3 mesoporous nanospheres via [C12mim][BF4]-assistant synthesis *Sens. Actuators* B **241** 967–77

[76] Yang C M, Chen T C, Yang Y C, Meyyappan M and Lai C S 2017 Enhanced acetone sensing properties of monolayer graphene at room temperature by electrode spacing effect and UV illumination *Sens. Actuators* B **253** 77–84

[77] Liang X, Jin G, Liu F, Zhang X, An S and Ma J 2015 Synthesis of In_2O_3 hollow nano fibers and their application in highly sensitive detection of acetone *Ceram. Int.* **41** 13780–7

[78] Liu W, Xu L, Sheng K, Zhou X, Dong B, Lu G and Song H 2018 A highly sensitive and moisture-resistant gas sensor for diabetes diagnosis with Pt@In_2O_3 nanowires and a molecular sieve for protection *NPG Asia Mater.* **10** 293–308

[79] Zhang X, Dong Z, Liu S, Shi Y, Dong Y and Feng W 2017 Maize straw-templated hierarchical porous ZnO:Ni with enhanced acetone gas sensing properties *Sens. Actuators* B **243** 1224–30

[80] Wei S, Zhao G, Du W and Tian Q 2016 Synthesis and excellent acetone sensing properties of porous WO_3 nanofibers *Vacuum* **124** 32–9

[81] Zhang P, Qin H, Lv W, Zhang H and Hu J 2017 Gas sensors based on ytterbium ferrites nanocrystalline powders for detecting acetone with low concentrations *Sens. Actuators* B **246** 9–19

[82] Zhang Y, Zhou L, Liu Y, Liu D, Liu F F, Liu F F, Yan X, Liang X, Gao Y and Lu G 2018 Gas sensor based on samarium oxide loaded mulberry-shaped tin oxide for highly selective and sub ppm-level acetone detection *J. Colloid Interface Sci.* **531** 74–82

[83] Moon H G, Jung Y, Jun D, Park J H, Chang Y W, Park H H, Kang C Y, Kim C and Kaner R B 2018 Hollow Pt-functionalized SnO_2 hemipill network formation using a bacterial skeleton for the noninvasive diagnosis of diabetes *ACS Sens.* **3** 661–9

[84] Shen J Y, Zhang L, Ren J, Wang J C, Yao H C and Li Z J 2017 Highly enhanced acetone sensing performance of porous C-doped WO_3 hollow spheres by carbon spheres as templates *Sensors Actuators* B **239** 597–607

[85] Shanavas S, Ahamad T, Alshehri S M, Acevedo R and Anbarasan P M 2021 A facile microwave route for fabrication of NiO/rGO hybrid sensor with efficient CO_2 and acetone gas sensing performance using clad modified fiber optic method *Optik (Stuttg)* **226** 165970

[86] Vasagiri S, Burra R K, Vankara J and Patnaik M S P K 2022 A survey of MEMS cantilever applications in determining volatile organic compounds *AIP Adv.* **12** 030701

[87] Asri M I A, Hasan M N, Fuaad M R A, Yunos Y M and Ali M S M 2021 MEMS gas sensors: a review *IEEE Sens. J.* **21** 18381–97

[88] Mathew M, Radhakrishnan S, Vaidyanathan A, Chakraborty B and Rout C S 2021 Flexible and wearable electrochemical biosensors based on two-dimensional materials: recent developments *Anal. Bioanal. Chem.* **413** 727–62

[89] Zulkefli A, Mukherjee B, Sahara R, Hayakawa R, Iwasaki T, Wakayama Y and Nakaharai S 2021 Enhanced selectivity in volatile organic compound gas sensors based on ReS_2-FETs under light-assisted and gate-bias tunable operation *ACS Appl. Mater. Interfaces* **13** 43030–8

[90] Prabhu S N, Gooneratne C P and Mukhopadhyay S C 2021 Development of MEMS sensor for detection of creatinine using MIP Based approach—a tutorial paper *IEEE Sens. J.* **21** 22170–81

[91] Teshima N, Li J, Toda K and Dasgupta P K 2005 Determination of acetone in breath *Anal. Chim. Acta* **535** 189–99

[92] Binson V A, Subramoniam M and Mathew L 2021 Discrimination of COPD and lung cancer from controls through breath analysis using a self-developed e-nose *J. Breath Res.* **15** 046003

[93] Leoncini E *et al* 2014 Pilot study: volatile organic compounds as a diagnostic marker for head and neck tumours *Head Neck* **36** 1391

[94] Poli D, Carbognani P, Corradi M, Goldoni M, Acampa O, Balbi B, Bianchi L, Rusca M and Mutti A 2005 Exhaled volatile organic compounds in patients with non-small cell lung cancer: cross sectional and nested short-term follow-up study *Respir. Res.* **6** 1–10

[95] Lukman Hekiem N L, Md Ralib A A, Mat Hattar M A bt B, Ahmad F, Nordin A N, Rahim R A and Za'bah N F 2021 Advanced vapour sensing materials: existing and latent to acoustic wave sensors for VOCs detection as the potential exhaled breath BM for lung cancer *Sens. Actuators* A **329** 112792

[96] Amiri V, Roshan H, Mirzaei A, Neri G and Ayesh A I 2020 Nanostructured metal oxide-based acetone gas sensors: a review *Sensors (Switzerland)* **20** 1–25

[97] Baharuddin A A, Ang B C, Haseeb A S M A, Wong Y C Y H and Wong Y C Y H 2019 Advances in chemiresistive sensors for acetone gas detection *Mater. Sci. Semicond. Process.* **103** 104616

[98] Hwang S I *et al* 2021 Breath acetone sensing based on single-walled carbon nanotube–titanium dioxide hybrids enabled by a custom-built dehumidifier *ACS Sens.* **6** 871–80

[99] Alizadeh N, Jamalabadi H and Tavoli F 2020 Breath acetone sensors as non-invasive health monitoring systems: a review *IEEE Sens. J.* **20** 5–31

[100] Hong S, Wu M, Hong Y, Jeong Y, Jung G, Shin W, Park J, Kim D, Jang D and Lee J H 2021 FET-type gas sensors: a review *Sens. Actuators* B **330** 129240

[101] Chen H *et al* 2018 NiO–ZnO nanoheterojunction networks for room-temperature volatile organic compounds sensing *Adv. Opt. Mater.* **6** 1800677

[102] Dennis J O, Rabih A A S, Md Khir M H, Ahmed M G A and Ahmed A Y 2016 Modeling and finite element analysis simulation of MEMS based acetone vapor sensor for non-invasive screening of diabetes *J. Sens.* **2016** 9563938

[103] McGinn C K, Lamport Z A and Kymissis I 2020 Review of gravimetric sensing of volatile organic compounds *ACS Sens.* **5** 1514–34

[104] Righettoni M, Tricoli A and Pratsinis S E 2010 Si: WO_3 sensors for highly selective detection of acetone for easy diagnosis of diabetes by breath analysis *Anal. Chem.* **82** 3581–7

[105] Cai X, Chen L, Kang T, Tang Y, Lim T, Xu M and Hui H 2017 A prediction model with a combination of variables for diagnosis of lung cancer *Med. Sci. Monit.* **23** 5620–9

[106] Sielemann S, Baumbach J I, Schmidt H and Pilzecker P 2000 *Quantitative Analysis of Benzene, Toluene, and m-Xylene with the Use of a UV–Ion Mobility Spectrometer* vol 4 (New York: Wiley)

[107] Li L, Wang Y, Chen C, Wang X and Luo J 2015 Comprehensive theoretical analysis and experimental exploration of ultrafast microchip-based high-field asymmetric ion mobility spectrometry (FAIMS) technique *J. Mass Spectrom.* **50** 792–801

[108] Li M W H, Ghosh A, Sharma R, Zhu H and Fan X 2021 Integrated microfluidic helium discharge photoionization detectors *Sens. Actuators* B **332** 129504

[109] Jayarathna T, Gargiulo G D and Breen P P 2019 Polymer sensor embedded, IOT enabled t-shirt for long-term monitoring of sleep disordered breathing *IEEE 5th World Forum on Internet Things, WF-IoT 2019 – Conf. Proc* 139–43

[110] Davies S 2019 Everything you wanted to know about smart health care *Early Years Educ* **20** x–xi

[111] Duda R O, Hart P E and Stork D G 2016 *Pattern Classification* 2nd edn (New York: Wiley), pp 0–41

IOP Publishing

Internet of Things in Biomedical Sciences
Challenges and applications
Varun Bajaj and Irshad Ahmad Ansari

Chapter 5

A comprehensive study on IOT applications in wearable healthcare devices

Samyak Hiteshbhai Kothari, Hiral Rajivkumar Shah, Jash Rupeshbhai Shah and Manan Shah

Wearable devices in healthcare refer to electronic devices that customers may put on their wrists, smartwatches, for example, and that are meant to gather the data of their personal fitness and health. Some wearable technology applications, including those for weight management and activity tracking, are meant to keep people healthy and avoid ailments. In the past few years, IoT, i.e. Internet of things, has come to be a pivotal technology in this century. The application of IoT in healthcare works in a variety of ways, encompassing illness prevention, disease treatment as a kind of healing, and disease monitoring as a form of healing. Wearable devices have been created as part of IoT to assist patients in receiving the appropriate therapy. The object and aim of writing this chapter is to convey understanding of the role of IoT in wearable technology; wearables with IoT capabilities offer people the data they need to improve their health. Many aspects of our lives are being redefined by IoT, including how we regulate and have automated our surroundings, how we shop, and how we access healthcare, among several other things. Wearables usher in a new digital and linked economy, in which individuals and organizations interact in new and deeper ways, gadgets communicate with one another, and customers have more freedom to pick what they want and need. A few of the outcomes of IoT in wearable devices are glucose trackers, wearables for heart attacks, asthma monitoring etc. We will discuss the advantages of wearable devices in healthcare and how IoT may be used to solve problems in the healthcare field, such as illness identification, monitoring, and treatment.

List of abbreviations

API	Application programming interface
AR	Augmented reality
BLE	Bluetooth Low Energy

BP	Blood pressure
BSN	Big switch networks
BUN	Blood urea nitrogen
CVD	Cardiovascular disease
D2D	Device-to-device
DDS	Data and device security
ECG	Electrocardiogram
EDA	Electronic design automation
EEMD	Ensemble empirical mode decomposition
EMA	European Medicines Agency
FCEWSN	Fog-aided computational efficient wearable sensor networks
FDA	Food and Drug Administration
GPRS	General Packet Radio Service
GPS	Global positioning system
GSM	Global System for Mobile Communication
GUI	Graphical user interface
HR	Heart rate
HTTP	Hypertext transfer protocol
IMF	Intrinsic mode function
IOC	Internet of computers
IOP	Intraocular pressure
iOS	iPhone operating system
IOT	Internet of Things
IPV4	Internet Protocol Version 4
IPV6	Internet Protocol Version 6
IT	Information technology
LCD	Liquid crystal display
LTE	Long-term evolution
MQTT	Message Queuing Telemetry Transport
MWN	Multi-hop wireless network
NFC	Near-field communication
NMPA	National Medical Products Administration
NTC	Negative temperature coefficient
NTER	National tax equivalent regime
OS	Operating system
OWL	Web ontology language
POC	Point-of-care
PPG	Photoplethysmography
QRS	Quasi random signal
RAD	Rapid application technology
SD	Standard deviation
SKT	Skin temperature
SLA	Service level agreement
SOA	Service oriented architecture
SpO2	Oxygen saturation
USB	Universal serial bus
W-BAN	Wireless Body Area Network
WBS	Wearable biosensors
Wi-Fi	Wireless fidelity
WIBMS	Wrist-worn integrated health monitoring device

WISE	Wireless Internet Solutions Expert
WMD	Wearable medical devices
WSN	Wireless sensor network

5.1 Introduction

Medical research and healthcare have greatly improved during the previous 10 years through the development of wearable medical devices. Wearable systems are gaining appeal as a personal health system because they enable seamless real-time tracking of human health on a frequent basis, even outside clinical situations [1]. The term 'wearable' alludes to a help environment that is either the human body or a thing of garments. Bandages, supports, eyeglasses, and contact lenses are examples of typical medical equipment that might be mentioned as wearable medical devices since they are worn and have a medical purpose. But in this case, we're talking about more advanced gadgets that combine mechanical operations with microelectronics, computing power, and, in some circumstances, intelligence [2]. With the aid of emerging technologies for identification, sensing, networking, storage and cloud services, wearable medical devices may be utilized to sense, record, evaluate, control, and intervene to maintain health [3]. These devices transmit live health data to the internet, where a healthcare practitioner may review it or respond.

Due to its enormous potential, over the past few years, there has been a significant increase in demand for wearables, notably for data collecting for cutting-edge health research. Wearables' accuracy and quality have increased recently, leading to an increase in clinically validated certifications [4]. Instead of patients going with the equipment, medical technology is advancing and making the devices wearable [5]. According to Loncar-Turukalo *et al*, wearable medical devices appear to play a significant role as start-up technology and as an important factor supporting the development of integrated healthcare [3]. Given the growing interest in health, well-being, illness prevention, and fitness and also the major shift toward healthcare that is personalized and controlled by individuals, wearable devices are becoming an attractive alternative platform for healthcare services. Additionally, the usage of wearable technology has given consumers new experiences not accessible through conventional healthcare-related goods and services due to the shift in the medical paradigm from illness treatment to preventive and health management. Wearable medical devices are being used by health-conscious individuals all over the globe.

E-health is the use of the internet for medical purposes. E-health delivers information on illness prevention, identifying early indicators of disease, and remotely monitoring the patient's state based on medical criteria. Furthermore, E-health links wearable sensors, smartphones, and online interfaces into a single system [2]. Wearable medical devices are handled the same as traditional medical devices since laws are focused on intended use rather than device size or platform. All wearable medical devices must be designed and manufactured in line with regulatory bodies such as the Food and Drug Administration (FDA), the European Medicines Agency (EMA), or the China National Medical Products Administration (NMPA). To avoid user dangers including external pollutants coming into contact with human flesh, radiation from electronics, and residue leaks during packing and processing, wearable medical equipment should be appropriately designed and produced [6]. People with acute or chronic incapacities can receive long-term help from wearable medical devices. Traditional medical assistance devices that provide specific medical functions include hearing aids and contact lenses. Information processing features including voice recognition, enhanced contextual awareness, alarms, and feedback are incorporated into more complicated systems [2]. A wearable medical device must have data collectors, sensors, input and output devices, wearable computers, and distant servers [7].

The actual world can be more easily integrated into computer-based frameworks thanks to IoT, which also improves efficiency and accuracy by enabling remote recognition and control of objects. IoT has been used in a variety of fields, including horticulture, home automation, traffic executives, conveyance executives, water supply executives, army executives, smart matrix, energy conservation, and so on [8]. The IoT platform is a set of components that let you distribute apps, collect data from afar, encrypt connections, and manage sensors. IoT is a hot topic with technical, social, and economic implications. IoT has significantly impacted world-wide communication thanks to cutting-edge protocols and algorithms [9]. It connects numerous devices, wireless sensors, household items, and technological devices to the internet. The main factor to take into account while creating an IoT-based device is ensuring the quality-of-service matrix, which includes cost, dependability, scalability, and data sharing confidentiality [10].

The new invention of IoT makes it possible to monitor a patient's health via wearable technology. Wearable sensors networks could be used to provide personalized healthcare. As a result, IoT appears to be a promising option for addressing the issues of large-scale personalized healthcare [11]. IoT-enabled wearables are intelligent gadgets that can be attached to or tattooed on the skin, sewn into clothes or other items, implanted into our bodies, or worn as external accessories. These wearables are changing from just being simple accessories to much more advanced and practical uses, and they're playing a bigger role in IoT technology [12]. Consumption of power is a key design factor for wearable IoT devices, as they are battery-powered. IoT in healthcare is a promising area for enhancing current technology and lowering costs across the board [13]. IoT is used in healthcare in a variety of ways, including disease detection as a preventative measure, disease treatment as a curative measure, and disease monitoring as a curative measure. Wearable technology has been created as a component of IoT to assist individuals in receiving the best care possible [14].

This chapter's goal is to provide a concept related to IoT-based wearable devices, its application, discussion related to wearable fitness activity trackers, biosensors, wearable blood pressure (BP) monitors, and wearable ECG, that is, electrocardiogram monitors, smart jewellery and challenges and the future spectrum of medical gadgets for wear.

5.2 Classification of wearable medical devices

There are several body areas where wearable medical devices can be used, such as the head, eyes, and limbs. These wearable medical devices keep track of many psychological and physical indicators that can be utilized to identify various disorders. Actually, wearable technology may be combined with a variety of sample

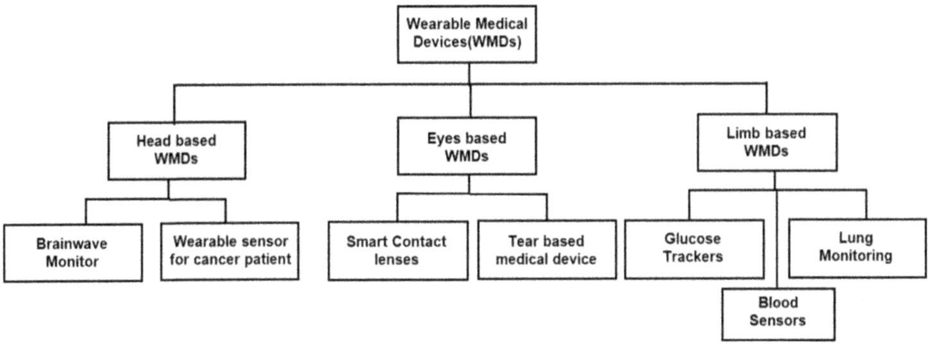

Figure 5.1. Classification of wearable medical devices.

systems to detect many chemical parameters in physiological fluids including saliva, blood, urine, perspiration, etc [15] (figure 5.1).

5.2.1 Glucose trackers

Diabetes is a chronic disease that develops once the body either cannot utilize insulin properly or the liver somehow doesn't generate enough of it. A hormone called insulin regulates glucose levels, which are used as a source of energy by tissues and organs [16]. The objective of the IoT-enabled glucose monitoring system for diabetic patients is to inform the treating physician and the patient's family of the patient's current blood glucose level. The system keeps the built-in Arduino glucose sensor shield that is now used to check blood sugar levels, but it will also upgrade to an IoT end-to-end solution that would alert healthcare professionals via smartphone when the blood sugar level exceeds the usual range [17]. The device uses a novel method to anticipate the rise and fall of glucose levels. The pattern is only produced by past readings. With the help of this number, it is possible to determine if a patient is just temporarily hospitalized or whether their condition is pre- or postprandial and so prevent inaccurate warnings. This device can help patients who cannot attend hospital appointments due to their health. The IoT-based glucose tracker would enable doctors to remotely monitor any circumstances using a cellular device with an internet connection.

5.2.2 Blood sensors

One of the applications of blood sensors is sensors for the disease of diabetes, i.e. blood glucose sensors. A group of metabolic diseases collectively known as diabetes are characterized by chronic increment in the blood sugar levels. Long-term diabetes care necessitates the participation of patients, as well as clinicians and family caregivers. With significant improvements in wireless and online technology, a variety of IoT-based diabetes management apps have been proposed. The majority of these applications are concerned with patient monitoring and technology-based decision making [18]. While some glucose sensors are not enzyme-based, the majority are. The first category includes sensitive things that are frequently utilized for both reliable diagnostic equipment in medical settings and daily self-sensing. The latter kind, and the boronic acid fluorescence sensor in particular, are straightforward and interesting. All sensors must thus offer accuracy, precision, and real-time detection [19]. Another application is sensors for detecting BP. BP is used to assess one's health status. On 26 August 2014, the IEEE adopted IEEE1708, a standard for wearing cuff-less BP monitoring devices, and the development of BP-based wearable devices is projected. Given this, BP should be visible at all times and in all locations, which can help raise health awareness [20]. One of the other applications is the use of magnetoelastic sensors for the monitoring of blood coagulation. Monitoring therapeutic anticoagulants requires precise measurement of blood coagulation time. Blood sample techniques are included in standard methodology for the assessment of blood clotting time, which calls for specialized experts. An innovative method based on magnetoelastic sensors has been used to monitor blood coagulation. In reaction in relation to imposed mass loads or a constant mass load with variable elasticity, the fundamental frequency of the ribbon-shaped magnetoelastic sensor oscillates linearly. Since the magnetoelastic sensors generate magnetic flux that may be detected by a pickup coil that is positioned far away, there is no requirement for direct physical connections. Blood coagulation causes a soft fibrin clot to develop, which alters the blood's viscosity. As a result, the magnetoelastic sensor's distinctive resonance frequency alters, allowing for continuous real-time monitoring of this biological process. A specific blood coagulation profile may be observed by tracking the signal output as a function of time [21].

5.2.3 Asthma monitoring

Continuous monitoring of symptoms, air flow obstructions, and exacerbations is necessary for asthma therapy. Doctors may advise using a peak flow meter, a self-monitoring gadget, depending on the severity of asthma in specific patients [22]. This instrument helps in monitoring alterations in asthma-related symptoms and signs throughout the day or over time. In order to monitor your progress with asthma, it can be useful to keep a diary that includes (1) the symptoms and indicators of asthma, (2) use patterns and schedules for various drugs, (3) the peak flow meter's readings, (4) the occasional triggers for asthma, such as allergens or activities. It is critical to continue keeping an eye on children with asthma. It will be important to carefully assess how asthma affects the child's daily activities, such as play and sports. With face-to-face follow-up and standardized surveys like the Asthma Control Questionnaire, which helps track asthma symptoms, children with asthma have demonstrated progress. After giving a child medication, parents should monitor their child's symptoms and contact the doctor if there are any changes in their mood or behaviour [23]. How well your lungs are functioning can be determined via lung function testing. This is used by doctors to identify asthma and track its development. Since you might not always be able to discern whether your asthma is under control only from your symptoms, monitoring asthma with lung function testing is beneficial.

5.2.4 Smart contact lenses

Smart contact lenses are a cutting-edge optical innovation created to expand human potential. There are several uses for smart contact lens technology, but many of them concentrate on how augmented reality (AR) capabilities of contact lenses can provide the human eye with a computer-like interface. Smart contact lenses have demonstrated tremendous potential for helping the clinical diagnosis and treatment of eye problems as flexible and wearable medical devices. They feature sensors to keep track of things like ocular fluid composition and intraocular pressure (IOP). They can offer useful biological data for the detection and management of disorders including diabetes, keratitis, and glaucoma. They can provide valuable biological information for illness detection and treatment at an early stage like diabetes, keratitis, and glaucoma. Modern contact lenses can be made from a variety of materials, such as silicone, 2-methacryloyloxyethyl phosphoryl choline, poly(methyl methacrylate), poly(ethylene terephthalate), poly(2-hydroxyethyl methacrylate), and poly(ethylene terephthalate) [24]. The future of smart contact lenses is very bright and effective. By monitoring the glucose in the user's tears, smart contacts may be able to measure the blood sugar levels of diabetics. Researchers have developed contact lenses that, over the course of many days or weeks, may administer medicine to the eye.

5.3 Wearable biosensors

Wearable biosensors (WBS) are now receiving a lot of interest due to their potential for personalized healthcare and personal health management. WBS have a record for fostering two-way communication between doctors and patients. Additionally, these tools make it possible to non-invasively and in real time quantify a variety of biochemical indicators in bodily fluids including saliva, perspiration, skin, and tears [25]. They are continuous biological datasets that, when incorporated into a smart analytics framework and can offer insightful knowledge about one's health. In order to gather and send data, smart biosensors in the area of medicine make use of current developments in microtechnology and wireless transmission. When used in combination with actuators, these technologies enable improved monitoring of patients. For instance, WBS are particularly successful in preventing and managing health risks and enable vital sign monitoring for everybody, including patients, infants, athletes and the elderly [26]. At first biosensing devices like glucometers and glucose test strips were made for single use only, but the development in WBS technology has made possible non-invasive and continuous monitoring in healthcare and biological applications. WBS are easily available and easy to use.

Due to their higher precision, efficiency, mobility, relatively low cost, and low power needs, biosensors have a lot of potential for wearable applications. Novel biosensor platforms for biofluid chemical analysis are available. This has unlocked new vistas for rational research, where a great deal of focus is now being placed on the development of a technology that would advance a variety of industries, including the industry of healthcare. A straightforward example is a biosensor used in pregnancy tests, where biologists have concentrated on biological aspects while engineers have focused on the technology of the apparatus for the check. Finally, experts are imparting knowledge and experiments to clients throughout the globe. It would be absurd to suppose that biosensor research is limited to a niche; the recent surge in the number of biosensors in the market is a demonstration of this [25]. Development in wireless electronics, biofluid sampling and flexible material has benefited such improvements in WBS. These have helped in reliability of WBS. These advancements contribute to healthcare cost reduction and realization of vision of healthcare. Overall, it can be said that WBS play a significant role in modern society as they enhance the standard of living in several fields such as healthcare, agriculture and environmental protection.

IoT has successfully altered the globe and had an impact on both personal and professional activities. Medical and healthcare is the most significant IoT sector, and it is poised to change the healthcare sector over the next ten years due to its enormous potential for a variety of applications, from hospital-centric to patient-centric. Thanks to IoT technology, which enables patients to contact their physicians, schedule appointments, and view their health information via online data transfer, patients are becoming more active in their care [27]. One of the impressive breakthroughs in science and technology is the creation of biosensors, which have evolved greatly from classic electrochemical biosensors to moment-in-time devices, labs on a chip, wearable nanobiosensors, etc [28]. Most systems have a straightforward wireless device connection. This results in the creation of a basic yet efficient network for data sensing, recording, and transmission. There is a noticeable trend in wearable IoT devices where sensors that are already in use are utilized to collect, send, and analyse data. Several prototypes with various sensors, including biosensors, have been constructed throughout time. Microcontrollers like the ARM7, STM32 Microcontroller, Arduino, Intel Galileo, and Raspberry Pi are also used in this industry. GSM (Global System for Mobile Communication), BLE (Bluetooth Low Energy), MQTT (Message Queuing Telemetry Transport), ZigBee and GPRS (General Packet Radio Service) were the communication protocols employed [8]. IoT is replacing the Internet of Computers (IoC) as the dominant form of internet connectivity since the majority of connected systems are made up of the people and the infrastructure that supports them.

Wearable biosensor	Advantages	Disadvantages	References
Skin-based	• Needleless • Economical	• Can cause skin irritation • Short-term stability • Requirement of fresh sweat as sample	[29]
Tear-based	• Portable • Intuitive while using • Continuous Monitoring	• Rely on reaction of enzymes • Not comfortable	[30]
Exercise-based	• Immediate analysis • Non-invasive while taking inputs	• Limited sample size • Not suitable for glucose monitoring without doing daily exercise	[29]
Drool-based	• Portable • Intuitive while using • Sensitive	• Viscidity of fluid is a challenge • Unhygienic	[31]

Mukhopadhyay *et al* stated that kidney clinical signs are often mild or absent until a major decrease of kidney function is noticed and/or a condition linked to kidney dysfunction becomes severe. Blood urea nitrogen (BUN) and creatinine are regarded as indicators for renal health. The creation of an IoT-enabled point-of-care (PoC) monitoring device method for the predictive and preventative control of creatinine from serum has been presented by the authors. A highest concentration of 50 ppm of creatinine in serum samples may be detected by the biosensing equipment within an allowable threshold. The findings were judged to be within an allowable threshold, with a deviation of less than 5%. The sensors were calibrated using standard laboratory procedures, however, because of ethical considerations, the efficiency and correctness level were not evaluated using real samples to determine pathology [32].

Pateraki *et al* demonstrated applications of how IoT and smart biosensors, which capture and analyse bio-signals without being invasive and enable early detection and treatment of potentially dangerous pathological problems, may be connected to create an environment for smart living solutions There are still many challenges to overcome in terms of the data privacy, aggregation of data and data integration, and sound decision making, so it is critical to increase the use of data processing and analysis methods, as well as the development of models of machine learning that can easily manage bio-signal datasets and begin determining the appropriate steps to be taken [26].

Madukwe *et al* presented a middleware external software platform that was used in a medical IoT application for remote patient monitoring. The idea behind the edge computing paradigm is to ensure an increase in application quality, with processing and storage resources being moved to the network's edge. The edge of the network is currently used by this work to perform functions like filtration and aggregation, temporary storage, visual analytics, alarm system, and user experience that are typically handled by centralized data centres in the cloud. Edge analysis just lightens the load on cloud analysis, not completely replacing it. Therefore, both edge and cloud computing should be included in IoT systems for maximum efficacy [33].

The latest developments in the design of transistor-based biosensors are discussed by Nagamine *et al*, along with specifics on interfacing architecture for non-invasive sweat gathering and analysis. The appealing and affordable smart medical gadgets will be made possible by an ultrasensitive transistor-based multi-biosensing. A flexible hybrid electronics system consists of both the printed optoelectronic devices and standard silicon technology. With the assessment of sweat rate and continuous sweat monitoring at rest of chemicals for further accurate sweat analysis, a hydrogel touchpad is integrated into a microfluidic device. The connection with sweat elements and illnesses is made clearer by omics analysis of sweat, which is being researched concurrently. These investigations should make it possible to diagnose many disorders that are related with variations in bodily fluid composition earlier than usual and to provide individuals with fact-based health advice [34].

Hamidi *et al* built a rehabilitation framework that incorporates IoTs centred on things, SOA (service oriented architecture) techniques, cross-optimizing techniques, and the basics of illness resource management distribution. Utilizing IoTs technology, a technique for automating the rehabilitation scheme, authors then showed the smart rehabilitation. Technology growth figures and relative technological maturity are studied using Fisher–Pry curves, S shaped curves. The early findings imply that the suggested system is productive and successful. The continued advancement of a rehabilitation system (rehabilitation) and the simplicity of information exchange in this field are two distinctive features of this framework, which together account for the remarkable roles played by ontology and the internet of objects in this process and their flawless performance [35].

5.4 Blood pressure monitoring

There's been a lot of interest in potential new company innovations in the medical industry. Particularly serious illnesses and conditions including strokes, heart problems, and kidney and liver disorders can be brought on by increased BP. Preventing the progression of disease has become more crucial as the population ages quickly and Western diets become more prevalent [20]. Recent recommendations that urge the use of out-of-office readings in terms of improving the supervision of hypertensive patients clearly illustrate how important out-of-office BP readings have become in recent decades for BP control. Nowadays, there seems to be a lot of work put into the design of electronic devices since both the science world and business are interested in inventing compact wearables to assess biological data. Some of these devices have previously been certified, and they operate utilizing a range of technologies and ways to measure BP [36]. According to the 2017 American Heart Association recommendations for hypertension, there is a roughly 90% lifetime probability of acquiring stage two hypertension, which is measured at or below 140 mm Hg systolic or 90 mm Hg diastolic. Furthermore, it has been demonstrated that rigorous BP management considerably lowers cardiovascular illness and all-cause mortality linked to BP [37].

Although swimmers can utilize the system, the suggested gadget does not show data to them. The measurement values can also be shown on the rescuer's smartphone as an alternative. If irregularities in heart rate and BP are found, the rescuer can analyse the situation and, if required, deliver the first aid required to relax the swimmer [38]. BP has been monitored by auscultation that has used the mercury sphygmomanometer for more than a generation in primary care and scientific study. In a relatively cost-effective manner, mHealth treatments provide an opportunity to improve both hypertension testing and continuing care. Numerous studies have demonstrated that treatments that combine additional assistance, such as educating patients, support networks, and group behavioural treatment with patient self-monitoring BP wearable devices, are likely to effectively regulate, thus also lessening BP [39].

To improve the effectiveness of hospital administration, several apps are being developed and put into use today. An IoT BP monitor was created to assist medical workers to remotely monitor patients' BP. This will improve how physicians decide based on clinical status instantaneously and decrease the reliance of patients on medical personnel. For elderly or disabled people who may find it difficult to come to the hospital to check on their health, an IoT BP monitor is especially helpful [40]. The WSN (wireless sensor network) system might be used as a potential option for heart patients who need a constant monitoring device. The WSN system can keep an eye on the person's body temperature, BP, pulse and heart rate. For critically ill patients, it can even maintain a real-time ECG using different sensors [8].

Method	Periodicity	Accuracy	Wireless	References
Volume clamp	Continuous	Disputable	Not yet	[41]
Blood flow	Per beat	Disputable	Available	[42]
Pulse wave	Per beat	Disputable	Available	[43]
Stroke volume	Per beat	Disputable	Available	[44, 45]
Blood flow	Per beat	Disputable	Available	[46, 47]

Hashim *et al* demonstrated a BP monitoring program's hardware and software architecture. The Raspberry Pi, which controls the entire system, is capable of detecting information from the BP gadget and transmitting it over the web so that users may examine it in Telegram and mail applications. The wrist-mounted BP monitor is linked to Raspberry Pi via a USB (Universal Serial Bus) wire. After that, the Raspberry Pi is linked to a Wi-Fi (Wireless Fidelity) dongle to access the internet. Data must be sent over the internet via a network link. The remainder is classified as hypertensive, stage 1, or stage 2. Based on the data, an overview is generated by the computer by each person's systolic measurements, taking into account whether they are normal, low, or high. The most accurate readings are acquired whenever the user is seated and holding a straight object in one hand. Additionally, the system can combine a variety of wireless technologies, including Wi-Fi, device-to-device (D2D) communications and multi-hop wireless networks (MWN) [40].

A proposal with four stages of development was given by Norsuriati *et al.* Stage 1 converts an analogue signal to a digital signal using input from PPG (photoplethysmography) sensors. The technique for estimating BP was created in stage 2 using the MATLAB R2019a programme. The ThingSpeak application and the MATLAB R2019a programme must be connected to the internet in stage 3 to allow for real-time observations. The fourth stage is used to monitor how the system performs when measuring BP and displaying the results in the ThingSpeak and ThingView applications. PPG signals have a frequency range of 0.5–4 Hz. To eliminate the harmonic distortion on the PPG signals, the filter's cut-off frequency is set to 4 Hz. Since the oscillometric cuff that produced arm stiffness after multiple readings was no longer utilized, this is convenient for all hypertension patients [48].

The objective of the development by Singh *et al* is to provide a flexible management framework that enables a network to easily integrate a variety of sensors. The technology was created with sending BP values in consideration. This can be utilized in most regions because it is affordable and mobile. The cuff must be inflated using a KPM27H mini air pump and a pipe. Between the air pump and the cuff, the valve controls air flow. The valve and the air pump are both under the direction and instruction of the H-bridge motor driver. Due to the project's low cost of less than a thousand Rupees, the project's economic goal has been met. Systolic BP values for the applicants who did not have any cardiovascular disease (CVD) or BP-related health complications varied from 110 mm Hg to 135 mm Hg. A patient with hypertension had measures done, and the results varied from 150 to 160 mm Hg [49].

Perdana *et al* state from experiment that the MPX5050DP sensor's BP monitoring findings have a low inaccuracy and, of course, precise measuring findings. In this experiment MPX5050DP is connected with IoT by Firebase as the dataset. Firebase's performance is quite excellent as long as the patient's data speed is equally fast, however, this IoT network still has a rather large latency because of serial transmission from Arduino to Nodemcu. The relative inaccuracy calculated was 3.83% for systole, 2% for diastole, and an average end-to-end delay of 13.943 383 33. In the future, we can add an NFC (near-field communication) introducing a module to the gadget so that more people can use the BP monitoring device with MPX5050DP sensor, which will aid with a clients' routine health screening [50].

Wan *et al* demonstrated the wearable IoT cloud-based health monitoring system named Wireless Internet Solutions Expert (WISE) framework which is a unique health tracker that offers real-time patient monitoring and permits internet access to data. The WISE body area network, the WISE cloud, and the WISE Users comprise three core parts of the WISE system. Without the need of a cell phone, WISE enables quick Wi-Fi transfer of data through W-BAN to the web. The real-time pulse and temperature records may be shown on a compact, small-in-size wearable LCD (liquid crystal display), to let users easily navigate the Wireless Body Area Network (W-BAN) signals. The real-time data will be shown after the WISE system is started [51].

Maddison *et al* performed an experiment in which BP data from wearable, ambulatory, and house tracking devices were evaluated and compared. Over the course of 24 h, they concurrently monitored the patients' BP utilizing wearable and ambulatory equipment in addition to a standardized digital BP tracking device. In fact, patients' BP was monitored over the course of 7 days using both at-home and wearable equipment. 20 healthy volunteers (mean age is 20.3 years, SD is 5.4 years, $n = 10$ females, $n = 10$ males) reported a total of 9090 BP measures. At the time of inclusion, the mean standard deviation (SD) systolic and diastolic blood pressure readings were 112.35 (9.79) mm Hg and 73.75 (9.14) mm Hg, accordingly [52].

All participants in the trial conducted by Golbus *et al* received an Apple Watch Series 3 or Series 4 as well as the MyDataHelps research mobile application and an Omron Evolv Cordless Blood Pressure Monitor. Respondents were required to perform daily or weekly activities, such as taking their BP at home and performing relaxation techniques, while wearing their wristwatch for 12 h or more each day. Over the course of 90 days, individuals submitted 172 (SD 50) BP readings and 31 329 (SD 24 620) heart rate readings, for a total of 1107 320 BP and 202 198 347 heart rate measures. The average systolic BP was 122 mm Hg (SD 10) and the average diastolic blood pressure was 77 mm Hg among the 167 312 (15%) readings with a systolic BP more than 140 mm Hg or a diastolic BP greater than 90 mm Hg (SD 8) [53].

5.5 Wearable fitness trackers

Wearable fitness trackers (also known as activity trackers) are IoT-enabled gadgets that keep a track of the physical fitness of the wearer. They are generally worn on the wrist as a bracelet. Fitness trackers can measure characteristics such as steps walked, distance travelled, average speed, and calories burnt. Heart rate and sleep quality may also be monitored by several fitness and activity monitors [54]. A standard wearable or health tracker connects to a companion app that runs on a smartphone through Bluetooth, and it could also feature Wi-Fi, LTE (long-term evolution), and GSM technologies for direct network connectivity.

Layers of architecture of a fitness tracker:

- *Sensing layer:* This layer is in charge of gathering information from sensors such as footsteps count, heart rate, body temperature, variations in the XYZ axis in relation to Earth's gravity, ambient magnetic strength, and direction in relation to Earth's magnetic field, which can be used to calculate the speed and elevation of the movement.
- *Network layer:* This layer is in charge of power management, monitoring of device and device control, quality of management of the service, and IPV6 (Internet Protocol Version 6) and IPV4 (Internet Protocol Version 4) transmission, addressing and routing.
- *Storage and processing layer:* This layer handles processing of data and data storing that the sensor layer sends to the device's databases or via an application programming interface (API) and push messages to the paired smartphone or the cloud for storage.
- *Service layer:* This layer is in charge of guaranteeing that the data is always visible on the screen, displaying it in an engaging user experience, and sharing it with other services or mobile apps on Android or iOS (iPhone Operating System) devices.

Fitness trackers are important since they can give a clear picture of a person's health wearing them. Some wearable fitness trackers enable users to establish daily fitness objectives and track their progress toward those objectives. This helps people achieve their daily exercise objectives and holds them accountable for doing so. A more sophisticated form of fitness trackers, smartwatches provide much more than just fitness tracking [54].

A few impact creators explain the benefits of using a wearable fitness tracking device:

- They monitor our heart rate, breathing, exercise, and other things. Ramneek Kalra, IEEE member explains that with the use of sensors built into their chips —software algorithms operating on the software layer—wearables are assisting us in tracking our activity levels, breathing patterns, and heart rates. We can carry out this monitoring using a variety of methods, including photoplethysmography for BP, accelerometer sensing for movement, and sharing of breathing and heart rates. Edge computing, IoT and cloud computing are some of the technologies that are most frequently used with wearables.

- We can monitor our exercises by our selves. Aiyappan Pillai, senior IEEE member says thanks to the epidemic, fitness has significantly increased in popularity. However, social-distancing regulations have limited access to gyms and other community sports facilities of a similar nature. In these situations, wearables are a godsend for monitoring one's activities. One might stay under acceptable levels of stress by having real-time feedback while exercising and monitoring vital signs and changes. Exercises might be recommended with more assurance for patients with lifestyle, chronic, or other disorders since accurate feedback mechanisms would assist prevent injury.
- They give us a fuller view of our health.

  Ramalatha Marimuthu, IEEE senior member explains that activity monitoring aids in raising people's awareness of the value of maintaining a healthy balance between exercise, sleep, and eating behaviours. However, wearables aren't just for the healthy; folks with conditions like obesity and heart disease are the ones who benefit from them the most. While training, athletes may also sustain ailments, which the wearables may assist track through exercise logs and other self-tracking techniques. Through applications and messages, which the user may access without even taking the gadget out of their pockets, the devices with self-tracking functions assist health-conscious people in keeping track of their own fitness levels. The main benefit of these wearables is that they provide a comprehensive picture of one's health in one location, saving time and money (table 5.1).

The following components are found in fitness trackers:

1. Data regarding the number of steps taken or the heart rate is gathered by sensors. The accuracy of an activity tracker increases with the number of sensors it contains. These are a few of the sensors found in activity trackers:
   - All trackers employ accelerometers to calculate the number of steps taken. The majority of activity trackers employ sophisticated three-axis accelerometers to more accurately estimate the user's location in three dimensions. Accelerometers and gyroscopes can be used together to account for orientation and angular velocity.
   - The path and terrain where the activity was conducted may be mapped using GPS (global positioning system) in activity trackers.
   - Heart rate sensors make it easier to monitor heart rates while exercising. For the most accurate heart rate readings, optosensor, galvanic skin response sensor, or bioimpedance sensor can be employed.
2. To enable usage by algorithms, the raw data gathered by sensors is combined and transformed into a common format.
3. Data are transformed into useful information and statistics by algorithms.
4. Information and data are presented in a user-friendly fashion, such as charts or graphs, using apps on a smartphone or computer. When a person is about to miss their daily target, apps can remind them to exercise. Additionally, they may connect to social media to post the user's fitness accomplishments.

Table 5.1. Wearable fitness trackers.

Year	Product	Water-safe	Style	Measures	Connectivity	References	Performance
2003	Garmin Forerunner 201	Yes	Wristband	Distance, time, speed, heart rate	GPS-based	[55]	Inconsistent performance
2006	Nike+ iPod Fitness kit	N/A	iPod device	Works as a pedometer i.e. measures distance/steps	Sensor to be embedded in shoes, Wireless sense–receiver combination	[56]	Design may compromise security, may lead to privacy issues, acceptable accuracy
2009	Fitbit Classic	No	Clip-on	Distance, motion, body movements while sleeping	An accelerometer	[57]	Not very accurate performance
2013	Fitbit Flex	Water-resistant	Wristband	Distance, sleep	Wireless—syncs over Bluetooth 4.0	[57]	Inconsistent sleep tracking
2013	Pebble Watch	Yes, up to 50 meters	Wristband/ kind of a smartwatch	Distance/steps, sleep	Wireless—Bluetooth enabled	[58]	Stable performance

Hong states that wearable technology is acknowledged as a prominent area of client devices in IoT business applications. For this study, activity trackers (also known as fitness trackers) are types of wristbands chosen from a wide range of wearable technology. The goal of the study is to establish customer requirements for activity trackers, which is the first NTER (National Tax Equivalent Regime) item, and then connect those needs to the activity tracker's marketing combination, which consists of the following four Ps (pPrice, place, product and promotion), with a concentration on the first three. A survey of Korean university students was undertaken for this study to determine their existing and future demands for activity monitors. Activity trackers have more potential needs than other IT (information technology) devices, according to the results of the four P's classification of needs. The market success of IoT applications depends on both IoT technology and user demands across several business areas. If not, there would be little market acceptability and IoT applications would not produce the promised outcomes in terms of commercial factors. The study highlighted possible uses for activity trackers and detailed how they vary from other electronic gadgets in traditional marketing methods. The majority of participants are more acquainted with smart watches than they are with activity trackers, and they prefer to purchase them from reputable merchants. The design elements, with the exception of distinctiveness, did not differ much between males and females. The present market price is pretty close to the market accepted price of $150. More than $250 will face stiff resistance in the market, per the findings. Additionally, the results of the exploratory study offer a conceptual framework that links client demands with activity tracker attributes. The success of new product development is impacted by several variables, including management and engineering viewpoints [59].

Li *et al* state that the use of fog-aided computational efficient wearable sensor networks (FCEWSNs) in systems for monitoring of health for sports and athletics utilizing IoT is suggested in this research. Additionally, the sensor data is transferred to the ethernet module of the IoT-connection systems, and the authenticated user can access it online to monitor the athletes' health. Our evaluation technique uses a queue and can ascertain at the very least of processing power necessary to meet the service level agreement (SLA) (both fog and cloud nodes). The results of the experiments offer a complete IoT- and cloud-based computing architecture enabling IoT and cloud-based infrastructure applications for the healthcare industry. They provide a platform for the medical data transmission from medical equipment to distant servers and/or cloud computing services. The vast cloud-based investigation, particularly fog-based computational technologies with standardized designs, spawned fog-based studies in healthcare applications. The real-time alert generating with important event measurement increases the usefulness of the suggested system. Equations in mathematics to assess the effectiveness of the IoT devices, public, private, and fog cloud nodes levels of the healthcare system. The FCEWSN method proposed is quite effective in spotting unexpected situations for athletes. When compared to other techniques now in use, the sensor's performance is relatively high [60].

Dawson *et al* made an in-depth forensic analysis to provide forensically significant artefacts from the TomTom Spark 3 GPS fitness watch and its accompanying Android app. Their forensic analysis and methodologies identified, extracted, analysed, and reassembled user activity data in a criminal investigation using non-forensic, commercial forensic, and a non-forensic manufacturer-independent analytical platform tool designed for endurance sports. They present forensic metadata that incorporates information from a smartwatch's hardware, earlier user behaviours, and voice recordings. They made it using the app's own databases and activity files, which include data on prior user actions on an Android mobile device. The results of the study show the existing forensic technology's shortcomings and inspire forensic software developers to create forensic software programs and strategies capable of decoding all pertinent data generated by wearable IoT-based devices. Forensic investigators need to resort to these results in order to support criminal investigations. This research aids forensic investigators to analyse artefacts derived from smartwatches and fitness trackers that serve as a significant reference for the forensic tool creators constructing software programmes that are capable of decoding all data that is critical offered by the wearable IoT devices [61].

Canhoto and Arp state, however, that these benefits of fitness trackers will not materialize unless users embrace and continue using these devices, rather than discarding them soon after purchase. Our research examines the potential influences of the user, the surrounding environment, and the characteristics of the device on the acceptance and sustainable usage of the health and fitness wearables. We learn that the elements defending the first are distinct from those who support the latter. For example, adoption depends on elements that make the potential of the device collect the activity data clearly, yet continuous usage depends on portability and durability. Despite the study's sample size's somewhat constrained age range of 25–32, the needs and goals of the participants point to a market with a lot of space for growth. Since the main non-medical consumer group in Germany are people are interested in sports and fitness wearables, they looked for participants at fitness centres and internet discussion forums. This was an effective tactic because the goal of their exploratory research was to look at current users. The study's main focus was on German wearables early adopters, which produced a sample that was both youthful and enthusiastic about using these tools to enhance one's fitness. Specialized fitness wearables are now growing in popularity and market share. Wearables' attraction, however, may wane as they go through subsequent phases in a product's life cycles and begin to be used by demographics that are less enthused about acquiring new technology. Our study found that a variety of factors have an impact on adoption and continued use of the wearables. Other factors were identified by their investigation that directly affect continuous use (e.g. learning through observation). Additionally, even while some variables have an effect on both adoption and continued use, the impact is caused by a variety of traits. For instance, functionalities connected to activity tracking versus functionalities connected to data accuracy [62].

Zhou and Piramuthu explain that wearable fitness trackers are becoming more and more popular with people, thus it is important to make sure that any privacy and security flaws are kept to a minimum. They examine potential solutions to these problems. A wearable fitness tracker called Fitbit has uncovered a number of vulnerabilities. They also went a step further and suggested ways to fix the discovered vulnerabilities, creating FitLock in the process. FitLock is not impervious to flaws, though. This in no way implies that all wearable fitness tracker gadgets with a direct connection to an online social network are open to security or privacy problems. As IoT devices proliferate, reachability should caution us to carefully consider any linked security and privacy weaknesses. This is particularly important when private information is at stake (like healthcare). The goal of this essay is to use it to increase awareness of this. Using FitLock as an illustration, potential flaws are demonstrated [63].

Kang *et al* explain that although fitness trackers are initially intended to monitor a user's health, their data is crucial for confirming the validity of a suspect's deposition answers or the victim's actions close to the time of the occurrence. 'Fitbit Alta HR' and 'Xiaomi Mi Band 2' are two examples of fitness trackers that let consumers examine measurement of the data that is on the linked mobile devices. They evaluate the functionalities of both the wearables, decide which data must be collected and offer digital forensics analysis techniques for each file. The processes can produce records that are very important to criminal investigations because of interaction between fitness bands and mobile devices. As a result, the linked gadget can provide pertinent data. The majority of the data is managed by the trackers using Android SQLite3 databases. In the instance of the Fitbit Alta HR, the user's account on a Fitbit server may be used to access the similar data that was downloaded in the associated mobile phone. The victim's death time may be estimated by using the victim's step count, heart rate, sleep cycle, and GPS data (with the timestamp) in addition to the suspect's statement being verified. Each vendor creates its own apps for connecting with the fitness tracker. As a result, there are differences in the file formats, names, and other aspects of how the apps manage the data [64].

5.6 Smart jewellery

The goal of the project has been to create a wearable prototype object that responds to environmental and bodily stimulation to generate playful interactions. These interactions are expressed through activating elements like color-changing chromic smart materials and light interactions made possible by electronic sensing techniques [65]. The initiative focuses on creating smart jewellery that children with impairments may wear to have their temperature and heart rate constantly monitored. The jewellery is made from recyclable materials and has a design influenced by Nature that resembles a marine monster frequently seen in cartoons. The user's biometric data is delivered to your phone through Bluetooth and uploaded to the cloud data centre server via an app on your phone when the user wears the smart jewellery [66]. Some examples of smart jewellery are Bellabeat Leaf Urban, which we wear on our wrists, clips, and necks to monitor our activity, sleep, and stress levels, among other things. RinglyLuxe is a smart ring that we wear on our fingers to measure our activities, including steps taken, distance travelled, calories burnt, etc. We wear joule earring backings as earring backs and use them to continuously measure our heart rates [67].

Smartwatches are becoming more and more common among wearables. These gadgets resemble conventional jewellery in the form of bracelets, rings, and necklaces but have technology built in that allows them to measure essential activity, health, and other data. While hybrid gadgets like Fossil's Q watch straddle the border between smart jewellery and smartwatches [65]. The combination of fashion and technology in these smart jewels is the secret. By monitoring your movements and analysing calories burnt, movement speed, and even sleep patterns, they can maintain tabs on your exercise regimen and general health. Wearables may have a significant impact regardless of one's age, gender, or race population health and well-being. Most significantly, wearables might help with improvement independent of race, financial class, or region, access to prompt care and treatment. A wide variety of rings, bangles, lockets, necklaces, earrings, and bracelets fall under the category of 'smart jewellery,' which can be readily synchronized with a smartphone. Smart jewellery has distinct qualities and skills that make it possible to monitor daily activities like sleep, stress, and many others. If a user has smart jewellery on them, they can measure their health problems wherever they are. Since the jewellery is portable, stylish, fashionable, lightweight, and simple to carry, it has an edge over other wearable technology. Among the main producers of smart jewellery are Oura, Ringly, Totwoo Fashion Technology, McLear Ltd, Bellabeat, and other well-known companies.

The growth of smart IoT wearable technologies has recently been dominating the digital lifestyle. With the use of IoT technology, intelligent jewellery that has a communication function may also have a linkage network function added to it. The main technology of the research and development of smart jewellery is the integration of sensor technology, wireless communication technology, and the microprocessor to realize the multifunction of the jewellery. The most popular wireless communication technologies utilized in smart jewellery are Bluetooth and NFC. A comprehensive IoT-based smart jewellery system uses data from the user's environment for collecting, storage, analysis, and individualized health plans. With the help of a smart jewellery gyro sensor, an exercise act, an exercise session, sleep time and activities are tracked. Through the usage of smart jewellery healthcare applications, users may long-term detect their health state and symptoms. Global IoT development firms have begun creating smart rings to improve our daily routines. Smart rings with IoT integration can replace fitness trackers. Smart rings may be used to monitor sleep as well as other factors including saturation of blood-oxygen saturation and heart rate. These sensors can record the data on pulse strength, heart rate, and saturation of blood-oxygen (table 5.2).

Kang *et al* stated that the idea behind smart jewellery is a piece of multipurpose technology that can interact with the wearer. With the introduction of the Apple Smart Watch in 2015, wearable technology advanced quickly. In the meantime, wearing technique became the primary growth path for jewellery accessories. As a result, it is intended to employ sensors identification to add intelligent function and design to trendy jewellery while taking into account human interaction. They begin by outlining the service oriented high level design of the framework and web ontology language (OWL) ontology models. Additionally, they link the approaches with other event-based processing agents in order to develop a plug-in-based adaptable framework. As long as they have smart jewellery on them, individuals in the personal healthcare space may measure their health status everywhere. Additionally, the platform is built to be installed on a cloud server, making all of its features accessible through interfaces. Through the smartphone application, we also display the status of the services. The programme offers a customized service to the consumer and assesses the danger before displaying the recommended actions for each ailment [65].

Khan stated that the primary purpose of this research is to present all of the most recent technologies, their associated trends, and information in the fields of IoT and digital jewellery, as well as a research proposal on the impact of IoT on this industry. In addition, parents are reluctant to send their daughters to work at night or anywhere far from them owing to recent adverse instances involving female children. The use of digital jewellery and IoT can overcome these issues. Digital jewellery will represent the advancement in digital technology that fully integrates computer components with the human form. The fundamental idea behind the digital jewellery concept is to maintain good fashion sense while having the convenience of wireless, wearable computing [72].

Sogi *et al* put together a device that will safeguard women, a wearable watch-like gadget that may be worn on the wrist. When in danger, the victim can press a button on the gadget to activate a camera built on a Raspberry Pi that will capture a picture of the attacker. Physical objects may connect with one another via the internet using IoT, regardless of distance. The suggested solution uses real-time, portability, and security to send alarm messages to the user's loved ones and the closest police station. The authors of this article have proposed a prototype of a device that employs a flex sensor and a fall detection sensor, both of which are unreliable since they can accidentally be activated by the victim. Providing women with the protection they deserve is the main goal of this study [73].

Fernández-Caramés and Fraga-Lamas stated that IoT-based clothing and smart wearables have the potential to make a significant impact by balancing usefulness with the joy that fashion brings. A new era in retailing is predicted by the potential of the smart textiles, which can communicate with smartphones to analyse physiological data like heart rate, temperature, respiration, stress, movements, accelerations, or even the hormone levels. This article talks about the primary needs for the creation of smart, IoT-based clothing and gives an illustration of the possible long-term effects of smart clothing on the business models. In order to make the idea of the Internet of Smart Clothing a reality, this article offered instructions for upcoming IoT smart garment designers and developers [74].

Klaib *et al* stated that eye tracking using IoT and cloud technology improves interactions when a person is not able to or doesn't want to make use of their hands to manage home appliances. Eyes may be the greatest option for those with neurological and muscular limitations in order to improve their user experience

Table 5.2. Sensors used in smart jewellery.

Sl. No.	Sensor	Use	Device	Accuracy	Reference
1	Gyroscope	The sensors enable the bracelets to continually gather user activities and vital data	Smart Bracelet	Extremely accurate and stable	[68]
2	Accelerometer	The sensors enable the bracelets to continually gather user activities and vital data	Smart Bracelet	Identifying sedentary behaviour was the most difficult, whereas detecting modest physical activity was the easiest	[69]
3	EDA-sensor	For monitoring emotions, sensations, and cognition, as well as stress levels	Smart Ring	89% accuracy when distinguishing calm condition from distressed condition	[69]
4	SpO2 sensor	For monitoring blood-oxygen levels	Smart Ring	SpO2 readings are accurate to within ±2% and ±3%, respectively, between 50% and 80% and 80% and 100%	[70]
5	Glucose sensor, and NTC thermistor	To monitor body temperature	Smart Ring	Precision of NTC thermistors' temperature measurements is quite high (±0.1 °C)	[71]

[6]. Therefore, an IoT-enabled eye tracker that employs a system that records the user's movements of eyes to correctly capture where they are looking and for how long they are gazing there may be the best option for the elderly and users with special needs. Additionally, software methods for processing of the images, filtering of the data, eye movements recording, and pupil detection are used. There are several methods for monitoring the eyes, including the Scleral Search Coil Approach and the Infrared Oculography Approach. Due to the employment of numerous cameras that record high speed pictures to show the user's eye and projectors that create a pattern of infrared light on the user's eyes, the Tobii eye tracking system was chosen in this study to construct the prototype [75].

Verma *et al* stated that one of the most popular subjects right now in the healthcare industry is the IoT, which has been suggested as a potential feature for the improvement of the technologies already in existence that decrease the effective cost of healthcare in all of its forms. IoT in biomedicine is viewed as vital for an hour to give medical assistance to individuals for detecting, managing, monitoring, and responding from the system after receiving data. This significantly lowers the cost of healthcare. IoT in healthcare might provide improvement in a patient's care, thanks to numerous smart devices including ultrasound, portable x-ray machines, smart beds, glucose metres, BP monitors, and thermometers. Body garments, heads (helmets and spectacles), wrists (bracelets and watches), and somatosensory modulators, such as body and foot sensory control devices, are the current categories of IoT-based portable devices. These wearables have grown to be an integral part of IoT technology, and they are evolving from simple accessories to include more specialized and practical capabilities [27].

Piekenbrock focused on putting the traditional component first and focus on changing the look itself. This thesis seeks to understand how the wearer's surroundings are affected emotionally. Compared to rings or bracelets, necklaces are viewed by the user as being far more personal. Additionally, the look of smart jewellery shouldn't be different from non-smart jewellery. The gadget has the ability to play produced abstract animations and music. Wearers can also select a different mode because it is wirelessly connected to an Android mobile phone. Some biometric and environmental data can be read by the necklace's sensors to trigger animations and music [76].

5.7 ECG monitoring system

Wearable ECG machine monitoring is one of the most popular and often employed techniques in the healthcare sector as a result of the pervasive computer environment [82]. The deaths from chronic and cardiovascular diseases (CVDs) has grown during the previous 10 years in every country on Earth (table 5.3). CVDs are diseases that affect the heart and blood vessels. The blood vessels are affected by vascular diseases, for example coronary artery disease. A few conditions that impact the heart includes arrhythmias, failure of heart, cardiomyopathy, rheumatic heart diseases, stroke, and heart attacks. The ECG is a standard test used to examine and diagnose CVDs [83]. The ECG signal is one of the most basic pieces of medical or healthcare data. It uses voltage between electrode pairs to monitor the heart's electrical activity. ECG is regarded to be the greatest tool to monitor and identify aberrant heart rhythms since it shows the heart's general rhythm. Additionally, the procedure is affordable and painless, and the heart rate may be calculated from the R–R peak interval. In this multidisciplinary field of healthcare and ubiquitous computing, the ECG has become one of the most referenced signals due to its advantages, such as convenient measurement and informative application [82].

ECG monitoring technologies are becoming more and more prevalent in the literature at an exponential rate. The two main issues in modern healthcare are continuous monitoring of heart rate and instant detection of heartbeat. According to experimental data, ECG signal analysis along with continuous monitoring might improve the diagnosis, management, and prevention of several CVDs. Due to the introduction of smart enabling technologies, ECG monitoring systems, which have been created and utilized extensively in the healthcare industry over the previous few decades, have drastically changed over time [83]. At least, three electrodes—two electrodes and one (virtual) ground—must be placed in various locations around the heart in order to assess the ECG. In reality, the physical form of the ECG monitor is restricted from being reimagined as a wearable device since the complete 12 lead ECG is made up of 10 separate electrodes that are fixed in place. We may categorize the wearable ECG monitor as it currently exists into three main sorts of devices based on their physical characteristics and locations where measurements are taken: shirts, wristwatches, and chest belts [82]. One of the crucial factors to consider when assessing exercise performance is heart rate. A signal obtained by a wearable ECG monitor serves as the foundation for one type of heart rate detection technique. Body movement will obstruct the ECG signal during exercising. Heart rate estimation and motion artefact cancellation are the two main foundations of heart rate detection investigations [84].

IoT solutions have been established in the healthcare industry as a result of the concept's quick development. With the help of these technologies, medical parameters may be remotely monitored while a patient is at home, and the data can be sent to experts for examination. Monitoring the ECG is one of the most significant IoT-based applications that may be used. One of the suggested architectures makes use of a gadget with three electrodes that communicates with Wi-Fi, Bluetooth, and ZigBee to connect to the internet (for the last two a smartphone is used as gateway). The MQTT middleware protocol is used to transport data to the internet. The patient, their family, and the doctor may access the data using a GUI (graphical user interface) interface that is saved in the cloud (via HTTP (Hypertext Transfer Protocol) requests or MQTT subscriptions) [85]. IoT has a wide range of applications in the medical industry. Healthcare personnel may assess, identify, and treat patients in distant areas with the use of telecommunications technology and remote information collection. A tiny ECG monitoring gadget that can capture heart rates and waveforms and communicate the information to a database and web server was the goal of one research. Using an Arduino microcontroller and a single-lead heart rate monitor sensor, an ECG collection device was created. The ECG data processing, analysis, and uploading application is coded using MATLAB and C# programmes. The gathered data is displayed in a GUI display that was C# written, as well as in a webpage. The process started with a quick design of the system and utilized rapid application technology (RAD). The development of the hardware and software systems involved a prototype cycle. Once complete, the system is assembled to create a whole IoT-based ECG monitoring system [86].

Ungurean and Brezulianu explain that through the use of a mobile tele-electrocardiograph and independent patient acquisition of ECG signals, an IoT-based architecture may be utilized in healthcare to monitor signals from ECG without a specialist's assistance. The primary characteristics of the mobile device are discussed, along with how these characteristics fit into the suggested IoT architecture. The essay also addresses the integrity, confidentiality, and authenticity security concerns that may arise while utilizing this system. The article discusses and refers to certain

Table 5.3. Comparison of features of different ECG monitors from different literature.

Reference	Signal acquisition	Signal pre-processing	Feature extraction	Processing	Visualization	Signal selection	Compression	Data storage	Modelling	Encryption
[77]	No	Yes	No	Yes	No	No	No	No	Yes	No
[78]	Yes	No	No	Yes	No	No	No	No	No	No
[79]	Yes	Yes	No	Yes	No	No	No	No	No	Yes
[80]	Yes	Yes	Yes	Yes	No	No	No	No	Yes	No
[81]	Yes	Yes	Yes	Yes	No	No	No	Yes	Yes	No

IoT solutions for the medical industry that have been written about in the literature. It also covers the architecture of the proposed system and illustrates how a mobile ECG device may be integrated into the system. It also addresses the primary security issues with the suggested design and suggests solutions. The application of the idea of patient remote monitoring within the framework of the IoT paradigm is what distinguishes the offered approach. A middleware system that uses the data and device security (DDS) protocol was also employed for data transfer via the internet. Data on security, integrity, and security that have been implemented utilizing the DDS requirements are another novel addition. The results of the ECG signals are not as accurate as those made at the doctor's clinic, which is a drawback. Based on the data gathered by the mobile device, the medical expert can assess whether more precise measures are required. As a consequence, the technology can identify individuals who require extra testing at the doctor's clinic [85].

Prawiro and Lin state that although these contaminated signals may not always be categorized as noise, they might be present during the collection of ECG measurements. In this work, we employ a strategy to process signals to separate the step signal from the signal of ECG. The recommended method has been created, tested, and evaluated using the ensemble empirical mode decomposition (EEMD) method to extract data from ECG using accelerometer's data as the reference step counter. The important concept is to select the proper intrinsic mode function (IMF) for the delineation of the gait signal in the ECG and to determine the accuracy of the identification of the gait signal using the step counter acquired from accelerometer data. To evaluate the accuracy of the gait detection, this experiment makes use of five training subjects. We evaluate the detection accuracy reached using the suggested methods, IMF 6 and IMF 7. Using the belt-tightening scenario of a 100% length of chest circumference, the proposed method achieves average detection accuracy of 91.93% and 94.72% for training and testing individuals, respectively [87].

Constant *et al* show the use of a wearable-IoT framework by presenting pulse-glasses as a wearable sensor that continuously keeps on collecting HR data from a wearer's face and sends it to a cloud platform via a mobile phone. They designed wearable, cloud-connected smart eyewear called pulse-glasses for covert and continual heart rate monitoring. The pulse-glasses' first design was 3D printed and uses a PPG sensor on one of the nose-pads to collect data of heart rate. They included more circuitry, such as an integrated board with BLE and a battery that is rechargeable, into the two temples of the pulse-glasses. In order to gather, display, and seamlessly save hear rate data from pulse-glasses on the cloud, they configured IoT functionality. The hardware upgrades for pulse-glasses, including IoT-based services and preliminary validation testing outcomes, are covered in this article. Their preliminary results are interesting and demonstrate the potential of pulse-glasses for cloud-connected BSNs (big switch networks). With regard to the algorithms that may detect and eliminate noise artefacts caused by head, facial, and body motions, they anticipate further improving pulse-glasses [88].

Jung and Kim in their study present the creation of a wearable, universal healthcare monitoring system that incorporates an ECG, a PPG, a skin temperature sensor, an accelerometer, and other technologies. The non-intrusive healthcare system in this concept was built on the W-BAN standard for wide area coverage and low battery consumption for RF transmission. This system uses ZigBee, a W-BAN technology, to link wearable physiological signal devices to the specialized mobile system. They were able to develop a variety of devices, such as wrist, chest wearables, and necklace wearables. To perform ECG measurements, the signal of ECG is converted into a digital signal with a rate of sampling of 100 Hz for detections of heart rate. Performance testing was done on the built-in ECG module using a commercial ECG simulator. For a variety of ECG outputs with a range of 30–200 bpm, the ECG module developed provided HR outputs with a 1% error range. Performance of the PPG module developed was verified using a commercial SpO2 simulator. To evaluate the effectiveness of SKT-skin temperature, the module developed was tested in a heated chamber at the temperatures that were raised from the range of 25 °C–40 °C in one-degree increments. The data obtained demonstrated high linearity and accuracy with a 1% error margin. The WIBMS (wrist-worn integrated monitoring device) checks whether the wearer is aware or not when it detects a fall incident by sounding an alert. The WIBMS then begins the important bio-signal measurements if the user doesn't respond within a certain amount of time (10 s) and notifies the preassigned caregivers of the emergency incident with the necessary details. The results over a variety of pulse rates recorded in PPG indicated accuracy with a 1% margin of error. Due to the WIBMS's limited bodily contact with the wrist region, the detected bio-signals have a low degree of fidelity [89].

Ha *et al* in their paper explain that the ubiquitous computer environment is transforming the healthcare sector, and wearable ECG measuring is one of the most often used strategies. Interdisciplinary viewpoints of the wearable ECG monitor make this more challenging. Reliability and performance of healthcare devices are crucial issues for their broad use. In this article, they suggest assessment standards that take into account both the characteristics of ECG measurement and ubiquitous computing. Depending on the assessment technique, several degrees of experimental analysis are carried out using our wearable ECG monitors. Reliability and performance of sensing are two of the basic challenges to the general adoption of ubiquitous healthcare technology. Wearable ECG monitors likewise face these challenges. The interdisciplinarity of IT technology and medical engineering in the dependability problem adds to its complexity. In other words, the proper evaluation procedure should take into account both of the two factors simultaneously. Even if the information from the gadget is intended to be used as medical diagnostic or at the very least for information of healthcare, they claimed that they have noticed that there are no standard protocols to validate the functionality of ECG monitor in the case of wearable and wireless circumstances. As a result, they suggest assessment criteria that take into account both the characteristics of ECG measurement and ubiquitous computing. In order to address wearability concerns, they begin by offering a wearable ECG monitor, which is designed in four distinct varieties. Then, They carried out a variety of data assessment levels, including wireless communication, ECG signal waveform analysis, and heart rate analysis. In order to report reliable results in accordance with different exercise intensities, they recruited a sizable number of volunteers with a variety of ages, especially for the dependability of HR. They assess the effectiveness of the ECG monitor during these assessment procedures with the goal of boosting both customer and supplier trust in wearable medical technology [82].

Lv and Guo explain that their research intends to enable real-time ECG signal monitoring and collection during IoT-focused athletic events. Its responsibility is to gather the physiological signals from an ECG and convey the information about those signals via wireless transmission technology. This study investigates an IoT-focused, real-time electrical signal collection and monitoring system for a sports competition process centre. Given that the QRS (quasi random signal) detection algorithm is the core algorithm, low power consumption is critical for ECG platform processing. In order to address the drawbacks of low-power implementation, the features of the time domain detection method that make it susceptible to noise, and in order to reduce the complexity and memory requirements of the transform domain technique, this work proposes a low-power QRS detection approach for waveform prediction. Almost 94.99% of wavelet transform values are found to be below the threshold of 31.25% of wavelet decomposition coefficients related to QRS waves by investigating wavelet decomposition coefficients using the wavelet transform approach. This study provides a time-domain land prediction approach. The core technology proposed in this study, in particular the ubiquitous buried device platform for ultra-low-power ECG processing has both scientific and practical importance for the development of wearable and electrical detection systems [90].

Yang *et al* explain that ECG monitoring is a critical method used to identify cardiac disorders that is extensively researched and used. However, almost all portable ECG monitoring devices now in use require a mobile application for data collection and presentation in order to function. In this study, they present a novel IoT-based ECG monitoring methodology. ECG data is gathered by a wearable monitoring node and wirelessly sent to an IoT-based cloud. The IoT cloud makes use of both the HTTP and MQTT protocols to provide users with visible and quick ECG data. The three main elements of the architecture of the IoT-based ECG monitoring system are the ECG sensor network, IoT cloud, and GUI. The web-based GUI does away with the need for mobile applications and gives users a flexible, mobile OS-independent method to examine the ECG data. The diagnostic outcomes from the ECG signal must be more precise in order to provide a more accurate diagnosis of the condition. It is thought that long-term, simple ECG monitoring might greatly lessen some of the present healthcare problems [91].

5.8 Conclusion

Numerous facets of human activity are greatly influenced by digital and information technology, which enhances the quality of our lives. Thanks to the widespread use of IoT platforms enabling sophisticated monitoring services and intelligent inferring systems, health systems are witnessing a true technological revolution that is fundamentally altering how medical services are given [2]. Wearable gadgets are presently at the centre of almost every IoT conversation. Because of the expected huge increase in the number of older persons until 2020, the need for self-health monitoring and preventative medicine is expanding and developed technology can truly cut total preventative and monitoring expenses. So we want to provide insights into the role of IoT in wearable devices through this chapter, as well as the capabilities that wearables with IoT provide individuals with the data they need to monitor their health [1]. The chapter discusses the classification of wearable medical devices and briefly discusses a number of these devices, including smart contact lenses, blood sensors, glucose monitors and asthma monitors, in the context of the IoT. A few more wearable medical devices are also presented in depth, including wearable biosensors, BP monitors, fitness trackers, smart jewellery, and ECG monitoring systems, where the chapter discusses the significance and impact of the device. Additionally, it highlights the IoT component in the gadgets. By looking at several articles that have been published on a certain device, it also reviews earlier efforts on such devices. The chapter's overall goal is to explain IoT in wearable medical devices as well as its significance and effects.

References

[1] Nasiri N 2019 *Wearable Devices: The Big Wave of Innovation* (London: IntechOpen)
[2] Fotiadis D I, Glaros C and Likas A C 2006 Wearable medical devices *Wiley Encyclopedia of Biomedical Engineering* (New York: Wiley)
[3] Lu L Z J, Xie Y, Gao F, Xu S, Wu X and Ye Z 2020 Wearable health devices in health care: narrative systematic review *JMIR Mhealth Uhealth* **8** e18907
[4] Huhn S *et al* 2022 The impact of wearable technologies in health research: scoping review *JMIR Mhealth Uhealth* **10** e34834
[5] Aksahin M 2017 Ergonomics importance of wearable medical devices *Ergon. Int. J.* **1** 000124
[6] Jiang N, Mück J E and Yetisen A K 2020 The regulation of wearable medical devices *Trends Biotechnol.* **38** 129–33
[7] Hemapriya D *et al* 2017 Wearable medical devices—design challenges and issues *2017 Int. Conf. on Innovations in Green Energy and Healthcare Technologies (IGEHT)*
[8] Mamdiwar S D *et al* 2021 Recent advances on IoT-assisted wearable sensor systems for healthcare monitoring *Biosensors* **11** 372
[9] Sinha P G 2021 *Introduction to IoT* (unpublished)
[10] Pradhan B, Bhattacharyya S and Pal K 2021 IoT-based applications in healthcare devices *J. Healthc. Eng.* **2021** 6632599
[11] Gatouillat A *et al* 2018 Building IoT-enabled wearable medical devices: an application to a wearable, multiparametric, cardiorespiratory sensor *Proc. of the 11th Int. Joint Conf. on Biomedical Engineering Systems and Technologies (BIOSTEC 2018) (Funchal)* 109–18
[12] Haghi M, Thurow K and Stoll R 2017 Wearable devices in medical Internet of Things: scientific research and commercially available devices *Healthc. Inform. Res.* **23** 4–15
[13] Dian F, Vahidnia R and Rahmati A 2020 Wearables and the Internet of Things (IoT), applications, opportunities, and challenges: a survey *IEEE Access* **8** 69200–11
[14] Surantha N *et al* 2021 A review of wearable Internet-of-Things device for healthcare *Procedia Comput. Sci.* **179** 936–43
[15] Iqbal S M *et al* 2021 Advances in healthcare wearable devices *npj Flex. Electron.* **5** 9

[16] Valenzuela F *et al* 2020 An IoT-based glucose monitoring algorithm to prevent diabetes complications *Appl. Sci.* **10** 921
[17] Ramly R, Abu Bakar Sajak A and Syahmi M 2020 IOT-based glucose monitoring system http://dx.doi.org/10.13140/RG.2.2.33859.63522
[18] Sankalp Deshkar T R Aa V G M 2018 A review on IoT based m-health systems for diabetes *Int. J. Emerg. Technol. Innov. Res.* **5** 49–54
[19] Wang H-C and Lee A-R 2015 Recent developments in blood glucose sensors *J. Food Drug Anal.* **23** 191–200
[20] Arakawa T 2018 Recent research and developing trends of wearable sensors for detecting blood pressure *Sensors* **18** 2772
[21] Puckett L G *et al* 2003 Monitoring blood coagulation with magnetoelastic sensors *Biosens. Bioelectron.* **18** 675–81
[22] Gibson P G 2000 Monitoring the patient with asthma: an evidence-based approach *J. Allergy Clin. Immunol.* **106** 17–26
[23] Cheriyedath S 2019 Monitoring asthma *News-Medical* www.news-medical.net/health/Monitoring-Asthma.aspx (Accessed 17 May 2023)
[24] Ma X *et al* 2021 Smart contact lenses for biosensing applications *Adv. Intell. Syst.* **3** 2000263
[25] Sharma A *et al* Wearable biosensors: an alternative and practical approach in healthcare and disease monitoring *Molecules* **26** 748
[26] Pateraki M *et al* 2020 Biosensors and Internet of Things in smart healthcare applications: challenges and opportunities *Wearable and Implantable Medical Devices* ed N Dey *et al* ch 2 (New York: Academic), pp 25–53
[27] Verma D *et al* 2022 Internet of things (IoT) in nano-integrated wearable biosensor devices for healthcare applications *Biosens. Bioelectron.* X **11** 100153
[28] Singh K R B *et al* 2021 Nano-enabled wearable sensors for the Internet of Things (IoT) *Mater. Lett.* **304** 130614
[29] Kim J, Campbell A S and Wang J 2018 Wearable non-invasive epidermal glucose sensors: A review *Talanta* **177** 163–70
[30] Tseng R C *et al* 2018 Contact-lens biosensors *Sensors* **18** 2651
[31] Zheng X *et al* 2021 Smart biosensors and intelligent devices for salivary biomarker detection *TrAC Trends Anal. Chem.* **140** 116281
[32] Prabhu S *et al* 2020 IoT-associated impedimetric biosensing for point-of-care monitoring of kidney health *IEEE Sens. J.* **21** 14320–9
[33] Madukwe K, Ezika-nee Anarado I and Iloanusi O 2017 Leveraging edge analysis for Internet of Things based healthcare solutions *IEEE 3rd Int. Conf. on Electro-Technology for National Development (NIGERCON) (Owerri, Nigeria)* 720–5
[34] Nagamine K and Tokito S 2021 Organic-transistor-based biosensors interfaced with human skin for non-invasive perspiration analysis *Sens. Actuators* B **349** 130778
[35] Hamidi H and Fazeli K 2018 Using Internet of Things and biosensors technology for health applications *IET Wirel. Sens. Syst.* **8** 260–7
[36] Konstantinidis D *et al* 2022 Wearable blood pressure measurement devices and new approaches in hypertension management: the digital era *J. Hum. Hypertens.* **36** 945–51
[37] Bard D M, Joseph J I and van Helmond N 2019 Cuff-less methods for blood pressure telemonitoring *Front. Cardiovasc. Med.* **6** 40
[38] Salah W A and Sneineh A A 2018 Development of pulse and blood pressure monitoring system *2018 IEEE Symp. on Computer Applications and Industrial Electronics (ISCAIE)*

[39] Zhang Y *et al* 2020 Adherence with blood pressure monitoring wearable device among the elderly with hypertension: the case of rural China *Brain Behav.* **10** e01599
[40] Hashim N *et al* 2020 IoT blood pressure monitoring system *Indones. J. Electr. Eng. Comput. Sci.* **19** 1384
[41] Birch A A and Morris S L 2003 Do the Finapres and Colin radial artery tonometer measure the same blood pressure changes following deflation of thigh cuffs? *Physiol. Meas.* **24** 653–60
[42] Uemura K, Kawada T and Sugimachi M 2019 A novel minimally occlusive cuff method utilizing ultrasound vascular imaging for stress-free blood pressure measurement: a-proof-of-concept study *IEEE Trans. Biomed. Eng.* **66** 934–45
[43] Ding X and Zhang Y-T 2019 Pulse transit time technique for cuffless unobtrusive blood pressure measurement: from theory to algorithm *Biomed. Eng. Lett.* **9** 37–52
[44] De Cort S C *et al* 1991 Cardiac output, oxygen consumption and arteriovenous oxygen difference following a sudden rise in exercise level in humans *J. Physiol.* **441** 501–12
[45] Chen Y-H *et al* 2014 Soft, comfortable polymer dry electrodes for high quality ECG and EEG recording *Sensors* **14** 23758–80
[46] Xiong G *et al* 2011 Simulation of blood flow in deformable vessels using subject-specific geometry and spatially varying wall properties *Int. J. Numer. Methods Biomed. Eng.* **27** 1000–16
[47] Ma Y *et al* 2018 Relation between blood pressure and pulse wave velocity for human arteries *Proc. Natl Acad. Sci.* **115** 11144–49
[48] Norsuriati M S, Norehan Mohd Sobri M S, Zaidatul Hafiszah H, Mohamad Nazib A, Wan Suhaimizan W Z, Ashok V and Muhammad Mahadi A J 2021 Development of IoT based cuffless blood pressure measurement system *J. Phys.: Conf. Ser.* **2071** 012030
[49] Singh B *et al* 2019 Blood pressure monitoring system using wireless technologies *Procedia Comput. Sci.* **152** 267–73
[50] Shihab K, Perdana D and Sussi S 2020 Design and implementation of IoT based blood pressure monitoring tools *Int. J. Simul. Syst. Sci. Technol.* **21** 03
[51] Wan J *et al* 2018 Wearable IoT enabled real-time health monitoring system *EURASIP J. Wirel. Commun. Netw.* **2018** 298
[52] Islam S M S *et al* 2019 Validation and acceptability of a cuffless wrist-worn wearable blood pressure monitoring device among users and health care professionals: mixed methods study *JMIR Mhealth Uhealth* **7** e14706
[53] Golbus J R *et al* 2021 Wearable device signals and home blood pressure data across age, sex, race, ethnicity, and clinical phenotypes in the Michigan Predictive Activity & Clinical Trajectories in Health (MIPACT) study: a prospective, community-based observational study *Lancet Digit. Health* **3** e707–15
[54] Govil N 2020 Wearable Fitness Trackers as an IoT Application, IoTDunia.com
[55] Mackett R *et al* 2007 Setting children free: children's independent movement in the local environment ed R Mackett, B Brown, Y Gong, K Kitazawa and J Paskins *Setting Children Free: Children's Independent Movement in the Local Environment* (London: Working paper. CASA Working Papers (118). Centre for Advanced Spatial Analysis (UCL))
[56] Saponas T *et al* 2006 Devices that tell on you: the Nike+iPod sport kit (unpublished)
[57] Sushames A *et al* 2016 Validity and reliability of fitbit flex for step count, moderate to vigorous physical activity and activity energy expenditure *PLoS One* **11** e0161224
[58] Foo M 2014 An analysis of the pebble smartwatch as an alternative interface to the smart phoneAustralian National University

[59] Hong S-K 2015 An explorative study on the features of activity trackers as IoT based wearable devices *J. Internet Comput. Serv.* **16** 93–8

[60] Li S *et al* 2020 Computational efficient wearable sensor network health monitoring system for sports athletics using IoT *Aggress. Violent Behav.* 101541

[61] Dawson L and Akinbi A 2021 Challenges and opportunities for wearable IoT forensics: TomTom Spark 3 as a case study . *Forensic Sci. Int. Rep.* **3** 100198

[62] Canhoto A and Arp S 2016 Exploring the factors that support adoption and sustained use of health and fitness wearables *J. Market. Manag.* **33** 1–29

[63] Zhou W and Piramuthu S 2014 Security/privacy of wearable fitness tracking IoT devices *2014 9th Iberian Conf. on Information Systems and Technologies (CISTI)*

[64] Kang S, Kim S and Kim J 2020 Forensic analysis for IoT fitness trackers and its application *Peer Peer Netw. Appl.* **13** 564–73

[65] Kang Y-J, Yin L and Choi D 2016 Smart jewelry system for health management based on IoT *J. Korea Inst. Inform. Commun. Eng.* **20** 1494–502

[66] Alwis L S and Vones K 2018 *Smart Jewellery: The Future of Health Monitoring. U!REKA* (Frankfurt: Urban Research and Education Knowledge Alliance)

[67] Godfrey A *et al* 2018 From A to Z: wearable technology explained *Maturitas* **113** P40–7

[68] Casson A J, Vazquez Galvez A and Jarchi D 2016 Gyroscope vs. accelerometer measurements of motion from wrist PPG during physical exercise *ICT Express* **2** 175–9

[69] Lynch B A *et al* 2019 Accuracy of accelerometers for measuring physical activity and levels of sedentary behavior in children: a systematic review *J. Prim. Care Commun. Health* **10** 1–8

[70] Solà J *et al* 2006 SpO2 sensor embedded in a finger ring: design and implementation *Conf. proceedings: ... Annual Int. Conf. of the IEEE Engineering in Medicine and Biology Society. IEEE Engineering in Medicine and Biology Society. Conf., 2006.* vol 1 4295–8

[71] Kamišalić A A-O *et al* Sensors and functionalities of non-invasive wrist-wearable devices: a review *Sensors (Basel)* **18** 1714

[72] Khan R 2019 A research and chronicle on Internet of Things and digital jewellery *Int. J. Innov. Eng. Manage. Res.* **8** 74–85

[73] Sogi N *et al* 2018 SMARISA: a Raspberry Pi based smart ring for women safety using IoT *2018 International Conference on Inventive Research in Computing Applications (ICIRCA) (Coimbatore)* 451–4

[74] Fernández-Caramés T M and Fraga-Lamas P 2018 Towards the internet of smart clothing: a review on IoT wearables and garments for creating intelligent connected e-textiles *Electronics* **7** 405

[75] Klaib A *et al* 2019 IoT smart home using eye tracking and voice interfaces for elderly and special needs people *J. Commun.* **14** 614–21

[76] Piekenbrock M 2019 Smart jewelry: appearance-changing necklaces and emotions *Thesis* Aachen RWTH Aachen University

[77] Vernekar S, Vijayasenan D and Ranjan R 2016 A novel for robust detection of heart beats in multimodal data using neural networks and boosted trees *2016 Computing in Cardiology Conference (CinC) (Vancouver)* 1137–40

[78] Jeong D and Kim S-J 2008 Development of a technique for cancelling motion artifact in ambulatory ECG monitoring system *Convergence Information Technology, Int. Conf. on* vol **1** 954–61

[79] Nawal M and Purohit G N 2014 ECG based human authentication: a review *Int. J. Emerg. Eng. Res. Technol.* **2** 178–85

[80] Banaee H, Ahmed Mu Fau-Loutfi A and Loutfi A 2013 Data mining for wearable sensors in health monitoring systems: a review of recent trends and challenges *Sensors (Basel)* **13** 17472–500

[81] Oresko J J *et al* 2010 A wearable smartphone-based platform for real-time cardiovascular disease detection via electrocardiogram processing *IEEE Trans. Inf. Technol. Biomed.* **14** 734–40

[82] Ha K, Kim Y, Jung J and Lee J *et al* 2008 Experimental evaluations of wearable ECG monitor *Annu. Int. Conf. IEEE Eng. Med. Biol. Soc.* **2008** 791–4

[83] Serhani M A-O *et al* ECG monitoring systems: review, architecture, processes, and key challenges *Sensors (Basel)* **20** 1796

[84] Prawiro E A P J and Lin Y-H 2018 Step estimator based on a wearable ECG monitor *Mob. Inf. Syst.* **2018** 8240687

[85] Ungurean I and Brezulianu A 2017 An Internet of Things framework for remote monitoring of the healthcare parameters *Adv. Electr. Comput. Eng.* **17** 11–6

[86] Ortiz K *et al* 2018 IoT: electrocardiogram (ECG) monitoring system *Indones. J. Electr. Eng. Comput. Sci.* **10** 480–9

[87] Prawiro E A P J and Lin Y-H 2017 ECG-based gait signal delineation as step counter estimator using EEMD: preliminary results *Int. J. Electr. Electron. Data Commun.* **5** 1–4

[88] Constant N *et al* 2015 Pulse-glasses: an unobtrusive, wearable HR monitor with Internet-of-Things functionality *2015 IEEE 12th Int. Conf. on Wearable and Implantable Body Sensor Networks (BSN) (Cambridge, MA)* 1–5

[89] Jung J and Kim D *et al* 2010 Wireless network of collaborative physiological signal devices in a U-healthcare system *Advanced Computer Science and Information Technology. AST 2010 Communications in Computer and Information Science* vol 74 (Cham: Springer) pp 76–88

[90] Lv W and Guo J 2021 Real-time ECG signal acquisition and monitoring for sports competition process oriented to the Internet of Things *Measurement* **169** 108359

[91] Yang Z *et al* 2016 An IoT-cloud based wearable ECG monitoring system for smart healthcare *J. Med. Syst.* **40** 286

IOP Publishing

Internet of Things in Biomedical Sciences
Challenges and applications
Varun Bajaj and Irshad Ahmad Ansari

Chapter 6

Integration of IoT and chatbot for spreading awareness on cancer using Engati

Nikhil Kumar Parida, Roopa Golchha, Apoorv Joshi, Uday Pratap Singh and Mridu Sahu

In this current era, human–machine interactions are growing exponentially, and this can be experienced in our daily lives where artificial intelligence (AI)-enabled systems help to organize and accommodate daily demands and queries. One such entity is a chatbot, software specially designed to carry out conversations with humans. These conversations can be text-based or speech-based. Although the concept of chatbots came around in the late 20th century with the first chatbot called ELIZA, these chatbots have become mainstream today with the emergence of AI, intelligent Internet of Things (IoT) devices, and machine learning (ML). With the integration of IoT-enabled devices with chatbots with ML, we can quickly reduce the number of cancer deaths worldwide. Many chatbots are currently being deployed on various platforms, such as websites and social media platforms that are helping users to accomplish basic tasks. Cancer can be a fatal disease affecting people directly and indirectly. In this chapter, a chatbot named Canci is created using Engati, a no-code chatbot platform. This initiative aims to benefit those who are impacted by providing them with awareness about cancer.

6.1 Introduction

Cancer is a term that refers to a class of diseases that can affect any area of the human body and in which body cells grow out of control, leading to the formation of tumors that are harmful to the body [1]. According to WHO predictions, approximately 10 million people will die worldwide in 2020 [2]. On the other hand, these statistics can be changed if we take care of ourselves, take precautions, and catch it early enough.

So, it is crucial to promote public knowledge about this illness [3, 4]. For this, we deploy an automated question–answer system, such as a chatbot. We designed a

doi:10.1088/978-0-7503-5311-3ch6

cancer-based question answering system, a chatbot that uses a no-code platform, Engati. In the proposed chatbot, the system analyses an expected type of question and then searches the predefined database for all possible responses. The questions used as a database in this paper are: organs affected, surgery, chemotherapy, stage of diseases, and patient fitness condition [5, 6]. AI chatbots are software that uses natural language processing (NLP) to replicate human-like conversations. Organizations are increasingly turning to AI chatbots to automate business activities like customer support, sales, and human resources [7].

6.1.1 Chatbot in IoT

IoT is a rapidly expanding network of smart technologies that have revolutionized our lives by combining devices and automating regular operations through internet connectivity. In various application domains, IoT devices provide seamless connectivity and diversity. IoT has gained massive importance in the last few decades because it allows things to communicate with each other at a minimal cost. Today, IoT is used in almost every industry, like healthcare, education, entertainment, etc. The goal of such IoT systems, along with contributing to making smart environments, is to improve the value and productivity of human life by addressing issues related to practical living conditions. To connect physical objects with computer and networking capabilities for applications and services across various use cases, the internet has played a crucial role as a worldwide backbone.

The development of platforms and frameworks that can synchronize chatbot apps within IoT platforms and frameworks is largely driven by this simplicity of integration. IoT cloud solutions already in existence address data source and transmission constraints. However, a significant issue with current IoT systems is providing the user with information about the different associated devices (sensors, objects, etc) in a straightforward manner that is easy to comprehend. This necessitates context, which is attained by empowering chatbots to identify the real purpose of user inquiries and gather and process data from their surroundings. Additionally, chatbots may be readily programmed to retrieve information in real-time from a vast worldwide network of information thanks to the internet, which might enhance the context. Practically speaking, chatbots make it easier to consume information by switching from several screens, heavy data, and complex images to simple conversational interfaces that may provide highly contextualized, understandable information while interacting with the chat app itself. The entire potential of the IoT may be realized by reaching this high degree of abstraction, which can provide actionable intelligence with domain and user knowledge.

6.1.2 Advantages of AI-chatbot

- Trainable: AI-powered chatbots can be trained to learn and grow over time, and they respond to input without complaint or delay. Every communication they have with their users improves their ability to perform tasks as they become smarter, more efficient, and more productive.

- Dependable: AI-powered chatbots are dependable because they never sleep. They hardly miss an incoming message and work around the clock. Talking to everyone in every time zone, in every language, and everyone who interacts with them.
- Scalable: In terms of the number of dialogues and users, an AI-powered bot is scalable, i.e. the performance of a chatbot does not depend upon the number of users. It may converse with a single individual as well as thousands and delivers the same performance as well as efficiency.
- On-brand: An AI-powered chatbot never gets irritable, never arrives at work frustrated, and always follows your brand's norms and tone. It will speak in the same tone as your brand, and it will become your brand's voice [7].

6.2 Literature survey

Today our dependency on technology is on the rise and it will increase with the development of technologies like the one we are considering in this paper, i.e. the chatbot. Of course, we cannot limit ourselves to any chatbot but it will surely make it much simpler for a novice to get a piece of basic information about the subject. Here are different chatbots used by many people all around the world.

i. Disha: Disha is the chatbot system developed by IRCTC. It is available in both Hindi and English language, where passengers can ask any query related to the schedule of the train, PNR Enquiry, Seat availability and other services offered by the Indian Railways, thereby facilitating ease of conversation for users [8].
ii. Fandango: This chatbot is mostly used in movie ticket booking, users can also use this chatbot to find what is showing in cinemas which saves a lot of time when someone is making a last-minute plan for any show [9].
iii. IPal: IPal was launched by ICICI bank in 2017, for queries related to the banking services of their customers. According to ICICI bank, IPal addressed six million queries in a span of eight months [10].
iv. Replica: Need a friend, here is a chatbot for you. It is an impressive piece of technology that can mimic human emotion and provide users with personal comfort. Replica's main aim is to give users a safe space in the digital world [11].

Chatbots are not limited to any particular service; they are widely used in different sectors with different personalization. Just as chatbots have many advantages, they have a few disadvantages too. Some features of the chatbot are liked by many users, some are not, so we categorize these features on the basis of the advantages and disadvantages of the chatbots [12].

Similarly, the development of IoT cannot be neglected and many scientists have worked with IoT for the betterment of cancer monitoring and cure. The rising prevalence of cancer sickness is becoming a burden on various communities. This is large because of a lack of appropriate medical infrastructure and high medication prices. The scenario is significantly worse for people with complex cancers. Which need ongoing observation in order to improve evaluations and therapy decisions.

Table 6.1. List of sensors and their respective roles. Reproduced with permission from [13]. Copyright © 2020 ACM.

Sensor	Role of sensor
Enzymatic sensor	Blood glucose level
Immunosensor	Protein level and DNA template strand
Nano sensor	Detection of leukemia
Temperature sensor	Detect temperature of patient
Pulse sensor	Detection of leukemia

Furthermore, prompt cancer detection and therapy can resolve several cancer difficulties The developments in embedded systems, wireless networking, and remote data collection will help with cancer therapy and greatly help in monitoring the situation. This project demonstrated a three-layer design for cancer detection systems where they developed a lightweight watch-like device to monitor a patient's pulse, heartbeat, temperature etc, and that data is directly sent to the monitor so that the data can be monitored by the doctor or concerned party. The set of sensors used in the device is also written below in table 6.1 [13].

6.2.1 Motivation

The chatbots are available 24 × 7, so a person can ask any question, at any time and receive a quick response. One can ask any simple question that is generally overlooked by most people while utilizing the services which are answered by the chatbot in a very simple manner. Chatbots are extremely rapid, with the ability to respond to most queries by accessing a database through which they can quickly access and respond to any user [14]. It is possible that sometimes it may take a bit longer to reply due to server load, but generally, the conversation between a user and a chatbot is incredibly smooth, and people feel very comfortable conversing with them. Users may simply file a complaint, and if they have a problem with a service, the chatbot will provide a remedy in a very simple manner [15]. The main benefit of chatbots (as inferred from figure 6.1) is that it offers multi-platform support. It can be used for serving different purposes like in the social media and entertainment industry.

Various platforms and channels where chatbots can be deployed are Telegram, Twitter, different websites, Facebook, etc.

6.2.2 Industries benefitting from chatbots

i. Insurance: Insurance is a sector where chatbots respond to user queries like term plan maturity date related to personal insurance and provide personalized advice. Some chatbots used in the insurance sector are A-ware, Myra, Boing, Mili etc [16].

ii. E-commerce and retail: Here, we use chatbots for different purposes like tracking the products delivery date availability of any products and many

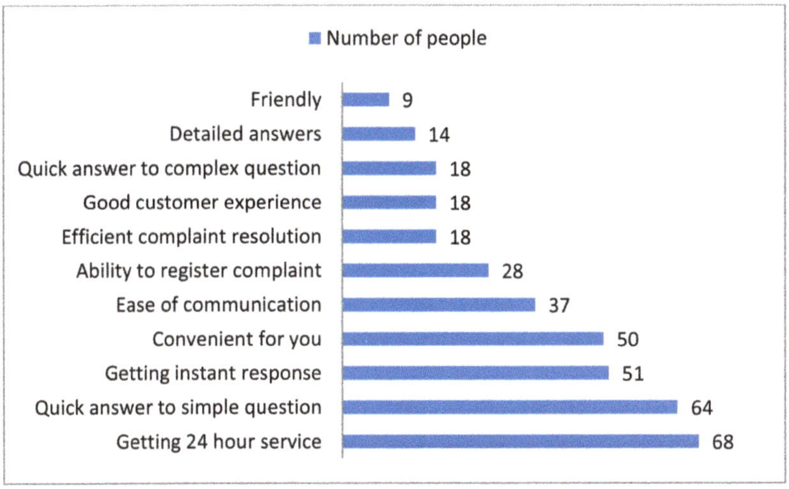

Figure 6.1. Benefits of a chatbot.

more related to the e-Commerce market. Some chatbots used in e-Commerce and retail sectors are Slackbot, Shopbot, etc [17].

iii. Logistics: In logistics, chatbots help to track the shipment, delivery related queries of any product and services. Some chatbots used in logistics are Botcare, UPS etc [18].

iv. Medical field: In the medical industry, we mostly need details like blood bank availability, ambulance services, medical treatment symptoms and many more, so these chatbots help customers by providing relevant information. Some chatbots used in this medical field are Florence, Giant etc [19].

v. Healthcare: In healthcare, we generally maintain and improve the health of any individual by various diagnosis treatments, symptoms analysis, cure of injury, illness or any other mental or fitness injury. Thus, we can develop chatbots for any disease by considering the basic frequently asked questions about their symptoms, prevention and cure and making it accessible for all so that they can get the basic idea about the disease and track their activity accordingly [20].

Considering the scenario of COVID-19, we can make a chatbot for awareness. It can contain all the basic queries like the data related to the number of people infected, how many are locally infected, symptoms of the diseases, precautionary measures, myths, etc these can be answered by a chatbot and also explain in terms of real-time statistics so data given by the bot is up to the mark with less error in it.

6.3 Methodology

Before designing any chatbot, the following are some courses of action that can be considered to provide the customer with the best experience:

- The chatbot should be accessible in the user's chosen language.
- Presenting it in layperson's terms and with the most engaging and simple user interface possible.
- Adding all possible multimedia services that make the experience more human.
- Instead of using the same old canned responses, uses reply templates.
- Using Live Chat in conjunction with automation.
- Not allowing customers to repeat themselves.
- Providing valuable analytics and insights is a priority.
- Routing conversation intelligently.
- Integration with customer relationship management.

In order to continue with these behaviors, we must design our system in the most efficient and effective manner possible. Let's take a glance at the key logic behind the backend's design which is depicted in figure 6.2. NLP provides the system with the capability for communication with users or any other machine using human natural languages. Natural language understanding (NLU) and natural language generating (NLG) are two aspects of NLP [14].

The NLU system examines the various elements of language. The NLG system, on the other hand, converts natural language input into a meaningful representation. The Engati platform comes with its own unique NLU engine that is pre-installed. This allows chatbots produced on this platform to answer user queries more accurately, yet it necessitates significant effort to keep the platform simple to construct and train chatbots. As a result, data and AI are required to effectively train a chatbot [21].

AI enables a chatbot to learn from the questions and information it receives. Because training a chatbot is an evolving process, the data must be saved in order for the chatbot to continue learning, which is also known as self-learning. Three

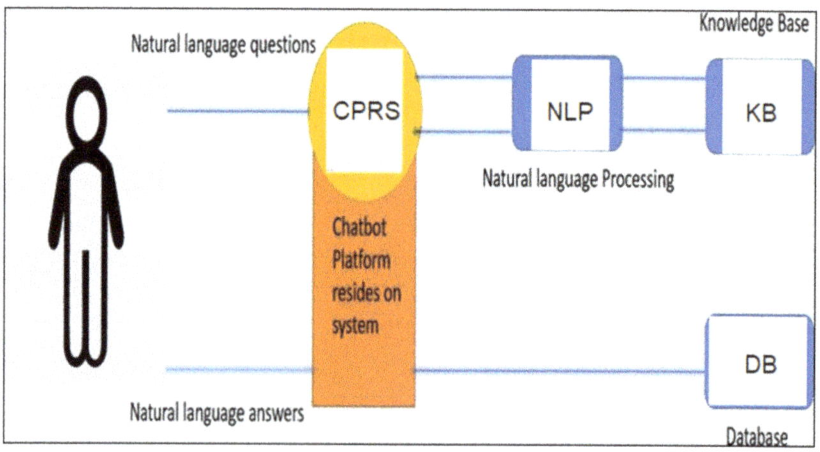

Figure 6.2. Working of the chatbot.

approaches are employed to understand natural language: parsing, semantic interpretation, and knowledge-based structures.

6.3.1 Core components of a chatbot

1. FAQs: Frequently asked questions (FAQs) are the standard queries relevant to a product or a service. These specify how bots can interact with humans. The number of alternatives we offer to the user is determined by how many trained responses matched the query and the distribution pattern of their scores. The system also selects the best well-formed statement/phrase from the collection of possibilities and presents it as the alternative.
2. Intent: It specifies the user's preferences or goals in the conversational flow. We can understand the motive behind a specific user input using intents.
3. Entity: Entities are crucial in recognizing and extracting precise and relevant data from natural language input. Entities are the key focused values extracted from the user query and they serve as a baseline for generating the user query's response.
4. Stopwords: Stopwords are phrases that are excluded from matching a query in NLP. Stopwords are frequently used terms like 'the,' 'and,' 'a,' and others that add little to text comprehension, therefore removing them minimizes noise and improves accuracy. Custom Stopwords can also be introduced to the NLP engine's training and improve its effectiveness.
5. Synonyms: Synonyms are words that have the same meaning or function. Synonyms are assigned the same value when matching a FAQ for a legitimate and improved response. It could also be used in cases involving common misspellings, abbreviations, etc.
6. Paths: Paths are the actions that a bot takes to make a conversation more interesting and dynamic. It refers to the several types of flows that a bot can generate.

6.3.2 Basic model of chatbot

The chatbot basically consists of a Core and Interface. Figure 6.3 illustrates the human-to-machine model of conversation. The Core is a database designed in RDBMS (Relational Database Management System). The Interface is used for accessing the core. The NLP pipeline is a sequence of steps that occur in perfect synchronization to process the query and words and deliver the best response. Each phase is aimed at achieving a certain goal, and the outcomes are then aggregated and reconciled to decide the chatbot's optimal response. RDBMS is a program set that is employed to define, manage, and process a database. It covers the knowledge storage and pattern-matching process. At a particular instance of time, a chatbot handles multiple sessions thus it needs to differentiate each conversation session and this is done efficiently using RDBMS [22].

The pattern template utilizes RDBMS to maintain the chatbot's main knowledge, allowing it to be accessed via Structured Query Language (SQL). Many built-in functions or procedures are available in the RDBMS, and these can be turned into

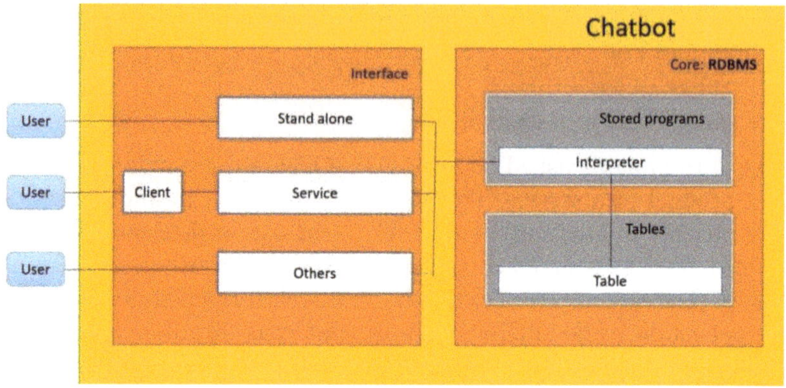

Figure 6.3. Human-to-machine conversation modeling.

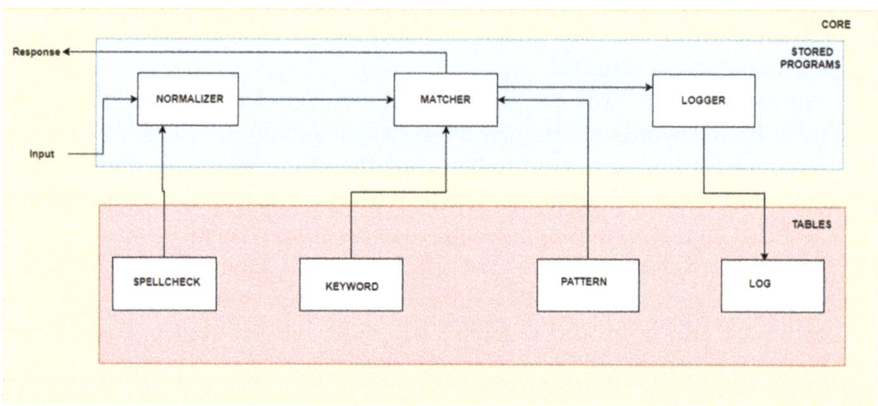

Figure 6.4. Chatbot core system.

user-defined stored programs [23]. The interface could be a stand-alone application or any service that supports other client programs to connect with the user, and it can also be expanded as needed. The boundaries of a chatbot are predefined. As for generating a better response, all user inputs must be freed from misspellings, and punctuation, so to accomplish this, a list of misspelled words and the corrections are stored in the tables of the database. In figure 6.4, the core systems and the conversion process in a chatbot are depicted.

For pattern-matching purposes, the stored program includes stored processes and functions. It contains a normalizer, matcher and logger.

- Normalizer: It corrects spellings and eliminates punctuation from user input and makes the desired changes to get the core components.
- Matcher: It is the main function that finds appropriate templates based on keywords and patterns.
- Logger: It is a procedure that stores the user's input and response to a query as a conversation history.

6.3.3 Integrating with APIs

Chatbots benefit immensely from integrations, and improving integration means enhancing chatbots. An integration, in the most general sense, is the collection of channels over which a chatbot can be deployed [24]. Here are a few examples of typical use cases:

- Data access: Integrations allow a chatbot to get information from a number of sources and use it to deliver more generalized responses.
- Transaction completion: Integrations allow a chatbot to complete a transaction that the user is interested in.
- Chatbots have to give fast responses so we use lightweight AI-enabled techniques to design the response system.

6.3.3.1 Representational State Transfer (REST)

This is a software architectural style that is intended to assist in the design and development of the World Wide Web framework. Performance, scalability, simplicity, visibility, portability, and dependability are some features of REST [25]. This is implemented by following REST principles such as client–server design, statelessness, cacheability, layered systems, code-on-demand support, and a uniform interface (figure 6.5).

To facilitate large-scale adoption, the REST architectural style is developed for network-based applications for personal devices. As a result, the connection between the user agent (client) and the origin server must be as lightweight as possible. This is accomplished by building a layer of abstraction on the server and hiding the underlying implementation details (file server, database, etc).

6.3.3.2 JavaScript Object Notation (JSON)

It is the most often used lightweight and web-based data transfer format on the internet. Engati provides the ability to connect to any system via REST APIs that employ JSON [26]. Using the JSON API plugin, we can now retrieve interactive

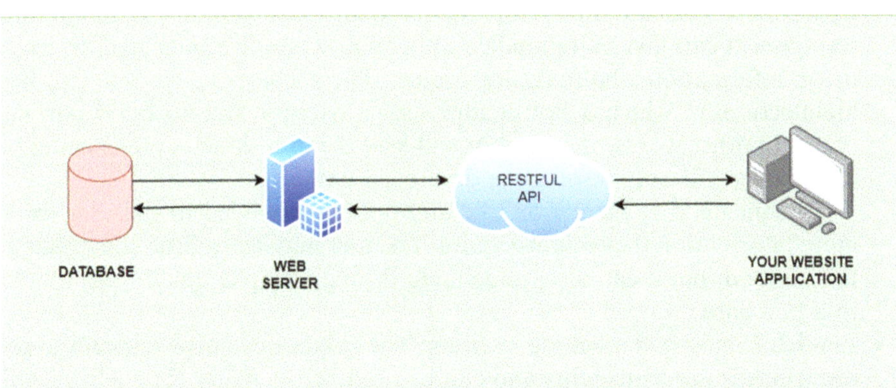

Figure 6.5. Simple representation of working of REST.

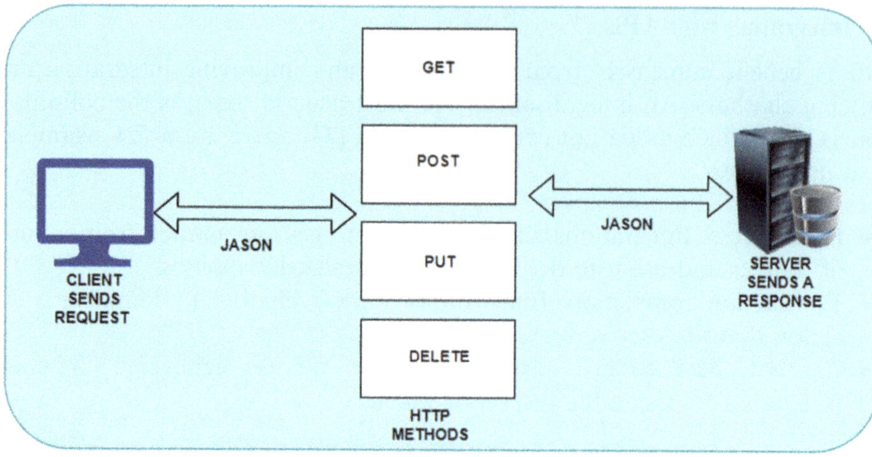

Figure 6.6. Working architecture of JSON API.

answers from our backend service or other cloud apps [27] (figure 6.6). Engati allows calling REST APIs using the following methods:

- GET: This technique is used to read data from a database.
- POST: This is a mechanism for updating data.
- PUT: This is a mechanism for writing or updating data.
- DELETE: This is a mechanism for deleting the entire collection.

Based on our criteria, we can make an API call using the most appropriate method. Engati JSON API node includes numerous options and templates that we can quickly adjust without writing a single line of code to finish our connection.

6.3.4 Chatbot maturity process

- **Level 1:** Rule-based interaction: The chatbot functions as a traditional notification assistant and can answer questions with a pre-programmed response. It can give us reminders about subjects we've indicated an interest in or information about future events. These chatbots have a tree-based architecture, in which a bot creator uses a decision tree to build particular paths. In other words, the chatbot will lead the user down a pre-existing path where they will only resolve the developed pathways.

  This means that there won't be any options provided to the user for any more information they might require. The user may feel a little constrained by this method, but it can also guide them through simple, quick steps that lead to a purchase.
- **Level 2:** Configured machine learning: The chatbot can now respond to some unexpected user statements and can be used across many channels, allowing for a multi-channel experience. At this level, the chatbot offers multi-language support. Chatbot uses state machine interactions with mood

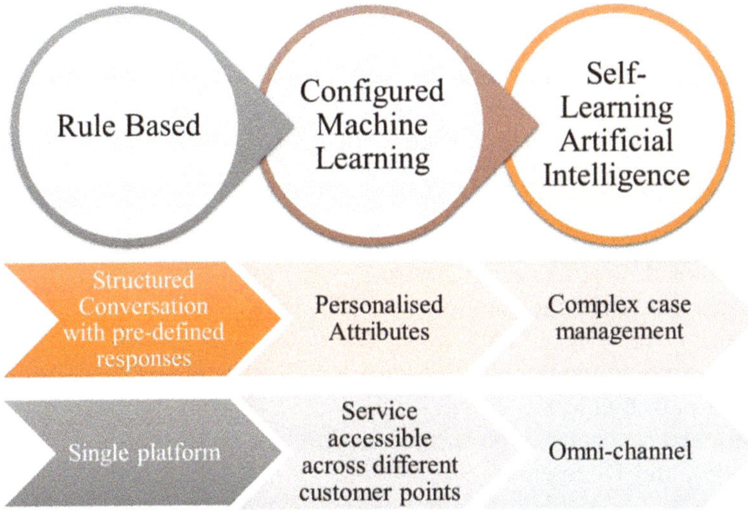

Figure 6.7. Chatbot maturity process.

detection techniques and has line-based intelligence with support from the training of NLP models.

Here the bot can initiate conversation, and API transactions, and have event listening and producing capabilities. The bot can also respond to the API intelligent queries.

- **Level 3:** Self-learning AI: Finally, the chatbot begins to understand the problem. It remembers our preferences and delivers customized and contextual recommendations. Figure 6.7 describes the various levels in the chatbot maturity process and various interactions, intelligence and integrations at each level. From a technical standpoint, a chatbot just represents the natural progression of a query–answer system that makes use of NLP. Answering questions in natural language is one of the most prevalent uses of NLP in end-use applications across several industries.

AI chatbots are unique because, after some initial training by the bot designer, they will learn how to respond to a user's question. Following their training, they are able to respond with information that is relevant to the user's inquiries. Users can receive correct answers from this type of chatbot even if their questions are phrased differently. It can provide users with a better experience the more it learns and is trained [28].

6.3.5 Chatbot flow in Engati

Without writing any code, the Engati platform enables us to design, train, and deploy a chatbot across numerous channels in minutes. It has the ability to be deployed in real time, which saves a lot of time while testing apps and features.

We can link our bot to any channel and quickly customize it, thanks to its omni-channel concept. It's simple to use, comprehensive and has a short learning curve. It gives us a lot of flexibility for interacting with the user. A bot's pre-configured ability to manage small talk is fantastic, as it keeps the conversation flowing. The platform's extensive metrics like user engagement and retention are impressive and eliminate the need for third-party tools like Bot Analytics.

To begin, plan beforehand and create a rough flow map of the conversation. After that, use Engati no-code visual flow builder to replicate it. The best idea while creating chatbot flow is to design separate paths for different scenarios. This will make it easier to understand the flow and edit it in the future. These paths can be connected using the Trigger Path node. Once done making the flow, proceed to polish the messages in the nodes and to test how the bot makes flow, test individual paths using a path builder.

In Engati, the chatbot can be trained in different ways that is with the help of FAQs, entities, and Docusense.

Engati allows us to deploy the chatbot we created to several channels. Most of those channels are shown below. We can collect the IoT device data and send it to the website where the chatbot is deployed. This will make it even easier to monitor the patient (figure 6.8).

With Engati's DocuSense technology, we don't need to upload these FAQs manually, and can automate the training process by just uploading the documents. The chatbot will use cognitive search to parse through the documents, it will pull answers directly from the documents and deliver them to our customers. The data which is used to train the chatbot is uploaded in tabular format. These are structured documents and this tabular data contains the information about entities and is uploaded in the tabular input section. The supported file formats are .xls, .xlsx and . csv for the dataset and .csv file upload mechanism to instantly train the chatbots with multiple FAQs. Figure 6.9 describes the flow diagram of the various paths and intents in the proposed chatbot.

In order to create a chatbot on this no-code platform we need to first create an account on Engati and simply follow the procedures mentioned there. First, it is necessary to know what are the core components and how to utilize them. After signing up there is an option named create bot, after clicking on it several templates will appear on screen; the user can use any of these present templates as their base

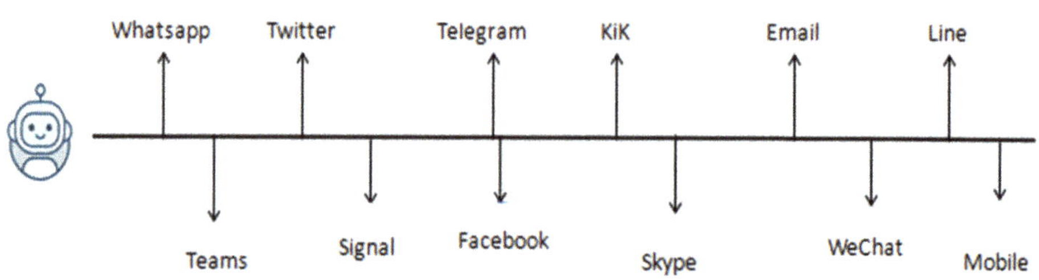

Figure 6.8. Chatbot deployment channels of Engati.

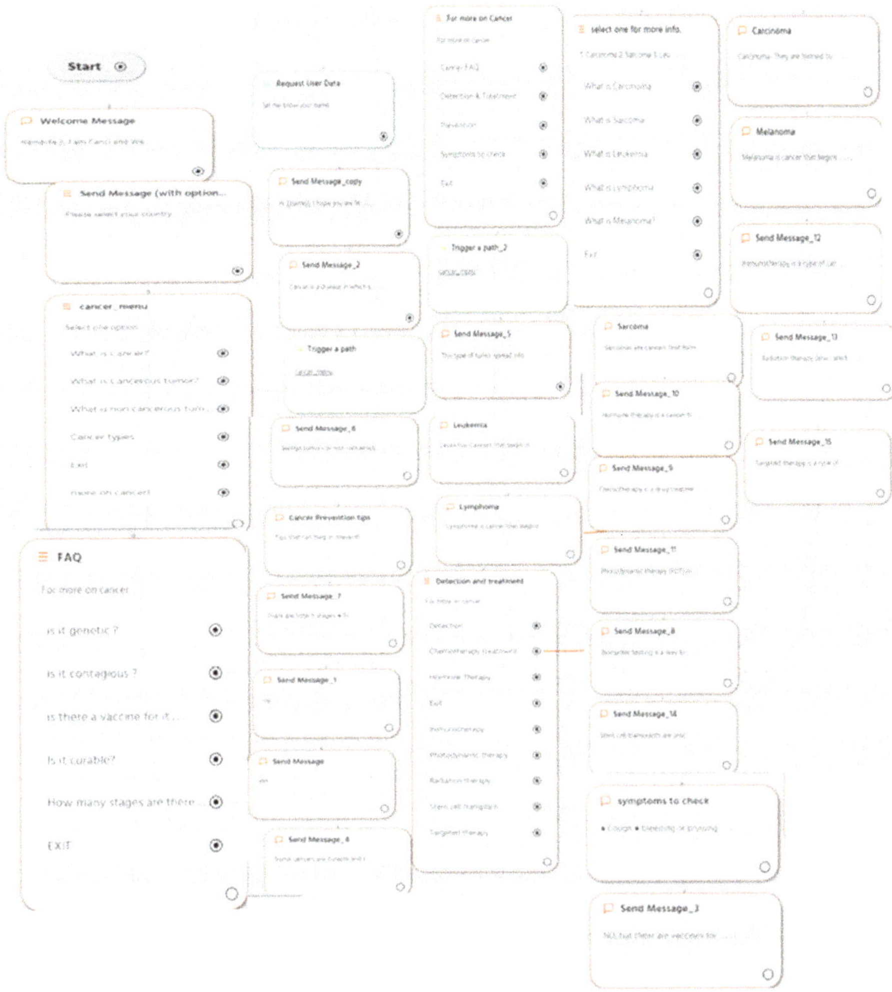

Figure 6.9. Flow diagram of the Engati chatbot.

and modify them. Users can create their own bots from scratch by clicking on the blank template. Users need to add new blocks (as shown in figure 6.9) and messages/questions should be written in those blocks and a response block created (which collect the input from the user) for the user to reply. It is important to maintain the correct flow so it is important to connect them appropriately. In the output, the user can add web links, images, audio files, video files etc. This will create a basic chatbot. Then they use the train option to train the chatbot and it is ready to deploy. While some deployment channels are free, some channels need money for deployment. In order to make a more advanced chatbot in Engati, it is required to add intents, entities and FAQs, and after training them they can pretty much answer every question related to them.

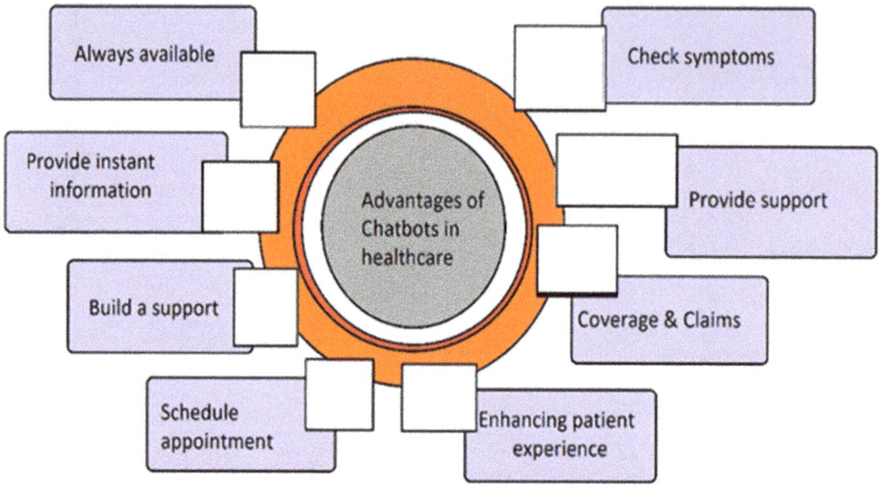

Figure 6.10. Chatbot usage in the medical field.

6.4 Case study

The healthcare business, in particular, has been severely impacted by the pandemic in 2019. However, AI's engagement has aided the industry in surviving the storm. The various AI applications bring patients' lives back from the edge, improve diagnosis and therapy, and assist healthcare providers in making quick judgments. Now, here we will see some of the chatbots that are enhancing the services of the healthcare sector. Firstly, we will see about COVIDAsha and secondly Cancer Dost.

Chatbots have become increasingly crucial in the fight against COVID in past years. Engati came up with a chatbot named 'Fight against COVID chatbot'. It gives accurate disease-related information. They give guidance on treatment at home so that the patient doesn't have to leave the house to see a doctor regarding their disease, and in serious cases, they refer the patient to a doctor with all of the patient's information so that the doctor can save time by getting all of the patient's information, making the entire process contactless and eventually preventing the spread. Finally, they provide access to necessary services such as medicine, oxygen cylinders, and ambulances. Figure 6.10 shows the active participation of chatbots in the medical field.

6.4.1 COVIDAsha

This was launched on 4 May 2021, with the capability of providing people with oxygen cylinders, medicines, and ambulance services, as well as guiding vendors in supplying these vital medical supplies to those in need. It connects registered vendors with people looking for medical-related supplies. It is available in seven languages which are English, Hindi, Gujarati, Kannada, Bengali, Telugu and Tamil. Professionals from top companies collaborated to develop this chatbot, which combines technology and data for assistance. The bot checks in with suppliers every few hours to see if they want to be shown as having stock or if they want their listing removed from the database. COVIDAsha makes use of the COVID-19 resources database created by RC Medicrew and the volunteer network [32].

Recently, one more functionality is added that is now providing information on the availability of vaccines as well. The chatbot saves your selected language and city to provide you with a real-time list of all centers where vaccine shots are available. It filters the results by age, dose, vaccination type, and district. When a previously unavailable slot becomes available, the page refreshes and sends notifications.

6.4.2 Hospido

During the pandemic, Hospido, India's first holistic cancer care platform, has developed a chatbot via which cancer patients may get the best treatment advice from India's top cancer professionals without having to visit hospitals.

Cancer Dost is an AI-enabled chatbot developed by the company that helps patients to learn more about their cancer and treatment solutions for free. The chatbot can help patients from all over the country and it is bilingual in Hindi and English. Through teleconsulting and in-person consultations, it also connects patients with renowned oncologists from the country's best hospitals. It also offers cancer patients home care, diagnostic tests, nutrition planning, and counseling support to help them along their entire journey of battling cancer.

It is a chatbot with a simple user interface that asks four key questions: organ affected, treatment (none, surgery, chemotherapy, or radiation), illness stage, and patient fitness.

The user input is then obtained using an online chatbot interface and transferred to a RESTful API-based application that is hosted on the company's server. The server employs a customized proprietary recommendation algorithm to search the exclusive knowledge repository built by top oncologists. The AI-driven system presents the most pertinent details regarding the patient's condition when a match is made. The user is then provided with this knowledge via the same chatbot to assist them in making knowledgeable treatment selections after consulting with their doctor. This chatbot would undoubtedly alleviate cancer patient's challenges in traveling to hospitals for their daily check-ups [33].

6.5 Results and discussion

A chatbot named Canci was created using the no-code Engati platform. Canci can answer questions specifically related to cancer and aids the user by providing different information related to cancer. The core components like intents, entities, paths and FAQs are perfectly coordinated to generate the best possible response as desired by the users. Canci has been designed to give information about all types of cancers, symptoms, diet plans, prevention tips, treatment details, and side effects of clinical treatments and can also provide the details of governmental and non-governmental institutions for further help to users. Several self-generated images of the Canci bot, describing the conversation flow are shown in figures 6.11–6.14.

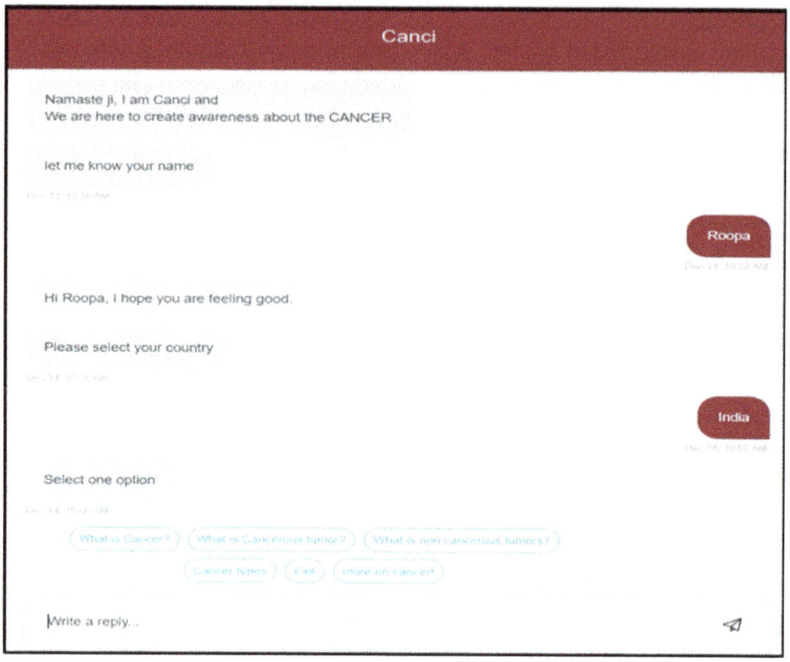

Figure 6.11. Engati chatbot asking basic details.

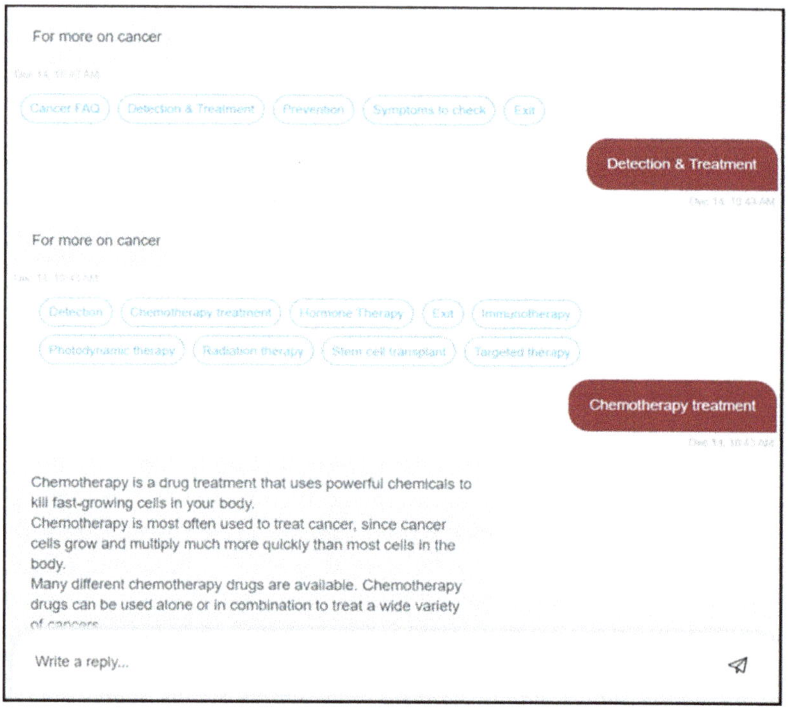

Figure 6.12. Engati chatbot providing relevant options to select from.

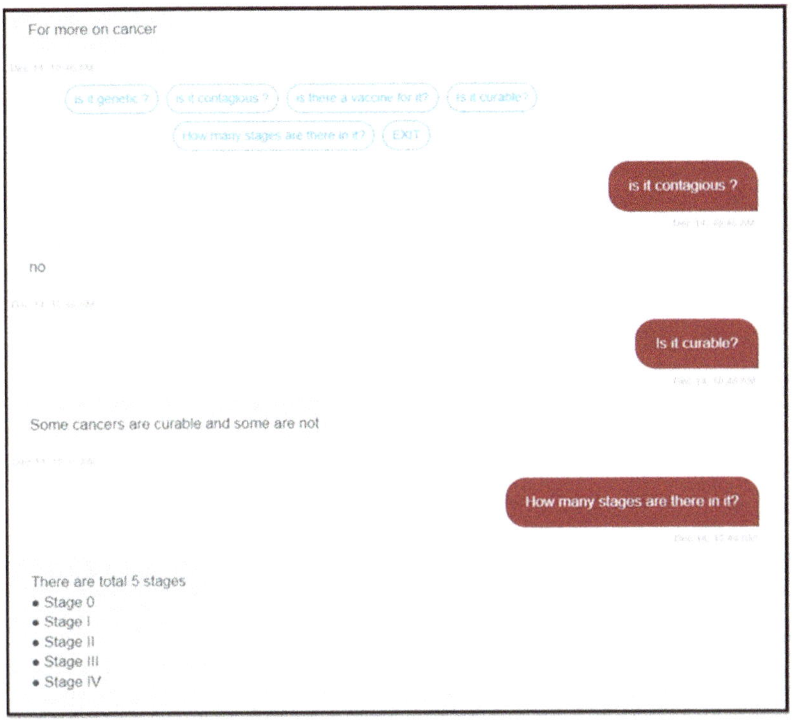

Figure 6.13. Engati chatbot answering cancer-related queries I.

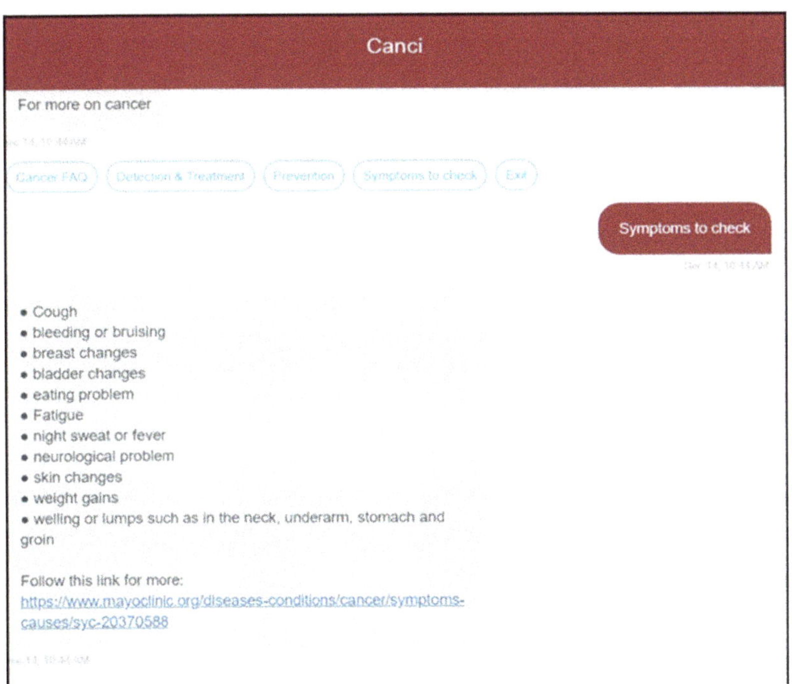

Figure 6.14. Engati chatbot answering cancer-related queries II.

6.6 Conclusion and future work

Chatbots are changing the face of business with the help of AI. They provide a wide range of applications in medical, hospitality, and various e-commerce platforms by reaching out to many audiences and providing speedy, quick, and round-the-clock responses. Although the dynamic nature of IoT has its share of challenges, it is poised to become integral to daily activities in the future. For this, IoT can be integrated with chatbots for their efficient working. Considering our chatbot model Canci, on Engati, we can say that this chatbot is efficient and helpful not only to cancer patients but also to their families. It will help them to have a basic idea about the disease and resolve some of their basic queries about the same, meanwhile creating awareness about this disease with the hope of saving lives in the future. Canci uses a model of NLP and AI to answer user queries efficiently. A lot can be added to this as the core technologies and concepts used behind chatbots are ever-evolving. We plan to provide information on NGOs and government organizations working in cancer research to benefit as many people as possible.

References

[1] Weinberg R A 1996 How cancer arises *Sci. Am.* **275** 62–70

[2] World Health Organization 2020 Report on cancer: setting priorities, investing wisely and providing care for all. *WHO Report* Available: http://apps.who.int/bookorders

[3] Hidalgo-Paniagua A, Millan-Alcaide A, Bandera J P and Bandera A 2019 Integration of the Alexa assistant as a voice interface for robotics platforms *Iberian Robotics Conf. (November 2019)* (Cham: Springer) pp 575–86

[4] Carlberg C and Velleuer E 2021 *Cancer Biology: How Science Works* (Berlin: Springer International Publishing)

[5] Amato F, Marrone S, Moscato V, Piantadosi G, Picariello A and Sansone C 2017 Chatbots meet eHealth: automatizing healthcare *Workshop on Artificial Intelligence with Application in Health (Bari, November 14, 2017)* 40–9

[6] Baez M, Casati F, Gaedke M and Dustdar S 2020 Remembering Florian Daniel *IEEE Internet Comput.* **24** 58–9

[7] Patel N and Trivedi S 2020 Leveraging predictive modeling, machine learning personalization, NLP customer support, and AI chatbots to increase customer loyalty *Empir. Quests Manage. Essences* **3** 1–24

[8] Srivastava V, Kishore S and Dhingra D 2021 Technology and the future of customer experience *Crafting Customer Experience Strategy* (Bingley: Emerald) pp 91–116

[9] Ask J A, Facemire M, Hogan A and Conversations H B 2016 The state of chatbots *Forrester. com Report* 20

[10] Kautikwar T 2020 *A study of role of emerging technology in current banking industry* https://vpmthane.org/jbcapp/upload/m6/170.pdf

[11] Ta V, Griffith C, Boatfield C, Wang X, Civitello M, Bader H, DeCero E and Loggarakis A 2020 User experiences of social support from companion chatbots in everyday contexts: thematic analysis *J. Med. Internet Res.* **22** e16235

[12] Zumstein D and Hundertmark S 2017 Chatbots—an interactive technology for personalized communication, transactions and services *IADIS Int. J. WWW/Internet* **15** 96–109

[13] Rehman O, Farrukh Z, Al-Busaidi A, Cha K, Park S and Rahman I 2020 IoT powered cancer observation system *9th Int. Conf. on Smart Media and Applications (September 2020)* 313–8
[14] Brandtzaeg P B and Følstad A 2017 Why people use chatbots *Int. Conf. on Internet Science (November 2017)* (Cham: Springer) pp 377–92
[15] Waghmare C 2019 Business benefits of using chatbots *Introducing Azure Bot Service* (Berkeley, CA: Apress) pp 147–65
[16] Nuruzzaman M and Hussain O K 2020 IntelliBot: a dialogue-based chatbot for the insurance industry *Knowl.-Based Syst.* **196** 105810
[17] Cui L, Huang S, Wei F, Tan C, Duan C and Zhou M 2017 Superagent: a customer service chatbot for e-commerce websites *Proc. of ACL 2017, System Demonstrations (July 2017)* pp 97–102
[18] Park S J, Lee Y P, Jeong W S, Choi Y T and Hong J W 2021 Big data/AI-based smart maritime logistics chatbot service *Proc. of the Korea Information Processing Society Conf.* (Seoul: Korea Information Processing Society) pp 1349–52
[19] Kaur M, Nazir N, Kaur N, Ali S F, Agarwal C, Dubey U, Gupta V, Sarwar A, Rakhra M and Dahiya O 2022 A web-based blood bank system for managing records of donors and receipts *2022 Int. Conf. on Computational Intelligence and Sustainable Engineering Solutions (CISES) (May 2022)* (Piscataway, NJ: IEEE) pp 459–64
[20] Nadarzynski T, Miles O, Cowie A and Ridge D 2019 Acceptability of artificial intelligence (AI)-led chatbot services in healthcare: a mixed-methods study *Digital Health* **5** 2055207619871808
[21] Panda S and Chakravarty R 2022 Adapting intelligent information services in libraries: a case of smart AI chatbots *Libr. Hi Tech News* **39** 12–15
[22] Gao J, Peng B, Li C, Li J, Shayandeh S, Liden L and Shum H Y 2020 Robust conversational AI with grounded text generation preprint arXiv:2009.03457
[23] Setiaji B and Wibowo F W 2016 Chatbot using a knowledge in database: human-to-machine conversation modeling *2016 7th Int. Conf. on Intelligent Systems, Modelling and Simulation (ISMS) (January 2016)* (Piscataway, NJ: IEEE) pp 72–7
[24] Behera R K, Bala P K and Ray A 2021 Cognitive chatbot for personalised contextual customer service: behind the scene and beyond the hype *Inf. Syst. Front.* 1–21
[25] Punjabi S, Sethuram V, Ramachandran V and Ravi S 2019 Chat bot using API: human to machine conversation *2019 Global Conf. for Advancement in Technology (GCAT) (October 2019)* (Piscataway, NJ: IEEE) pp 1–5
[26] Severance C 2012 Discovering javascript object notation *Computer* **45** 6–8
[27] Snodgrass E and Winnie S 2019 API practices and paradigms: exploring the protocological parameters of APIs as key facilitators of sociotechnical forms of exchange *First Monday* **24** 2
[28] Duijst D 2017 Can we improve the user experience of chatbots with personalisation *Master's Thesis* University of Amsterdam
[29] Gardiner A and Smith M A 2021 Conversational AI as an emerging technology *Proc. of the EDSIG Conf.* vol 2473 p 4901
[30] Kar R and Haldar R 2016 Applying chatbots to the internet of things: opportunities and architectural elements preprint arXiv:1611.03799
[31] Top 14 chatbots benefits for companies and customers. (n.d.)., https://research.aimultiple.com/chatbot-benefits/ (accessed 19 December 2022)

[32] A team that has never met each other, builds a chatbot, saves lives—The Hindu (n.d.). https://thehindu.com/sci-tech/technology/a-team-that-has-never-met-each-other-builds-a-chatbot-saves-lives/article35017505.ece (accessed 19 December 2022)

[33] [Startup Bharat] How Hospido is helping cancer patients from Tier II and III cities get treatment in their hom. (n.d.). https://yourstory.com/2020/09/startup-bharat-hospido-cancer-patients-healthtech-covid-19?utm_pageloadtype=scroll (accessed 19 December 2022)

IOP Publishing

Internet of Things in Biomedical Sciences
Challenges and applications
Varun Bajaj and Irshad Ahmad Ansari

Chapter 7

IoT solutions for fighting antimicrobial resistance

Dang Ngoc Tung, Nguyen Cuong and Nguyen Thi Thu Hoai

Antimicrobial resistance (AMR) is a growing problem of medicine which can endanger public health globally. This phenomenon is defined as the unrespondence of pathogens to antimicrobial drugs, resulting in difficulty and even failure in clinical treatment. Apart from disability and death, AMR also leads to longer hospital stays, higher treatment costs and stronger impact on personnel in the care of patients. Today, development of technology particularly information technology, has brought solutions to many challenges that humans face. Internet of Things (IoT), the interconnected network of intelligent devices having the ability to collect data, work in groups, process and exchange data with other devices, systems, or access the cloud, is a new achievement of information technology. It has shown great application potential in industry, business, infrastructure, agriculture, environment, pharmacy, and medicine. In this chapter, we will present IoT as a potential solution for controlling AMR via its ability in improving diagnosis, treatment, and surveillance of AMR. At the same time, how IoT benefits the development of pharmaceutical and AMR research is also discussed.

7.1 Internet of Things (IoT), history and evolution

You may or may not have heard of or understood the phrase Internet of Things (IoT). However, it is today a prevalent concept, the 4.0 industrial revolution is inseparable from people's daily life activities whether or not they have heard of or understood it, and it is rather an important and revolutionary aspect of human activities.

IoT can be described and understood as a connected network between 'things'. These 'things' can consist of any mechanical or electrical device with technologies that help connect and exchange data between these devices and systems over the internet. For example, your doorbell cam can be connected to either your phone or watch or any remote device that you carry through the network, thus you can monitor the doorbell cam, which allows you to answer your door from any remote location as well as be aware of any motion changes and suspicious activity on your doorstep.

This concept of making individual devices able to connect to each other by supplementing in intelligence and sensors was firstly discussed in the early 1980s. One attempt was carried out by a group of students at the Carnegie Melon University. They aimed to create a way to make a Coca-Cola vending machine on the campus report on its contents via a network so that they did not have to check the situation of the machine manually. Unfortunately, this attempt was complicated and the progress was limited.

Later, further similar attempts were conducted by many researchers across the world. However, it was not until 1999 that the term 'Internet of Things' was finally introduced by Kevin Ashton, a computer scientist. At that time, he proposed to put chips on products for tracking them over the supply chain. He reportedly mentioned one of the most significant words that exist for the human industry revolution, 'internet', in his proposal to attract executives' attention. This concept was then used until the present day.

Over the next decade, IoT technologies started to develop very quickly when more connected devices were introduced to the market, and so the evolution began. In 2000, LG introduced the first internet-connected fridge or smart refrigerator. This fridge can be controlled remotely using apps on smartphones for temperature, on–off mode, content report, cooking suggestions etc. Seven years later, the first iPhone was announced to the public. And by the following year, the number of connected devices reached billions and is continuously growing. In 2009, driver-free cars were firstly tested by Google and in 2011, Google's Nest smart thermostat hit the market, which allowed remote control of central heating.

7.2 Internet of Medical Things (IoMT), its importance and potential in healthcare

Internet of Medical Things (IoMT) is a part of the previously mentioned concept, IoT. IoMT is a collection of medical devices and applications that support a healthcare system by connecting to the healthcare IT system through an online computer network (figure 7.1).

IoMT's impact on the healthcare market is vastly significant, undeniable, and irreversible. According to a recent Deloitte survey [1], the overall IoMT market is expected to grow from $41 billion in 2017 to $158 billion by 2022.

In medicine, many IoMT developments, patents, and healthcare solutions might benefit healthcare systems [2–4].

Current applications of IoMT would include remote monitoring of patients with chronic or long-term conditions; tracking patient medication history or tracing the location of patients admitted to hospitals; patients' wearable health devices transmitting information directly to caregivers in real-time. Hospital beds are equipped with sensors to monitor patients' vital signs.

The applications of IoMT have proven to be significantly important to the healthcare system. This claim is more precise than ever as the system is now being

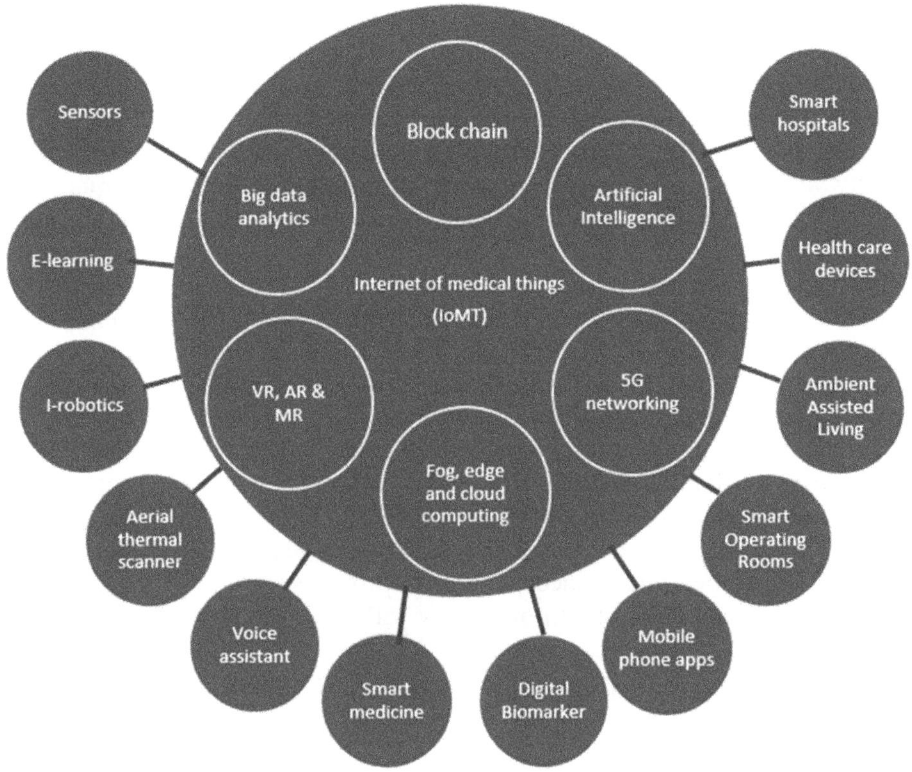

Figure 7.1. Graphical presentation of the infrastructure of IoMT.

put on such a high alert for the first time on a worldwide scale, facing the sudden explosion of COVID-19.

During the COVID-19 pandemic, the requirement of continuous monitoring of health conditions in the unpredicted huge number of patients during both pre- and post-infection stages is considered crucial. This has shown the flaws of the healthcare system because the system was not prepared, and this brought in a highly overloaded situation immediately. Medical practitioners around the world are suffering an extreme amount of workload as the amount of data they must process daily is massive during the pandemic. IoMT has helped reduced the tension vastly by helping medical experts to monitor the outburst speed situation as well as treating the disease by collecting and exchanging information about the disease from the patient and fellow experts around the globe more effectively.

The potential of IoMT is the same as IoT, limited only by the human imagination. With growing demand, these technologies will become less expensive, and everyone will be able to access them. Healthcare costs might be decreased, but only with greater efficiency as computing power and wireless capabilities develop, removing the need for in-person medical appointments. According to Goldman Sachs, IoMT will save the healthcare sector $300 billion in yearly costs, mostly through remote patient monitoring and improved prescription adherence [5].

Clinicians may monitor and treat patients remotely by placing kiosks that allow connectivity to care providers—addressing the rising demand from patients in rural towns as they struggle to attract and retain medical professionals.

The availability of electronic medical records enables certain documents to be eliminated, making the data associated with them more accessible and reducing the difficulty and inconvenience of document management. The large quantity of accessible data enables artificial intelligance (AI) to construct prediction models capable of automatically diagnosing illnesses or even predicting adverse medication reactions based on patient and drug information.

Robotic technology may also be used to help hospitals by programming and training robots/machines to operate on patient health information data obtained through the network among health professionals or by employing intelligent computing to function in the medical environment [6]. As they can carry medicine, food, and medical supplies, or collect samples from patients with minimum human interaction, this will aid in biological waste and disinfection management. They can even perform surgery with haptic-enhanced feeling, tissue identification, and real-time diagnosis. The decrease in hand tremor and better visibility given by high-definition three-dimensional video pictures improves surgical accuracy. This will allow surgeons from afar to perform surgery without regard for distance.

7.3 IoT and IoMT in fighting antimicrobial resistance

7.3.1 AMR, a global threat

Antimicrobial resistance (AMR) is the changing and adapting of microbes over time, making them more resilient against drugs. Thus, infections and diseases caused by these microbes are harder to treat and can be easier to spread, more severe, and possibly fatal [7]. This process can happen naturally, Antibiotic and antifungal exposure, as well as the propagation of those bacteria and their resistance mechanisms, can also drive increases in antimicrobial resistance [8].

As mentioned, the AMR process is a natural process and has been happening for millions of years, however, this natural process has become a major health crisis and even become one of the most concerning global threats according to WHO. This is because of the severe abuse and excessive use of antibiotics in recent decades, accelerating the process of creating drug-resistant pathogens or superbugs. Alongside the overuse and misuse of antimicrobials, microbes also have the ability to exchange genetic material including antimicrobial resistance traits resulting in spreading the resistance traits to other microbes more rapidly [8].

AMR, especially antibiotic resistance brings a lot of difficulties, challenging the current existing treatments in the healthcare system. As per conservative estimates, antibiotic-resistant bacteria alone now account for more than 500 000 annual mortalities [9–11]. Such antimicrobial methods as antibiotics have been the saving grace for humanity against microbes and have established themselves to be pillars in the modern health system. The importance of antibiotics is undeniable from basic healthcare to advance technology-supported medicine. But the pillars are in danger as the emergence of AMR is at an unexpectedly rapid rate. AMR leads to inefficiency in treating bacteria with the already existing and widely used antimicrobial methods such as antibiotics, increasing mortality, lengthening hospital stays, and costing more money to treat.

7.3.2 Challenges in fighting against AMR

The battle against AMR is challenging because it is very hard to monitor the rate of appearance and the state of current or possible resistant strains. Furthermore, there are other reasons that dampen the situation including:

- Large amounts and types of prescribed antibiotics;
- Trade and usage of antibiotics with no prescription;
- Patients not following the prescribed instruction;
- Overuse of antibiotics in agriculture and aquaculture;
- Ineffective infection control in generals;
- Poor hygiene and sanitation;
- Slow antibiotic developments.

The solutions are almost impossible for the current healthcare system. Not only must we control the number of antibiotics that medical practitioners prescribe for patients, but also assist them to have appropriate treatment decisions. More often, healthcare professionals must rely on shaky or inaccurate information to identify an infection and, as a result, either prescribe an antibiotic just in case or a broad-spectrum antibiotic in an empiric therapy when a particular medication could be more effective. These circumstances increase antimicrobial resistance and selective pressure [12]. Besides, monitoring patients to ensure they follow the antibiotic course correctly would put the system in an extreme overload of work.

The use of antibiotics in agriculture and aquaculture is one of the major contributions to creating resistant strains of microbes, as the antimicrobials are being exposed to the environment abundantly through farming without control [13] and need to be monitored strictly just like the situation of antibiotic usage in healthcare. Also, what kind of antibiotics are being used in the farming of each area in order needs to be monitored to prepare for the potential emergence of corresponding resistant strains. This also creates a massive workload for whoever should be responsible.

Poor infection control in the healthcare setting proves that the current system already cannot handle the situation due to shortage of manpower and poor monitoring setup.

The absence of new antibiotics being discovered is due to complicated reasons [14–16], which makes antibiotic development a diminishing return in investment, no longer a wise investment for investors compared to other fields of medicines [17].

7.3.3 Applications of IoT, IoMT in controlling AMR

With the help of IoT–IoMT, many of the causes can be handled, as monitoring and treating the situation would be easier and less taxing on health workers.

Web-enabled smart devices with wearables, medical equipment, consumables, and smartphones are essentially necessary for medical applications. Those devices would be prepared with up to durable standard IoT-interlinked sensors along with processing and communication software [18]. Such tools would be beneficial for programs that collect comprehensive healthcare information as well as for efforts for AMR infection prevention, diagnosis, and treatment. Additionally, they can even go beyond medical facilities like hospitals, nursing homes, doctor's offices, etc to assist with situations on farms and in the patient's own home, as well as with ecological monitoring (figure 7.2).

7.3.3.1 Real-time diagnosis

To be expected of the interference of IoT, individual real-time monitoring of biomarkers for humans or animals could be possible. IoT-connected diagnostic devices would allow us to monitor important bio features such as sweat, urine, blood, etc, as well as the ability to distinguish different sources of infections. With such information in real-time, not only would prescribing accuracy and precision increase significantly but the time to make the decision would be shortened, avoiding unwanted delays in treatment due to hesitation [19, 20]. Furthermore, personalized predictive algorithms for any potential complication (antibiotic shock, inflammation, relapse, allergy, stroke, etc) up to hours before even possible signs could be visible observed by collecting real-time data from the patients and setting the algorithms up beforehand [21]. In addition, the effectiveness of the antibiotics applied during treatment can be monitored in real-time, indicating if the therapy choice is correct and if AMR is present, allowing physicians to have more time to react and change their strategies depending on the situation more effectively.

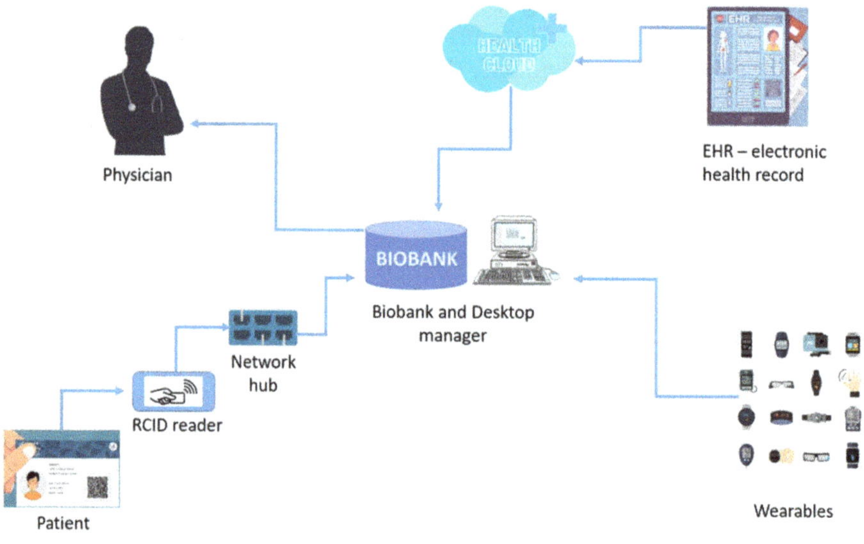

Figure 7.2. Revolution of IoT in medicare.

7.3.3.2 Treatment

The problem of patients following their antibiotic therapy course incorrectly could be improved. By employing IoT technologies in devices such as pill dispensers or wearables such as smartphones through apps, patients or their care providers would be notified when the next tablets of drugs are due, when and how to take and maybe a visual encouragement to 'finish the whole course to avoid complication and to have a healthy result' or warning 'the prescribed medicines are only to be used by patients'.

Poor hygiene and sanitation as well as poor infection control situations could be solved by attaching sensors to handwashing dispensers or similar devices to monitor handwashing compliance [22]. Caregivers can also be notified about their hygiene status when moving between patients, and places by using smartphone location or other types of IoT services. This would prevent caregivers and patients from unknowingly infecting one another by accident [23]. Infection prevention strategies specifically for hospitals could be handled by monitoring medical air disinfection parameters by IoT [24].

While simultaneously securing patient information, block chain-based IoT technology may be valuable for tracking patient health history and medication levels, including antibiotic treatment. Using a cryptographic technique known as hashing, the entries in the auto-updating system of 'blocks' that makes up the Block Chain are linked to one another. The previous record's cryptographic hash is contained in each record, forming a chain that prevents alterations to the records [25].

The coming of the 5G network will enhance the quality of IoT-based connectivity and healthcare systems. With this technological progress, IoT technologies would even be closer to our daily life as smart hospitals, smart vehicles, and smart homes will start to exist more and more, monitoring and protecting our health through IoT applications (biosensors, apps, telemedicine, wearables, etc) [26].

The implementation of IoT in the health system may not end the battle against antimicrobial resistance, but it is certainly the best weapon to ease the current and upcoming situation on a worldwide level.

Soon, the electronic health record (EHR) will replace the traditional patient's paper chart. For many hospitals worldwide, particularly in developed countries, a patient's health data records are completely digitalized and made available instantly and securely to those who are authorized.

However, even after being digitalized, the amount and standard of clinical data are rapidly ever changing and growing, including EHRs. Bigger data and digitalization does not mean automatically better care for patients, the management and usage of the data should also be optimized and used correctly in order to have better care for patients. Only implementing EHRs and computerized physicians order entry (CPOE) can rapidly decrease many avoidable errors and incidents but also introduce several more benefits according to studies [27, 28]. Therefore, a high-quality clinical decision-support system (CDSS) is essential if the healthcare systems are to achieve the full benefits of EHRs and CPOE.

More than often, clinicians are not aware of the patients' existing available data in EHRs, or how to access the data or do not have time to look for the data and are drowned in it. In many cases, a clinician must decide urgently during direct patient contact, ward rounds, etc… This means that many decisions are made within seconds or minutes, thus, even with digitalized data, clinicians are prone to make mistakes and errors and quality of treatment decision relies heavily on the experience and knowledge of the professional. Moreover, many subtle changes of patients before entering hospital, ward admission are overlooked as the clinicians likely focus on the patient current status. A CDSS however, takes into account all data available, making it possible to notice changes outside the scope of the professional and notices specific changes for a certain patient, within normal limits.

7.3.3.3 Improvement of antimicrobial usage

As mentioned above, the overuse and misuse of antimicrobials are among the main drivers of AMR. Optimizing the use of antimicrobials is one important target of the WHO Global Action plan. Since 2019, WHO has released the antimicrobial stewardship (AMS) program placing it as an integral component of the human health system. It emphasizes the importance of appropriate antimicrobial usage and provides tool kits for nations, particularly low and middle-income countries, to implement the AMS successfully (table 7.1).

Table 7.1. Key steps to establish a national AMS program, instructed for leadership at the national and institutional level [29].

Step	National level	Institutional level
1	Establish a governance structure, such as a national working group (TWG) that work on AMS	Perform analysis of healthcare facility core elements to identify problems and solutions regarding antimicrobial consumption (AMC) and/or use, prescription audits. Collecting information and analysing AMR surveillance data and existing AMS competencies at the facility.
2	Review what has been done and what is required and prioritize the national core elements	Setting up a sustainable AMS governance structure
3	Identify pilot healthcare facilities both public and private for initial AMS rollout	Identify resources and priority and prioritize the healthcare facility core elements
4	Develop a national AMS strategy[1] with national indicators	Identify AMS interventions
5	Dedicate financial and human resources as required	Develop a healthcare facility AMS action plan
6	Monitor and evaluate implementation of the national AMS strategy	Implement, monitor and evaluate AMS interventions
7	Support the optimized prescription of antimicrobials	Offer basic and continued educational resources and training on optimized prescription of antimicrobials

[1] Include community and/or primary care AMS programmes (not covered in this toolkit).

In the AMS program, WHO has acknowledged that IoT/IT can contribute to every level of the program including basic, intermediate, and advanced levels.

At the basic level, IoT/IT can help to generate databases on procurement and ward dispensing in pharmaceutical units as well as databases of AMR surveillance in different units.

At the intermediate level, calculation of antimicrobial consumption/AMC (e.g. in defined daily dose/1000 inpatients/day) can be performed and reported real-time and automatically. Besides, other important information can also be automatically provided for patients and clinicians such as alerts on time-sensitive automatic stop orders for surgical prophylaxis, specific antibiotic usage and electronic guidelines. Furthermore, apps for doing a point prevalence survey (PPS) in order to obtain auditing or prospective (real-time) or retrospective collection of antibiotic prescription data on hospitalized patients can also be feasible with the employment of IT. In PPS, the data are analysed and then fed back to the prescribers. This is laborious, thus in the beginning, it can begin with weekly or bimonthly quick audits during ward rounds, with real-time feedback to the prescribers, similar to a repeated and small-scale PPS.

At the advanced level, with the help of IT, CPOE system, clinical decision-support systems (commercial or self-developed) of different levels of complexity, point-of-care access to microbiological results from all units, computerized patient dispensing billing data, estimations of clinical outcomes related to antibiotic treatment, automatic submissions/reporting of computerized facility-level data to the national centre, apps for national, regional or facility; guidelines are feasible options to improve overall antimicrobial usage.

While AMS is dealt with at a strategic level, at point-of-care level or personalized level, the application of IoT is rather in supporting antimicrobial therapeutic drug monitoring (TDM). Obviously, the optimal use of antimicrobials is essential but challenging as it must minimize toxicity, and avoid the development of AMR while still reaching clinical response for patients. There are a number of factors that affect the success of an antimicrobial therapy, including variability in pharmacokinetics, pharmacodynamics, comorbidities, and polypharmacy. In this case, the development of biosensors offers potential solutions for dose optimization, thus optimal usage of antimicrobials. Thanks to technological advances, biosensors can be miniaturized, becoming portable and point-of-care devices that can facilitate real-time antimicrobial monitoring. (figure 7.3) [30]. The availability of biosensors would also assist in diagnosis and treatment, as mentioned in sections 7.3.3.1 and 7.3.3.2.

7.3.3.4 AMR surveillance

Many efforts have been made to cope with AMR, a global threat [31], at both global and national levels [32] such as Global Antimicrobial Resistance and Use Surveillance System (GLASS) [33]. Those efforts aim to build an Antimicrobial Resistance Surveillance System (ARSS) for real-time collecting, analyzing, integrating, and reporting AM data and trends.

However, there are challenges in antimicrobial susceptibility testing (AST), data collection, and integration. First, the conventional AST takes a very long time, up to

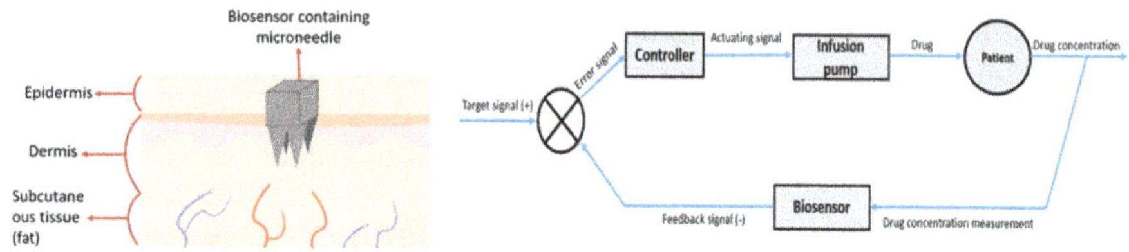

A) Biosensor containing microneedle penetrating skins to collect information on drug concentrations.

B) Closed loop controlled for automated, precision drug delivery.

Figure 7.3. Real-time drug monitoring. (A) Information on drugs inside the body like concentration is collected via biosensors containing microneedles penetrating the skin. (B) Automated and precise drug delivery can be performed via closed-loop control.

48 h, and intensive labor works for preparing growth media and serial dilution. Second, it takes time and effort to transport samples from rural hospitals to centralized microbiology laboratories. Finally, the national ARSS integrated data is from multiple laboratories with different surveillance components such as retail meat, farms, and human and animal clinics. Therefore, annual reports are usually released late, up to 1.5–2 years, and thus cannot reflect the current AMR trend [34].

Fortunately, the emergence of AI, IoT, and Omics technology potentially tackles the above-mentioned challenges, especially in the context of resource-limited regions.

An IoT-based ARSS typically possesses four components: sensing component; computational analysis and machine learning component; data transmission component; and cloud server and application component [35].

At the heart of the system, the sensing component performs either AST or AMR detection. To date, there are many methods with different approaches such as phenotypic, molecular, genomic, and biochemical utilizing different technologies [36]. However, in the context of rural hospitals/clinics lacking resources, hardware, and infrastructure, AI and mobile devices come into place.

The Kirby–Bauer disk diffusion test is the most popular method because it is simple, low cost, and easy to perform daily in the laboratory on a variety of scales. It places cellulose disks (pellets) containing antibiotics on agar plates which are inoculated with bacteria. After 16–24 h of incubating, the diameter of the inhibition zone around each disk is measured. The diameter of the inhibition zone from different combinations of organism–antibiotic signs Susceptible (S), Intermediate (I), and Resistant (R). Measurement of the diameter, the keypoint to determine the susceptibility, relies on proficient technicians due to the nature of the test [37]. Therefore, automatic reading systems which automatically measure the inhibition zone's diameters from acquired plate pictures have been introduced [38, 39]. To enhance quality and reduce turnaround time, the commercial systems typically integrate an expert system and automation modules which can read automatically antibiograms. However, these systems are not affordable to hospitals in general due to their requirement of infrastructure and hardware. Thanks to the advancement of

AI algorithms and hardware, smartphones that are easy to use and fully connected through 3G or Wi-Fi now can measure the diameter and are ready to send the data to the cloud for further analysis [40].

Another technology that is lightweight to implement in rural areas is to use intelligent sensors that leverage the microfluidic lab-on-chip technique and home-built image sensing system to perform AST. Its portability, low cost, and low labor work make it easy to be implemented in various locations, especially in rural regions which are resource-limited [34].

At the computational analysis and machine learning component, the images from lab-on-chip AST were used to train and validate the machine learning algorithms which are implemented either locally on a local computer or remotely on the cloud via smartphone. The outcomes of the machine learning algorithms are transmitted to the cloud server via Wi-Fi or 3G connections which is a so-called data transmission component. All the transmitted data from various regions are gathered, harmonized, and stored on the cloud server and application component. In this component, a portal presents the AMR dashboard to the end-users.

Notably, this architecture of the IoT-assisted ARSS is flexible and open to integrating data types and sources as many as possible thanks to big data technologies. For more details on different approaches and technologies used for antimicrobial susceptibility testing, consult an excellent review on innovative and rapid antimicrobial susceptibility testing systems conducted by van Belkum *et al* [36].

This real-time IoT-based ARSS can continuously monitor and promptly alert about the potential AMR pathogens' outbreaks, enabling early and effective prevention and intervention of an AMR crisis. With this IoT-based ARSS, the data of various kinds and from various sources is automatically and continuously gathered and analyzed therefore a prompt AMR report can be reported rather than an annual report in the conventional ARSS. Additionally, the cloud database of the IoT-based ARSS is accessible across different sectors both locally and nationally. Therefore, IoT-based ARSS is a potential and promising system that provides prompt alerts for the emergence of AMR pathogens, aids in the quick control of outbreaks, and makes the assessment of AMR interventions easier.

7.3.3.5 Development and discovery of new antimicrobials

In the past, the primary method for creating antibiotics was by searching soil-dwelling microbes for secondary compounds that inhibited the growth of pathogenic bacteria [41, 42]. This method however is now plagued by replication issues as the same molecules keep being repeatedly discovered [43]. This results in the slow development of new antimicrobials.

New techniques for antimicrobial discovery are required in light of the AMR issue in order to speed up the discovery of new antimicrobials and lower their related costs, making the development of the antimicrobial once again a smart investment for investors.

A new technology, AI, has been used to scan and find new medications. The idea of this method is to create and manipulate algorithms in order to find the connection between different genes and compositions by recognizing active reagents and observing their interaction with microorganisms [44].

AI started off with machine learning technologies, the computer operates with supposed 'raw data' to find patterns and construct algorithms [45, 46]. And so, the 'raw data' size and quality determine the efficiency and value of the algorithm [45, 46]. This technology manages to improve programs and predictions by computational power and rapid large quantities of information processing [45, 46].

Machine learning, however, still needs the help of humans in order to work. Deep learning technologies can go beyond, these technologies can understand complex concepts and manage to simplify the information, continuously learning from their own discoveries to discover even more, unknown to humans [47].

One noted example for using deep learning to discover new potential antimicrobials is the finding of halicin. Halicin is a compound that potentially could develop to be a new broad-spectrum antibiotic. It was identified by using *in silico* deep learning technologies by AI researchers at the MIT Jameel Clinic in 2019 [48].

According to Stokes *et al*, the *in silico* deep learning method used to discover halicin consists of three stages. First, a deep neural network model would be trained specifically to predict growth inhibition of a target pathogen, in this case *Escherichia coli*, with a collection of molecules (the collection used in finding halicin consists of 2335 molecules). Then, the potential lead compounds with activity against *E. coli* will be identified by applying the resulting model to various discrete chemical libraries, comprising millions of molecules. Finally, a list of candidates would be chosen from the compound ranking by the model's predicted score based on a pre-specified prediction score threshold, chemical structure, and availability constructed [44]. In addition to the finding of c-Jun N-terminal kinase inhibitor SU3327 (halicin) [49, 50], another eight potentially antibacterial compounds with structures different from known antibiotics were also found.

Halicin discovery result suggested the importance of machine and deep learning in antibiotic discovery by not only increasing the rate and accuracy of identifying new potential compounds but also reducing the cost of investment.

IoT can also ease the development and discovery of new antimicrobials with many offers as indicated below.

Deep neural network model training: According to Stokes *et al*, the biological outcome that is preferred after cells are exposed to compounds should be taken into more consideration. This is due to the number of bacterial phenotypes that could theoretically result in efficacious antibiotics [51, 52]. Their approach selected growth inhibition as the biological criteria to gather data for machine learning as this results in a reasonable proportion of active compounds relative to the size of the screening library, thus it can easily generate reproducible data. Future applications could incorporate phenotypic screening conditions to resolve this more thoroughly.

Composition of the training data: Utilizing training data with adequate chemical diversity in both active and inactive molecules is crucial. This is because if the selected molecules have similar structures, the model will be unable to generalize to new frames. In order to maximize the likelihood of effective generalization in new chemical domains, it is beneficial to have the broadest structural variety feasible during the training phase. Appropriate pharmacology/absorption, distribution, metabolism, and excretion (ADME)/toxicity properties for *in vivo* application are also important. A properly regulated training set with more implementations would enable more manageable predictions that avoided potentially unfavorable compounds at this early stage of using machine learning for antibiotic development, suitable for practical application. A database approved for usage as a drug library such as the FDA-approved drug library would be ideal to train model select molecules with appropriate pharmacology/ADME/toxicity.

Prediction prioritization: The criteria for each prediction should be suitable with the expectation of the researchers about the developing molecules, and compounds that are potentially new antibiotics. For example, in the case of Halicin discovery, prioritization of criteria includes having a high prediction score, structurally unique to clinical antibiotics, and unlikely to display toxicity [41].

7.4 Concluding remarks

With the development of the internet and technology, IoT is growing and obviously bringing significant change to every sector of life, including the medical sector (IoMT). To combat AMR, one big problem in the healthcare sector, IoT has offered various solutions, from real-time diagnosis, therapeutic drug monitoring, clinical decision-support system, patient data recording and maintaining, AMR surveillance to new antimicrobial discovery using IT. The extra solutions provided by IoT no doubt can help to control AMR at different levels and scales, thus effectively protecting public health from AMR threats. By implementing EHR to digitalize patient's data and CDSS to process them effectively, we can improve treatments, reducing errors, ultimately, preventing AMR from emerging.

References

[1] Deloitte 2018 Medtech and the Internet of Medical Things: how connected medical devices are transforming health care *Deloitte* https://www2.deloitte.com/content/dam/Deloitte/global/Documents/Life-Sciences-Health-Care/gx-lshc-medtech-iomt-brochure.pdf (accessed 1 August 2022)

[2] Qiu F 2021 Hospital archives intelligent management system based on 5G network and Internet of Things system *Microprocess. Microsyst.* **80** 103564

[3] Javed A R, Fahad L G, Farhan A A, Abbas S, Srivastava G, Parizi R M and Khan M S 2021 Automated cognitive health assessment in smart homes using machine learning *Sustain. Cities Soc* **65** 102572

[4] Islam S R, Kwak D, Kabir M H, Hossain M and Kwak K S 2015 The Internet of Things for health care: a comprehensive survey *IEEE Access* **3** 678–708

[5] Stern C 2021 Goldman Sachs says a digital healthcare revolution is coming—and it could save America $300 billion *Business Insider* https://businessinsider.com/goldman-digital-healthcare-is-coming-2015-6?international=true&r=US&IR=T (accessed 1 August 2022)

[6] Simoens P, Dragone M and Saffiotti A 2018 The Internet of Robotic Things: a review of concept, added value and applications *Int. J. Adv. Robot. Syst.* **15** 1729881418759424

[7] World Health Organization 2021 Antimicrobial resistance *WHO* https://who.int/news-room/fact-sheets/detail/antimicrobial-resistance (accessed 1 August 2022)

[8] Centers for Disease Control and Prevention 2022 How do germs become resistant? *Centers for Disease Control and Prevention* https://cdc.gov/drugresistance/about/how-resistance-happens.html (accesssed 1 August 2022)
[9] Phumart P, Phodha P, Thamlikitkul V, Riewpaiboon A, Prakongsai P and Limwattananon S 2012 Health and economic impacts of antimicrobial resistant infections in Thailand: a preliminary study *J. Health. Syst. Res* **6** 352–60
[10] Centers for Disease Control and Prevention—CDC 2013 Antibiotic Resistance Threats in the United States, 2013 *Centers for Disease Control and Prevention—CDC*
[11] CDC/EMEA Joint Working Group 2009 The bacterial challenge: time to react. A call to narrow the gap between multidrug-resistant bacteria in the EU and development of new antibacterial agents *Technical Report* European Centre for Disease Prevention and Control – ECDC and European Medicines Agency—EMEA
[12] NIH: National Institute of Allergy and Infectious Diseases 2011 Causes of antimicrobial (drug) resistance *NIH: National Institute of Allergy and Infectious Diseases* https://niaid.nih.gov/research/antimicrobial-resistance-causes (accessed 1 August 2022)
[13] Martin M J, Thottathil S E and Newman T B 2015 Antibiotics overuse in animal agriculture: a call to action for health care providers *Am. J. Public Health* **105** 2409–10
[14] Bartlett J G, Gilbert D N and Spellberg B 2013 Seven ways to preserve the miracle of antibiotics *Clin. Infect. Dis.* **56** 1445–50
[15] Gould I M and Bal A M 2013 New antibiotic agents in the pipeline and how they can help overcome microbial resistance *Virulence* **4** 185–91
[16] Wright G D 2014 Something old, something new: revisiting natural products in antibiotic drug discovery *Can. J. Microbiol.* **60** 147–54
[17] Piddock L J 2012 The crisis of no new antibiotics—what is the way forward? *Lancet Infect. Dis.* **12** 249–53
[18] Zhao L, Li H, Meng J and Li Z 2020 The recent advances in self-powered medical information sensors *InfoMat* **2** 212–34
[19] Stein M, Lipman-Arens S, Oved K, Cohen A, Bamberger E, Navon R and Klein A 2018 A novel host–protein assay outperforms routine parameters for distinguishing between bacterial and viral lower respiratory tract infections *Diagn. Microbiol. Infect.* **90** 206–13
[20] Shapiro N I, Self W H, Rosen J, Sharp S C and Filbin M R *et al* 2018 A prospective, multicentre US clinical trial to determine accuracy of FebriDx point-of-care testing for acute upper respiratory infections with and without a confirmed fever *Ann. Med.* **50** 420–9
[21] Bhatia M, Kaur S and Sood S K 2020 IoT-inspired smart home-based urine infection prediction *J. Ambient Intell. Humaniz. Comput.* 1–15
[22] Bal M and Abrishambaf R 2017 A system for monitoring hand hygiene compliance based on Internet of Things *2017 IEEE Int. Conf. on Industrial Technology (ICIT): Proc. (Toronto, March 2017)* (New York: IEEE), 1348–53
[23] Al Qathrady M, Helmy A and Almuzaini K 2016 Infection tracing in smart hospitals *2016 IEEE 12th Int. Conf. on Wireless and Mobile Computing, Networking and Communications (WiMob): Proc. (New York, October 2016)* (New York: IEEE), 1–8
[24] Yang L, Yao T, Liu G, Sun L, Yang N, Zhang H and Hou X 2019 Monitoring and control of medical air disinfection parameters of nosocomial infection system based on internet of things *J. Med. Syst.* **43** 1–7

[25] Nørfeldt L, Bøtker J, Edinger M, Genina N and Rantanen J 2019 Cryptopharmaceuticals: increasing the safety of medication by a blockchain of pharmaceutical products *J. Pharm. Sci.* **108** 2838–41
[26] Shafique K, Khawaja B A, Sabir F, Qazi S and Mustaqim M 2020 Internet of Things (IoT) for next-generation smart systems: a review of current challenges, future trends and prospects for emerging 5G-IoT scenarios *IEEE Access* **8** 23022–40
[27] Nebeker J R, Khawaja B A, Sabir F, Qazi S and Mustaqim M 2005 Internet of things (IoT) for next-generation smart systems: A review of current challenges, future trends and prospects for emerging 5G-IoT scenarios *Arch. Intern. Med.* **165** 1111–6
[28] Magrabi F *et al* 2016 Improving evaluation to address the unintended consequences of health information technology: a position paper from the Working Group on Technology Assessment & Quality Development *Yearb. Med. Inform.* **1** 61–9
[29] Antimicrobial Resistance Division, Surveillance, Prevention and Control, Global Coordination and Partnership, and Health Product Policy and Standards 2019 Antimicrobial stewardship programmes in health-care facilities in low-and middle-income countries: a WHO practical toolkit *World Health Organization* https://who.int/publications/i/item/9789241515481 (accessed 1 August 2022)
[30] Rawson T M, Wilson R C, O'Hare D, Herrero P, Kambugu A, Lamorde M and Holmes A H 2021 Optimizing antimicrobial use: challenges, advances and opportunities *Nat. Rev. Microbiol.* **19** 747–58
[31] HM Government/Wellcome Trust 2014 Antimicrobial Resistance: Tackling a crisis for the health and wealth of nations *AMR Review Paper* https://amr-review.org/sites/default/files/AMR%20Review%20Paper%20-%20Tackling%20a%20crisis%20for%20the%20health%20and%20wealth%20of%20nations_1.pdf
[32] Founou L L, Founou R C and Essack S Y 2016 Antibiotic resistance in the food chain: a developing country-perspective *Front. Microbiol.* **7** 1881
[33] Thakur S and Gray G C 2019 The mandate for a global 'one health' approach to antimicrobial resistance surveillance *Am. J. Trop. Med.* **100** 227
[34] Government of Canada 2018 Executive summary *Canadian integrated program for anti-microbial resistance survillance (CIPARS)* https://canada.ca/en/public-health/services/surveillance/canadian-integrated-program-antimicrobial-resistance-surveillance-cipars/cipars-reports/2018-annual-report-executive-summary.html
[35] Ma L, He W, Petersen M, Chou K C and Lu X 2021 Next-generation antimicrobial resistance surveillance system based on the Internet of Things and microfluidic technique *ACS Sens.* **6** 3477–84
[36] van Belkum A, Burnham C A D, Rossen J W, Mallard F, Rochas O and Dunne W M 2020 Innovative and rapid antimicrobial susceptibility testing systems *Nat. Rev. Microbiol.* **18** 299–311
[37] EUCAST 2023 EUCAST Disk Diffusion Test Methodology https://eucast.org/ast_of_bacteria/disk_diffusion_methodology/
[38] Lestari E S, Severin J A, Filius P M G, Kuntaman K, Duerink D O, Hadi U and Verbrugh H A 2008 Comparison of the accuracy of disk diffusion zone diameters obtained by manual zone measurements to that by automated zone measurements to determine antimicrobial susceptibility *J. Microbiol. Methods* **75** 177–81
[39] Hombach M, Zbinden R and Böttger E C 2013 Standardisation of disk diffusion results for antibiotic susceptibility testing using the sirscan automated zone reader *BMC Microbiol.* **13** 1–8

[40] Pascucci M, Royer G, Adamek J, Asmar M A, Aristizabal D, Blanche L and Madoui M A 2021 AI-based mobile application to fight antibiotic resistance *Nat. Commun.* **12** 1–10
[41] Clardy J, Fischbach M A and Walsh C T 2006 New antibiotics from bacterial natural products *Nat. Biotechnol.* **24** 1541–50
[42] Wright G D 2017 Opportunities for natural products in 21st century antibiotic discovery *Nat. Prod. Rep.* **34** 694–701
[43] Cox G, Sieron A, King A M, De Pascale G, Pawlowski A C, Koteva K and Wright G D 2017 A common platform for antibiotic dereplication and adjuvant discovery *Cell Chem. Biol.* **24** 98–109
[44] Stokes J M, Yang K, Swanson K, Jin W, Cubillos-Ruiz A, Donghia N M and Collins J J 2020 A deep learning approach to antibiotic discovery *Cell* **180** 688–702
[45] Mohri M, Rostamizadeh A and Talwalkar A 2018 *Foundations of Machine Learning* (Cambridge, MA: MIT Press)
[46] Jordan M I and Mitchell T M 2015 Machine learning: trends, perspectives, and prospects *Science* **349** 255–60
[47] Goodfellow I, Bengio Y and Courville A 2016 *Deep Learning* (Cambridge, MA: MIT Press)
[48] Trafton A 2020 Artificial intelligence yields new antibiotic. A deep-learning model identifies a powerful new drug that can kill many species of antibiotic-resistant bacteria *MIT News* **February 2020** https://news.mit.edu/2020/artificial-intelligence-identifies-new-antibiotic-0220
[49] De S K, Stebbins J L, Chen L H, Riel-Mehan M, Machleidt T, Dahl R and Pellecchia M 2009 Design, synthesis, and structure–activity relationship of substrate competitive, selective, and *in vivo* active triazole and thiadiazole inhibitors of the c-Jun N-terminal kinase *J. Med. Chem.* **52** 1943–52
[50] Jang S, Yu L R, Abdelmegeed M A, Gao Y, Banerjee A and Song B J 2015 Critical role of c-Jun N-terminal protein kinase in promoting mitochondrial dysfunction and acute liver injury *Redox. Biol* **6** 552–64
[51] Farha M A and Brown E D 2015 Unconventional screening approaches for antibiotic discovery *Ann. N. Y. Acad. Sci.* **1354** 54–66
[52] Kohanski M A, Dwyer D J and Collins J J 2010 How antibiotics kill bacteria: from targets to networks *Nat. Rev. Microbiol.* **8** 423–35

IOP Publishing

Internet of Things in Biomedical Sciences
Challenges and applications
Varun Bajaj and Irshad Ahmad Ansari

Chapter 8

IoT-based heart valve disorder detection using an amplitude and frequency modulated signal model

Mohan Bansal, Rajeev Sharma and Ajay Dagar

In this chapter, a novel IoT-based framework is proposed to detect heart valve disorders (HVDs) in humans using an amplitude and frequency modulated (AFM) signal decomposition model. The presented framework aims to detect and classify HVDs into different categories, namely aortic stenosis (AS), mitral regurgitation (MR), mitral stenosis (MS), and mitral valve prolapse (MVP), using a machine learning approach. To investigate and diagnose cardiac disorders, a phonocardiogram (PCG) signal best fits the proposed framework as it contains the most relevant information about the heart's functionality and auscultation. Additionally, the AFM signal decomposition model, already applied and tested on the speech/audio signal for various speech processing applications, is used in the proposed framework to extract feature vectors from the recorded PCG signals. Subsequently, the proposed IoT framework uses a Wi-Fi module to transmit the extracted features to the backend for further classification. Finally, an ensemble learning classifier detects the HVDs based on the transmitted feature vectors.

8.1 Introduction

Internet of things (IoT)-based systems utilize the diversity of interconnection and communication between multiple heterogeneous devices/sensors to work remotely and collaboratively to perform a specific task [1]. IoT-based systems are readily found in developing smart homes, commercial security solutions, military surveillance, weather forecasting and agriculture technology [2]. These IoT-based solutions can also be deployed in public places, such as markets, bus/railway stations, schools, and hospitals, to enhance security, accessibility, productivity and the overall user experience [3]. In this chapter, an IoT-based framework is developed to work in the hospital environment, focusing on enhancing the accessibility of human diagnosis.

doi:10.1088/978-0-7503-5311-3ch8

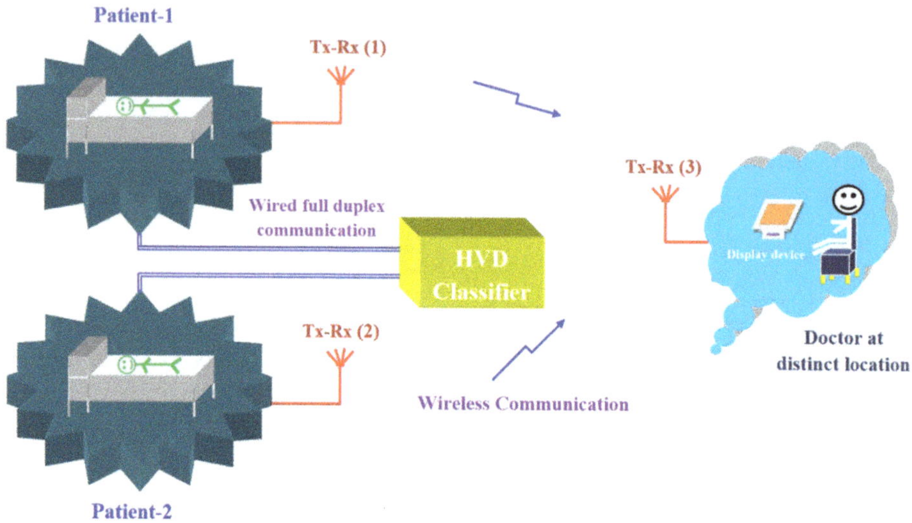

Figure 8.1. IoT framework for HVD classification.

The main objective is to develop an automatic heart diagnosis system that detects the patient's heart impairments and communicates the corresponding reports to doctors in real time. A diagrammatic representation of such an IoT-based framework is presented in figure 8.1. In the proposed IoT-based framework, multiple heart patients are continuously monitored for heart impairments, and real-time diagnostic reports are made available to the concerned doctors over the wireless medium sitting at a remote location.

HVDs are considered one of the prime causes responsible for cardiovascular diseases (CVDs) and, therefore, need to be detected in the early stages to minimize the mortality rate [4]. The vital information related to the heart's functionality and auscultation is mainly captured during *phonocardiography*, which results in generating the phonocardiogram, i.e. a PCG signal, which is widely used for diagnosing HVDs [5]. A dissimilar PCG signal is observed between a normal heart and an abnormal heart in terms of amplitude, time, frequency, intensity, homogeneity, and spectral content observed in their corresponding phonocardiograms [6, 7]. The observed characteristics of the heart's sound during phonocardiography may also differ based on the type of the heart disease.

The human heart consists of four valves [8]; aortic, mitral, tricuspid and pulmonary. The proper cardiac valve opening and closing ensures a healthy heart and corresponding mechanical performance [9]. When one or more of the four heart valves are damaged/flawed, the condition is called HVD. AS, MR, MS, and MVP are typical examples of HVDs [10].

A phonocardiogram is a graphical representation of the heart signal obtained using an electronic stethoscope. The generated PCG signal contains a variety of sounds, such as typical S1–S2 and S3–S4 sounds, also known as murmurs [11]. The S1 and S2 sounds occur due to the closure of the mitral/tricuspid valve, i.e. an atrioventricular valve, at the beginning of the systolic interval and, subsequently, the

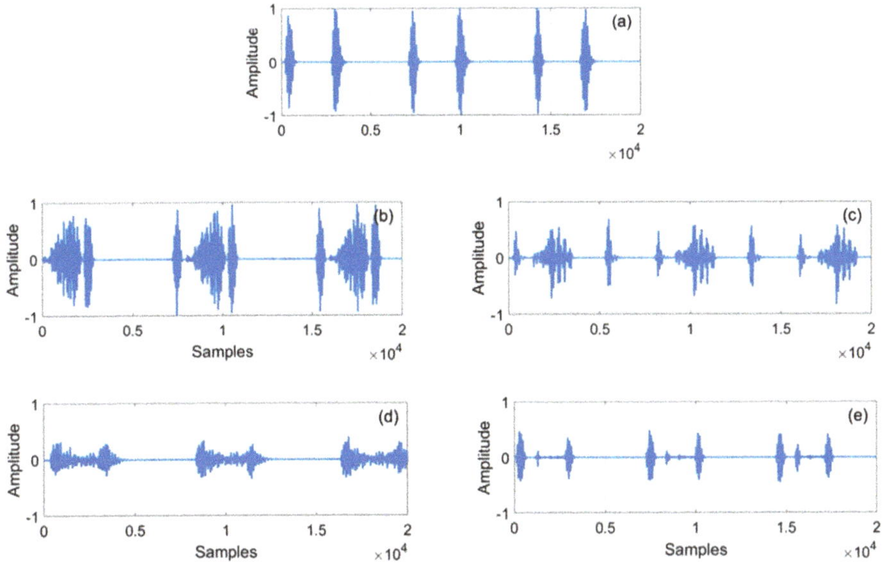

Figure 8.2. (a) Normal, (b) AS, (c) MS, (d) MR and (e) MVP PCG signals.

closure of the aortic/pulmonic valve at the start of the diastolic interval, respectively. The S3 and S4 are unusual heart sounds typically inaudible but observed on the phonocardiogram [12]. The placement of these murmurs in a phonocardiogram decides the abnormalities in a human heart. The categorical representation of these cardiac disorders is presented in figure 8.2.

Among many, transthoracic echocardiography (TTE) is one of the most used methods to detect HVDs [13]. The standard procedure involves moving the transducer onto various chest/abdominal wall locations to obtain multiple heart views. The transducer, similar in shape to a microphone, detects the echoes reflected from the various parts of the heart in response to the sound waves pumped into the chest [14]. The TTE is constrained by its moderate cost and lengthy examination time. Even with adequate training, sometimes it is difficult for medical practitioners to examine the recorded PCG signals and detect impairments [15]. In such cases, computer-aided automatic systems always have an advantage over the traditional methodology [16]. The current automated systems [17] employ supervised machine learning algorithms where the recorded PCG signals are fed as inputs and processed. As a result, these systems predict and classify the HVDs [18].

In this context, the state-of-the-art systems have extracted features from the PCG signals using the time-domain, the frequency domain, and the time–frequency (TF) domain approaches in collaboration with various classifiers for detecting HVDs [19–25]. Discrete-time continuous wavelet transform (DT-CWT) and dyadic wavelet transform (DWT) are the candidate methods that are widely used for analyzing and extracting features from the PCG signal [26, 27]. However, due to their low-resolution response to the sharp signals, DT-CWT and DWT domains likely contribute to an inefficient feature set. Therefore, the wavelet synchro-squeezed transform (WSST) method is used for feature extraction for sharp-edged and non-stationary signals, like PCG signals. In WSST, the wavelet coefficients are reassigned in the time–frequency domain, considering the instantaneous frequencies or energy values of a multi-component signal [21]. It has been employed to segment the heart sound signals from the PCG signal [23]. In [26], an automatic system to classify and distinguish the PCG signal of a normal and HVD heart is developed using a deep neural network (DNN) wherein feature sets are defined jointly using DWT and Mel frequency cepstral coefficients (MFCC). Similarly, the PCG signals are analyzed using wavelet packet decomposition (WPD) and continuous wavelet transform (CWT) for detecting HVDs. In [28], the authors extracted features using a tunable *Q*-factor wavelet transform (TQWT) and distinguished abnormal hearts, similar to [26]. A comprehensive review of the localization and classifications of the heart sounds are presented by Ismail *et al* [29].

Several recent studies rely on the fast-Fourier transform (FFT) [30, 31], the short-time Fourier transform (STFT) [32], the chirplet transform [33], the time–frequency decomposition (TFD) and probability density function (PDF) modelling [34] techniques for detecting HVDs from heart sounds. These methods have been widely used in conjunction with various classifiers, such as support vector machine (SVM) [26], convolutional neural network (CNN) [35], probabilistic neural network (PNN) [36], deep neural network [37],[38] and deep WaveNet model [39], to develop automatic systems that distinguish the normal and HVD heart sounds. The performance of these classifiers not only depends on the huge amount of training data but also on the correct feature selection. Therefore, it is required to develop a feature-based approach using an advanced signal processing method for accurate HVDs classification.

A PCG signal being non-stationary has varying amplitude and frequency components. For such non-stationary signals, the modulated signal model is more suitable for signal analysis [40]. The independent amplitude-modulated (AM) signal model and frequency modulated (FM) signal model are suitable for observing independent amplitude variations [41] and the frequency change [42], respectively. In the case of biomedical signals, like electroencephalogram (EEG) and PCG, it is more appropriate to represent both amplitude and frequency variations in the signal using combined AM and FM signal models [43], known as the AFM signal model [44]. The AFM signal decomposition model, already applied and tested on the speech/audio signal for various speech processing applications [45–51], is used in the proposed framework to extract features from the recorded PCG signals. The amplitude envelope (AE) and the instantaneous frequency (IF) of each component are individually analyzed using a discrete energy separation algorithm (DESA) to estimate the parameters of the proposed model [49, 52]. The extracted feature vectors are then fed to an ensemble classifier that detects and classifies the HVD and normal signal.

8.2 Proposed methodology

The proposed IOT-based framework for HVD detection consists of three stages: PCG signal acquisition, feature extraction and HVD classification [19]. The initial stage comprises echo/phonocardiography to acquire a preliminary PCG signal.

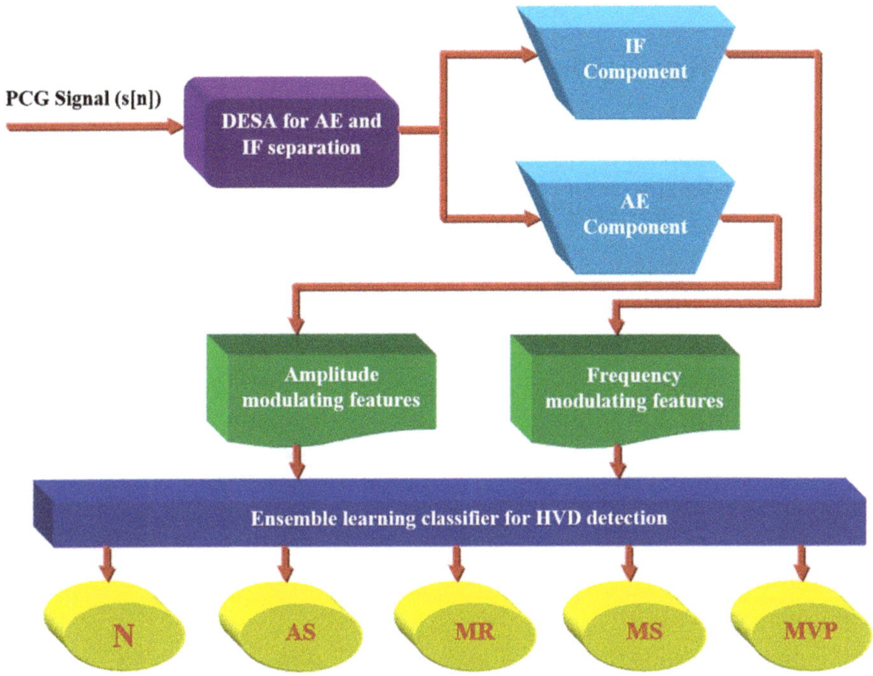

Figure 8.3. A systematic representation of the proposed HVD classifier.

Since the PCG signals are non-stationary, the parametric representation is compatible with an AFM signal model [48]. To extract features, the PCG signal is processed within a multi-tone AFM signal model, which decomposes the signal into AE and IF components using DESA [24, 49]. Subsequently, in the second stage, the features, also known as the modulating features, are then extracted from the AE and IF components, respectively. The most pertinent peaks in the spectrum of AM–FM components are used to choose highly discriminating features. In the final stage, these modulating features are used within the framework to train an ensemble learning classifier [53] to detect and classify the HVDs. A systematic representation of the proposed approach is illustrated in figure 8.3.

A detailed description of the proposed framework is presented in the subsequent subsections. Initially, the signal analysis using an AFM signal model is discussed. Subsequently, the modulating feature extraction followed by a supervised classification approach used within the proposed framework is presented in the ensuing subsections.

8.2.1 AFM signal model

For any non-stationary signals, like speech and PCG signals, the amplitude and the frequency components can be individually represented as a linear combination of sinusoidal basis functions forming a multi-tone AFM signal model. The parametric representation of a non-stationary signal $s[n]$ using the AFM signal model given by

$$s[n] = a[n]\cos(\phi[n]) \tag{8.1}$$

where $a[n]$ and $\phi[n]$ are the instantaneous AE and the instantaneous phase envelope represented as the linear combination of multiple sinusoids and are mathematically modelled as

$$a[n] = A\left(1 + \sum_{m=1}^{M} \mu_{am}\cos(\omega_{am}n + \theta_{am})\right) \tag{8.2}$$

$$\phi[n] = \left(\omega_c n + \sum_{p=1}^{P} \mu_{fp}\sin\left(\omega_{fp}n + \theta_{fp}\right)\right) \tag{8.3}$$

where A and ω_c are the fundamental parameters corresponding to amplitude and carrier frequency of the signal model, respectively. The amplitude envelope $a[n]$ and the phase envelope $\phi[n]$ consist of total M and P sinusoids with subscript 'm' and 'p' representing the mth-tone AM and the pth-tone FM, respectively. Additionally, these envelopes are represented by six other parameters ω_{am}, ω_{fp}, θ_{am}, θ_{fp}, μ_{am} and μ_{fp} corresponding to frequency, phase and modulation index of the mth-tone AM and the pth-tone FM.

Combining equations (8.1), (8.2) and (8.3), the non-stationary PCG signal $s[n]$ using the AFM signal model is mathematically represented as

$$s[n] = A\left(1 + \sum_{m=1}^{M} \mu_{am}\cos(\omega_{am}n + \theta_{am})\right)\cos\left(\omega_c n + \sum_{p=1}^{P} \mu_{fp}\sin\left(\omega_{fp}n + \theta_{fp}\right)\right) \tag{8.4}$$

where the IF component $\Omega[n]$ is obtained from the derivative of the instantaneous phase $\phi[n]$ and is given as

$$\Omega[n] = \frac{\mathrm{d}\phi[n]}{\mathrm{d}n} = \omega_c + \sum_{p=1}^{P} \mu_{fp}\omega_{fp}\cos\left(\omega_{fp}n + \theta_{fp}\right) \tag{8.5}$$

8.2.2 Feature extraction

Feature extraction is one of the most crucial steps in automatic classification. The accuracy of an automatic machine learning based system depends on efficiently extracting the features that represent the entire domain of interest. PCG, a non-stationary signal, has noticeable aspects in its time-varying amplitude and frequency [44]. As discussed in the previous section, these time variations, in amplitudes and frequencies, are modelled using the AFM signal model. The modulating parameters thus obtained, i.e., A, ω_c, ω_{am}, ω_{fp}, θ_{am}, θ_{fp}, μ_{am} and μ_{fp} are sufficient to capture the randomness present in both time-varying amplitude and frequency. Therefore, the proposed framework uses these modulating parameters as the features to represent the domain of interest, i.e., a recorded PCG signal.

In order to extract the features, a sampled PCG signal, $\{s[n]|n = 0, 1, \ldots, N - 1\}$, is initially utilized to obtain the AE and IF components using the DESA algorithm as defined in equations (8.2) and (8.5). Subsequently, the spectrum of AE and IF signals are separately analyzed to obtain frequency-related modulating features, i.e., ω_{am}, ω_{fp} corresponding to both time-variating amplitude and frequency. The complete feature vector containing the modulating feature set is later extracted by solving two independent linear-programming models representing the extracted AE and IF signals.

The detailed discussion and the mathematical modelling involved at every step during the feature extraction are presented in the ensuing subsections.

8.2.2.1 AE and IF component extraction

The PCG sampled sequence, $\{s[n]|n = 0, 1, \ldots, N - 1\}$, is used in the proposed framework to extract the independent AE and IF signals using a DESA algorithm. The DESA algorithm uses a Teager-energy operator, $T(\bullet)$, mathematically defined as [54]

$$T(s[n]) = s^2[n] - s[n-1]s[n+1] \tag{8.6}$$

The AE and IF signals obtained using the Teager-energy operator are mathematically given by

$$|\, a[n]\, | \approx \sqrt{\frac{T[s[n]]}{1 - \left(1 - \frac{T[d[n]] + T[d[n+1]]}{4T[s[n]]}\right)^2}} \tag{8.7}$$

$$\Omega[n] \approx \cos^{-1}\left(1 - \frac{T[d[n]] + T[d[n+1]]}{4T[s[n]]}\right) \tag{8.8}$$

where, $d[n]$ is a single delay differential operator defined as $d[n] = s[n] - s[n-1]$. The extracted $|\, a[n]\, |$ and $\Omega[n]$ signals are used to estimate the modulating features from two independent linear-programming models corresponding to AE and IF signals discussed in the following subsection.

8.2.2.2 Parameter estimation

In order to estimate the feature vectors, the amplitude envelope, as in equation (8.2), can be expanded by replacing the co-sinusoidal variation with its equivalent complex exponentials and is expressed as [49]

$$a[n] = A\left(1 + \frac{1}{2}\sum_{m=1}^{M}\mu_{am}[e^{j\theta_{am}}e^{j\omega_{am}n} + e^{-j\theta_{am}}e^{-j\omega_{am}n}]\right) \tag{8.9}$$

From the above equation, it can be observed that the AE spectrum will clearly include peaks at M modulating frequencies on either side. Therefore, it is feasible to extract AM-modulating frequency features, i.e., ω_{am}, $\forall\, m$, by choosing the pertinent frequency response peaks from the AE spectrum. The other modulating features, μ_{am} and θ_{am}, $\forall\, m$, within equation (8.9), are predicted by solving a linear-programming model formulated by the obtained amplitude sequence $\{a[n] | n = 0, 1, \ldots, N-1\}$. The linear-programming model using the amplitude sequence can be mathematically written as

$$\boldsymbol{a} = \boldsymbol{A}\boldsymbol{b} \tag{8.10}$$

where, $\boldsymbol{a}$ is the sample vector of size $N \times 1$, $\boldsymbol{b}$ is the parameter vector of size $(2M+1) \times 1$ and $\boldsymbol{A}$ is the projection matrix *of* size $N \times (2M+1)$, given by

$$\boldsymbol{a} = \begin{bmatrix} a[0] & a[1] & a[2] & \cdots & a[N-1] \end{bmatrix}^T \tag{8.11}$$

$$\boldsymbol{b} = \begin{bmatrix} A & \frac{A\mu_{a1}}{2}e^{j\theta_{a1}} & \frac{A\mu_{a1}}{2}e^{-j\theta_{a1}} & \ldots & \frac{A\mu_{aM}}{2}e^{j\theta_{aM}} & \frac{A\mu_{aM}}{2}e^{-j\theta_{aM}} \end{bmatrix}^T \tag{8.12}$$

$$\boldsymbol{A} = \begin{bmatrix} 1 & 1 & 1 & \ldots & 1 & 1 \\ 1 & e^{j\omega_{a1}} & e^{-j\omega_{a1}} & \ldots & e^{j\omega_{aM}} & e^{-j\omega_{aM}} \\ 1 & e^{j2\omega_{a1}} & e^{-j2\omega_{a1}} & \ldots & e^{j2\omega_{aM}} & e^{-j2\omega_{aM}} \\ \vdots & \vdots & \vdots & \ldots & \vdots & \vdots \\ 1 & e^{j(N-1)\omega_{a1}} & e^{-j(N-1)\omega_{a1}} & \ldots & e^{j(N-1)\omega_{aM}} & e^{-j(N-1)\omega_{aM}} \end{bmatrix} \tag{8.13}$$

The above projection matrix $\boldsymbol{A}$ is an overdetermined, as $N > (2M+1)$, and a known matrix, as ω_{am}, $\forall\, m$ are already obtained by analyzing the AE spectrum. Therefore, the least-squares solution of the linear-programming model, as defined in equation (8.10), will provide an estimate of the column vector $\boldsymbol{b}$ with its optimal value given as

$$\boldsymbol{b}^* = (\boldsymbol{A}^H\boldsymbol{A})^{-1}\boldsymbol{A}^H\boldsymbol{a} \tag{8.14}$$

This optimal value of $\boldsymbol{b}$ contains the mean amplitude A, the modulation indexes μ_{am} and the phase features θ_{am}, corresponding to amplitude envelope and can be obtained as

$$A = |b_1^*|; \quad \mu_{am} = \frac{2}{A}|b_{2m}^*|, \forall\, m; \quad \theta_{am} = \angle b_{2m}^*, \forall\, \mathrm{m} \tag{8.15}$$

Similar to AE, the IF envelope can be analyzed to obtain the FM-based modulating features. To analyze the IF spectrum, equation (8.5) can be re-written as

$$\Omega[n] = \omega_c + \frac{1}{2}\sum\nolimits_{p=1}^{P} \mu_{fp}\omega_{fp}[e^{j\theta_{fp}}e^{j\omega_{fp}n} + e^{-j\theta_{fp}}e^{-j\omega_{fp}n}] \tag{8.16}$$

From this expression, it is observed that IF spectrum will have pertinent frequency response peaks at P modulating frequencies, ω_{fp} , $\forall\, p$, on either side, and, therefore, these frequencies can be easily extracted. Similar to AE, the other FM modulating features, μ_{fp} and θ_{fp}, $\forall\, p$, are extracted by solving a linear-programing model, corresponding to IF envelope, given by

$$\boldsymbol{c} = \boldsymbol{W}\boldsymbol{d} \tag{8.17}$$

where, $\boldsymbol{c}$ is the sample vector of size $N \times 1$, $\boldsymbol{d}$ is the parameter vector of size $(2P + 1) \times 1$ and the matrix $\boldsymbol{W}$ is in the size of $N \times (2P + 1)$, given by

$$\boldsymbol{c} = \begin{bmatrix} c[0] & c[1] & c[2] & \cdots & c[N-1] \end{bmatrix}^T \tag{8.18}$$

$$\boldsymbol{d} = \begin{bmatrix} \omega_c & \frac{\mu_{f1}\omega_{f1}\mathrm{e}^{\mathrm{j}\theta_{f1}}}{2} & \frac{\mu_{f1}\omega_{f1}\mathrm{e}^{-\mathrm{j}\theta_{f1}}}{2} & \cdots & \frac{\mu_{fp}\omega_{fp}\mathrm{e}^{\mathrm{j}\theta_{fP}}}{2} & \frac{\mu_{fp}\omega_{fp}\mathrm{e}^{-\mathrm{j}\theta_{fP}}}{2} \end{bmatrix}^T \tag{8.19}$$

$$\boldsymbol{W} = \begin{bmatrix} 1 & 1 & 1 & \cdots & 1 & 1 \\ 1 & \mathrm{e}^{\mathrm{j}\omega_{f1}} & \mathrm{e}^{-\mathrm{j}\omega_{f1}} & \cdots & \mathrm{e}^{\mathrm{j}\omega_{fP}} & \mathrm{e}^{-\mathrm{j}\omega_{fP}} \\ 1 & \mathrm{e}^{\mathrm{j}2\omega_{f1}} & \mathrm{e}^{-\mathrm{j}2\omega_{f1}} & \cdots & \mathrm{e}^{\mathrm{j}2\omega_{fP}} & \mathrm{e}^{-\mathrm{j}2\omega_{fP}} \\ \vdots & \vdots & \vdots & \cdots & \vdots & \vdots \\ 1 & \mathrm{e}^{\mathrm{j}(N-1)\omega_{f1}} & \mathrm{e}^{-\mathrm{j}(N-1)\omega_{f1}} & \cdots & \mathrm{e}^{\mathrm{j}(N-1)\omega_{fP}} & \mathrm{e}^{-\mathrm{j}(N-1)\omega_{fP}} \end{bmatrix} \tag{8.20}$$

The above projection matrix $\boldsymbol{W}$ is an overdetermined, as $N > (2P + 1)$, and a known matrix, as ω_{fp} , $\forall\ p$ are obtained from IF spectrum, the least-squares solution of the linear model defined in equation (8.17) is given as

$$\boldsymbol{d}^* = (\boldsymbol{W}^H\boldsymbol{W})^{-1}\boldsymbol{W}^H\boldsymbol{c} \tag{8.21}$$

Similar to $\boldsymbol{b}^*$, the optimal value of $\boldsymbol{d}$ contains the central frequency ω_c, the modulation indexes μ_{fp} and the phase features θ_{fp},corresponding to IF envelope are obtained as

$$\omega_c = |d_1^*|;\ \mu_{fp} = \frac{2}{\omega_{fp}}\left|d_{2p}^*\right|,\ \forall\ \mathrm{p};\ \theta_{fp} = \angle d_{2p}^*,\ \forall\ p \tag{8.22}$$

The combined modulating features extracted for both AE and IF envelope are then used in the proposed framework as the feature set to train an ensemble classifier to automatically detect and classify the HVDs, if any.

8.2.3 Classification techniques

A machine learning technique called ensemble learning classifier [53] combines predictions from various models to enhance the prediction accuracy. In this context, a bagged trees ensemble learning classifier aggregates the performance of multiple individual decision trees, as illustrated in figure 8.4. The unique subsets of samples are fitted to each decision tree (DT) for training and prediction, and the class predicted by maximum number of trees, individually, is decided as the final prediction of a bagged tree classifier. This improves both the learning rate and the classification accuracy. Unlike decision tree classifiers, the overfitting problem is also significantly reduced. The robustness of a bagged trees classifier depends on the number of trees, thus resulting in higher classification accuracy.

In the proposed framework, the HVDs detection problem is formulated as a classification problem. The AFM signal model is used to extract the modulating features from the entire dataset of PCG signals before the classification. The dataset

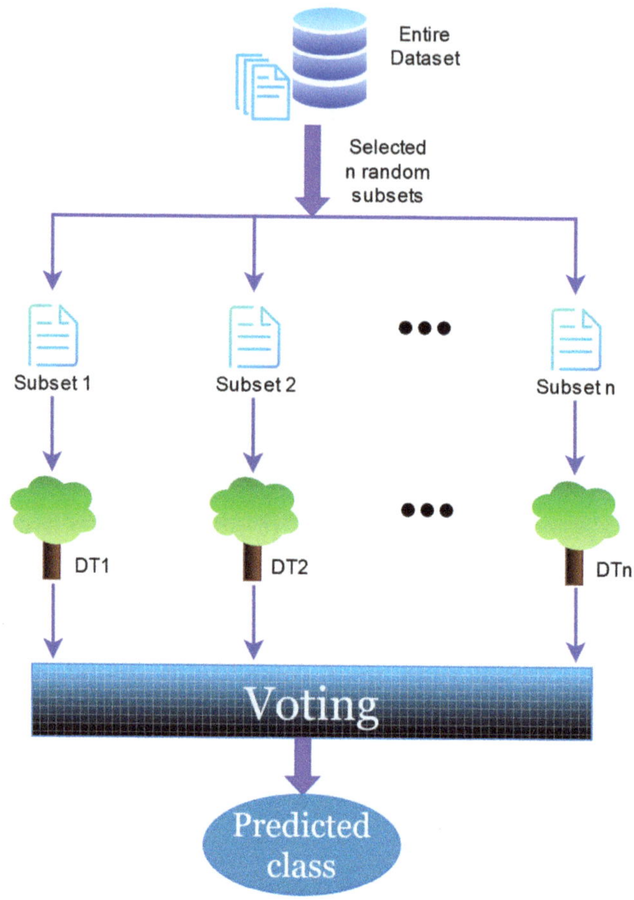

Figure 8.4. Bagged trees ensemble learning classifier.

is divided into training and testing by using k-fold cross-validation. The $k-1$ subsets are utilized to train the model and the remaining one set is utilized for model testing. Three cycles of the PCG signals are used to extract the feature vector, $\boldsymbol{x}_i$ and are categorized to a class y_i out of five possible classes considered in the framework. The ensemble classifier as discussed above is then used for HVD detection and classification.

8.3 Performance measures

8.3.1 Database

A public database [26] is used to gather the PCG signals. A total of 1000 PCG recordings in audio (.wav) file format from various patients are included in the database. The database consists of five different classes including 200 samples from normal class and 800 samples from four abnormal classes (AS, MR, MS, and MVP) are shown in table 8.1. Each PCG recording contains three PCG cycles in the dataset

Table 8.1. Database.

Binary class	Multiple classes	Number of signals in each class
Normal	N	200
	AS	200
HVD	MR	200
	MS	200
	MVP	200
Total		1000

recorded at 8000 Hz sampling rate. In this study, all PCG recordings from all five classes are taken into account for the detection of HVD. In this investigation, the PCG signal was filtered using a low-pass filter with a cut-off frequency of 1000 Hz.

8.3.2 Confusion matrix

A table containing the predicted and actual data is the confusion matrix [55]. It is used to demonstrate how well the classifier is performing. The correctly identified data for each class is displayed in the confusion matrix's diagonal entries. The confusion matrix is explained in the application of binary classification for HVD detection for the positive class as HVD patients and the negative class as normal patients. True positive (TP) refers to the number of actual HVD patients who are predicted to be HVD, while true negative (TN) refers to the number of actual normal patients who are predicted to be normal. The false negative (FN) is the number of actual HVD patients who are classified as normal, while the false positive (FP) is the number of actual normal patients who are classified as HVD.

8.3.2.1 Accuracy

The accuracy is defined by the proportion of successfully predicted data to all accessible datasets. The ratio of correctly classified samples to total number of samples can be used to calculate accuracy. It is a useful measure when applied to a balanced dataset, but when applied to an unbalanced dataset, the accuracy of an unbalanced dataset is heavily biased toward the higher sample class. To evaluate the performance of an unbalanced dataset, other matrices such as precision, recall, and $F1$-measure are used [56].

$$\text{Acc} = \frac{\text{TP} + \text{TN}}{\text{Total number of samples}}$$

8.3.2.2 Precision

The proportion of chosen data that are correctly classified for a class is known as precision. The ratio of TP to the total predicted positive class (TP+FP) can be used to calculate the precision value of the positive class. The precision for the HVD class will let us know what percentage of the total patients is actually made up of HVD detection.

$$\text{Prec} = \frac{\text{TP}}{\text{Total predicted as positive}}$$

8.3.2.3 Recall

The proportion of data correctly classified from a class of actual data is referred to as recall. The recall value for the positive class can be calculated using the ratio of true positive to total samples of the actual positive class (TP+FN). The recall will reveal the percentage of patients correctly identified as having HVD out of all actual HVD patients.

$$\text{Rec} = \frac{\text{TP}}{\text{Actual positive samples}}$$

For better classification, the recall and precision should be high (near to one). In actuality, a hybrid approach is preferred that is called $F1$-measure.

8.3.2.4 F1-measure

The $F1$-measure ($F1_{\text{mes}}$) is a composite metric that evaluates the precision–recall balance [57]. The harmonic mean of the precision and recall serves as the $F1$-measure.

$$F1_{\text{mes}} = \frac{2 * \text{Prec} * \text{Rec}}{\text{Prec} + \text{Rec}}$$

8.4 Results and discussion

This section presents the analysis of the results obtained from the proposed features and classification. In this study, 1000 PCG signals from HVD patients and normal people are analyzed. For categorization purposes, 800 samples from the HVD class and 200 samples from the normal class are employed. The first stage in the process is to analyze the PCG signal using an AFM signal model. The HVD samples are further divided into four additional categories: AS, MR, MS, and MVP, each with 200 samples. Because PCG signals are non-stationary, AFM model decomposition is used to effectively deal with PCG signal's non-stationarity.

In the experiment, two categories of classification problems are considered. The first category addresses the binary classification between normal and HVD signals. The second category involves multiclass classification, making a distinction between the five categories listed earlier. For both categories of classification task, the PCG signals are first represented using the AFM model. The representation of PCG signal using the AFM model makes it suitable to extract AE and IF using the DESA algorithm. Further, the modulating features are extracted from the AE and IF components. A total of 14 modulating features are computed and used as features

Table 8.2. Results of Kruskal–Wallis test on different features.

AE features	*p*-Value	IF features	*p*-Value
A	9.44×10^{-30}	ω_c	3.38×10^{-60}
ω_{a1}	1.16×10^{-117}	ω_{f1}	4.94×10^{-4}
ω_{a2}	1.47×10^{-108}	ω_{f2}	3.87×10^{-12}
μ_{a1}	2.43×10^{-72}	μ_{f1}	6.71×10^{-27}
μ_{a2}	2.16×10^{-19}	μ_{f2}	3.33×10^{-07}
θ_{a1}	4.44×10^{-23}	θ_{f1}	0.08
θ_{a1}	2.41×10^{-11}	θ_{f2}	0.16

for both binary and multiclass classification. The statistical significance of the features is tested statistically using Kruskal–Wallis test [58]. The nonparametric version of one-way ANOVA is considered as Kruskal–Wallis test, which is applicable to data with two or more groups. In this work, the mentioned five classes are considered as the groups for Kruskal–Wallis test. The statistical significance of features is shown in terms of its *p*-value as listed in table 8.2. It is evident that most of the features show statistical significance except two features of modulating phases θ_{f1} and θ_{f2}. The θ_{f1} and θ_{f2} are derived from IF obtained from PCG signals. All the features obtained from AE show significant discrimination abilities as evident from the *p*-values (table 8.2). The boxplot of the features obtained from AE of different PCG classes are also depicted in figure 8.5. It is evident that all the features obtained from AE have distinct median values and can be considered significant for classification. Similarly, the boxplots depicted in figure 8.6 show the distribution of the features computed from IF. It can be observed that most of the features obtained from IF have distinct median values except θ_{f1} and θ_{f2}. In the classification experiments, all the features are considered to create feature vector for classification. In the subsequent subsections, the classification experiment for both binary and multiclass classification are discussed in detail.

8.4.1 Binary classification

The aim for the binary classification is to show the effectiveness of the proposed method in separating normal signal from HVD signals. The classification results of binary classification using different ensemble classifiers are computed. The classification accuracy obtained using boosted trees, bagged trees, subspace discriminant (SSD), subspace *k*-nearest neighbors (SS-KNN), and RUS boosted trees classifiers are listed as shown in table 8.3. For the purpose of robust classification, the results are obtained with 10-fold cross-validation. The results indicate that the bagged tree classifier provides best classification accuracy for the normal and HVD class. On the other hand, the SSD results in the poorest classification accuracy. The classification performance is similar by boosted tree and SS-KNN classifiers. However, RUS boosted trees resulted in comparable results with Bagged tree classifier. The correctly

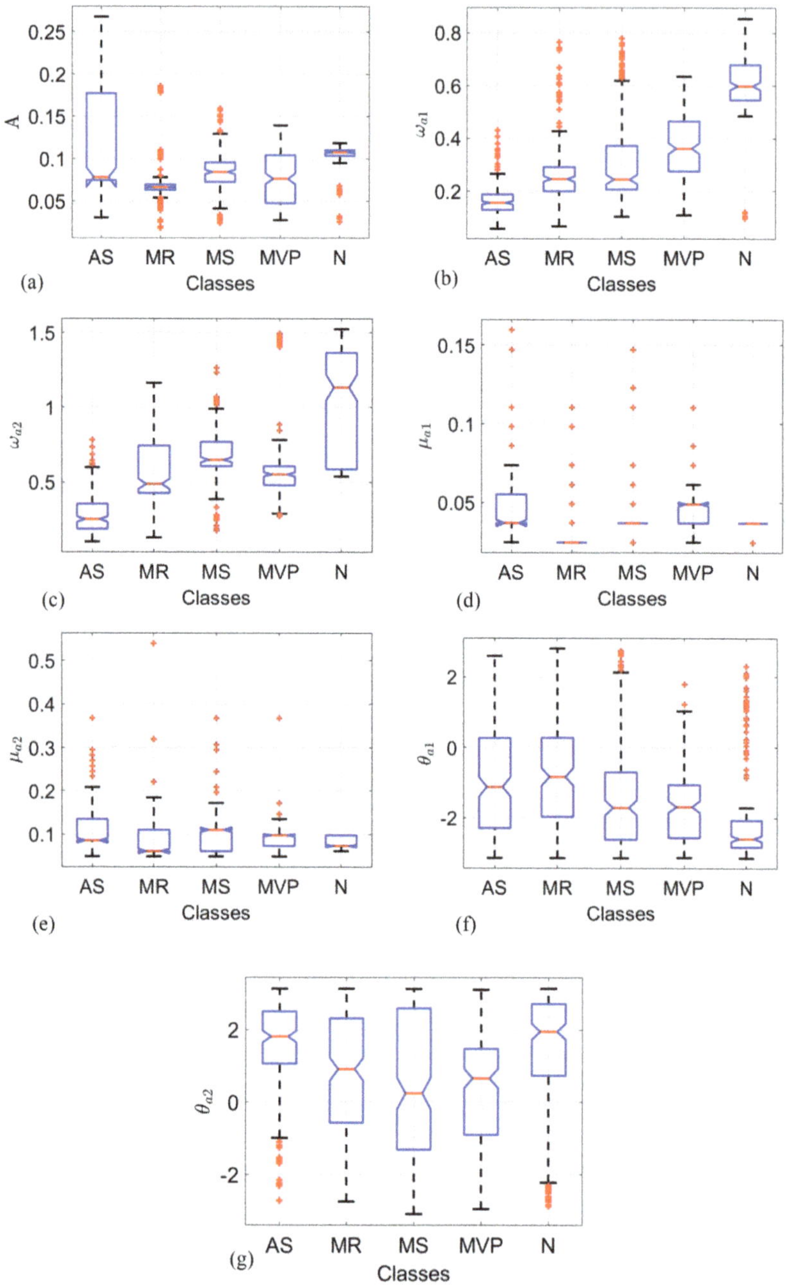

Figure 8.5. Boxplots of features obtained from AE components of PCG signals. (a) A (b) ω_{a1} (c) ω_{a2} (d) μ_{a1} (e) μ_{a2} (f) θ_{a1} (g) θ_{a2}

classified instances of normal and HVD patients are depicted in figure 8.7. The overall average accuracy using bagged trees classifier is 99.5% with 798 and 197 instances correctly classified for HVD and normal classes, respectively.

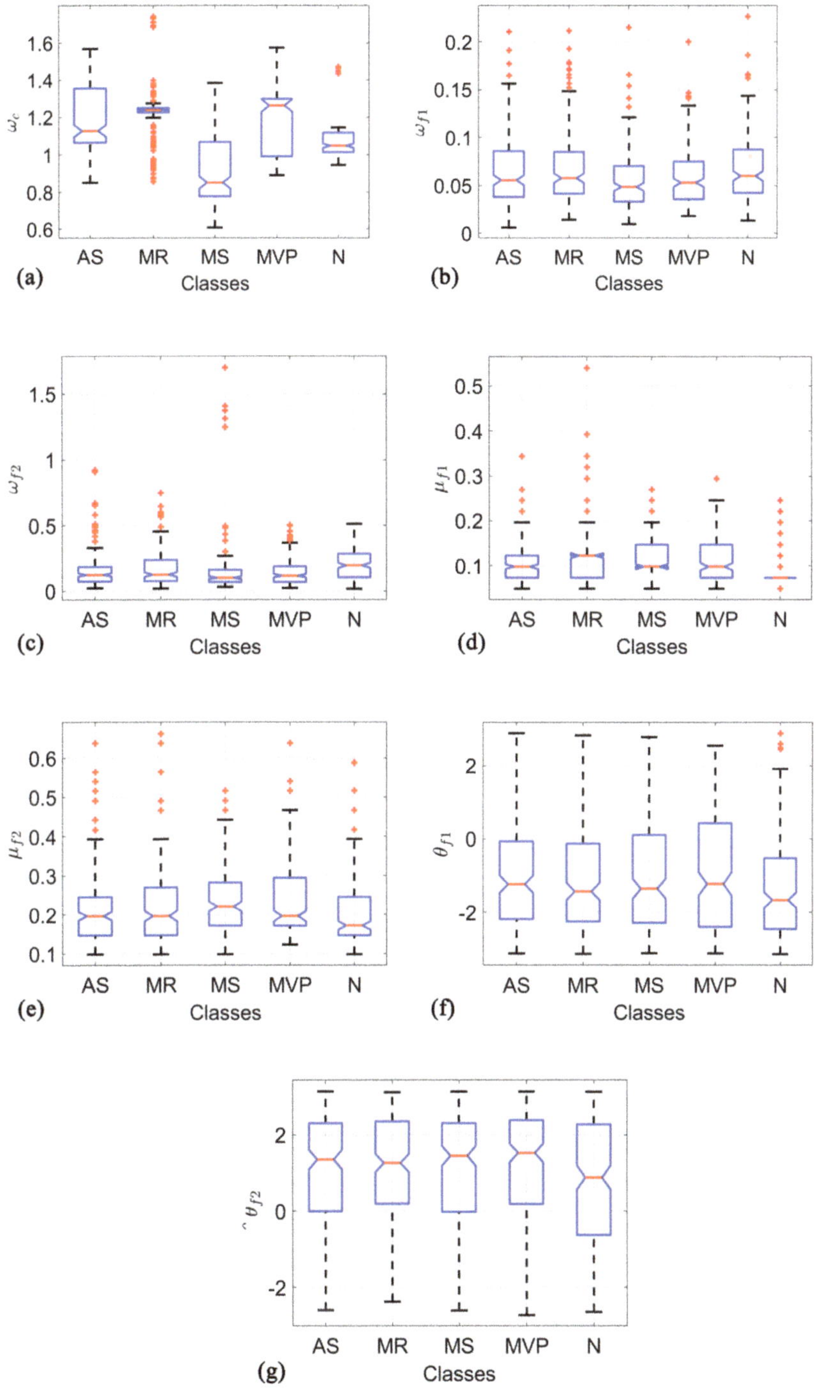

Figure 8.6. Boxplots of features obtained from IF components of PCG signals. (a) ω_c, (b) ω_{f1}, (c) ω_{f2}, (d) μ_{f1}, (e) μ_{f2}, (f) θ_{f1} and (g) θ_{f2}.

Table 8.3. Classification accuracy (%) of binary class using ensemble learning classifier.

Class	Boosted trees	Bagged trees	SSD	SS-KNN	RUS boosted tress
Normal	96.1	98.5	91.6	95.9	99.4
HVD	94.9	99.7	72.4	93.3	98
OA	95.9	99.5	88.1	95.4	99.1

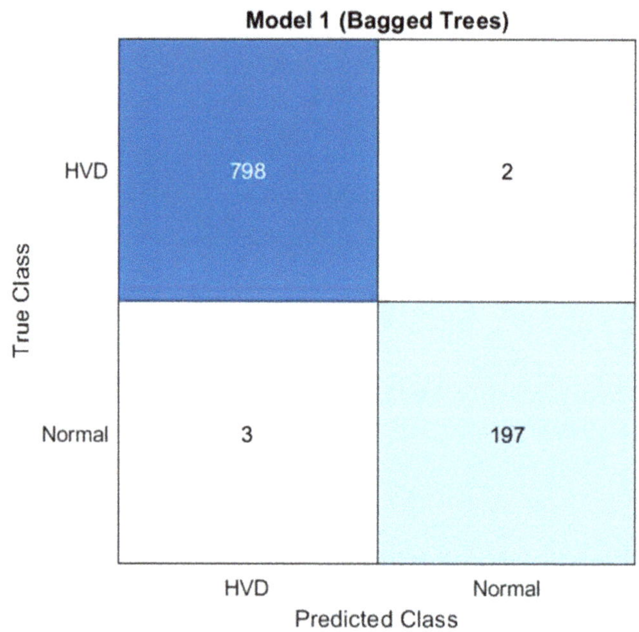

Figure 8.7. Confusion matrix for HVD detection in PCG signals.

In the binary classification, the number of samples is unbalanced. Usually, the accuracy of an unbalanced dataset is heavily biased toward the higher sample class. Precision, recall, and $F1$-score are calculated to overcome the issue of high biasing. In an unbalanced dataset, the higher the value of $F1$-score, the better the classification results. The precision, recall, and $F1$-score for the binary classification are 0.996, 0.9975, 0.9967 respectively. These parameters have values close to one, indicating the robustness of the proposed features for PCG classification.

8.4.2 Multiclass classification

The strength of the proposed method for distinguishing different categories of the HVD is described in terms of the performance of multiclass classification. The results obtained when the proposed features are used with boosted trees, bagged trees, SSD, SS-KNN, and RUS boosted trees classifiers are shown in table 8.4. The

Table 8.4. Classification accuracy (%) of multiclass using ensemble learning classifier.

Class	Boosted trees	Bagged trees	SSD	SS-KNN	RUS boosted trees
AS	83.1	91.4	76.3	78	87.6
MR	95.5	94.2	60.7	69.8	91.8
MS	91.4	97	63.4	86.1	78.3
MVP	86.5	92.2	68.1	74.3	84
N	98.5	99	70.6	86.8	97.3
OA	90.7	94.7	67.8	79	87.5

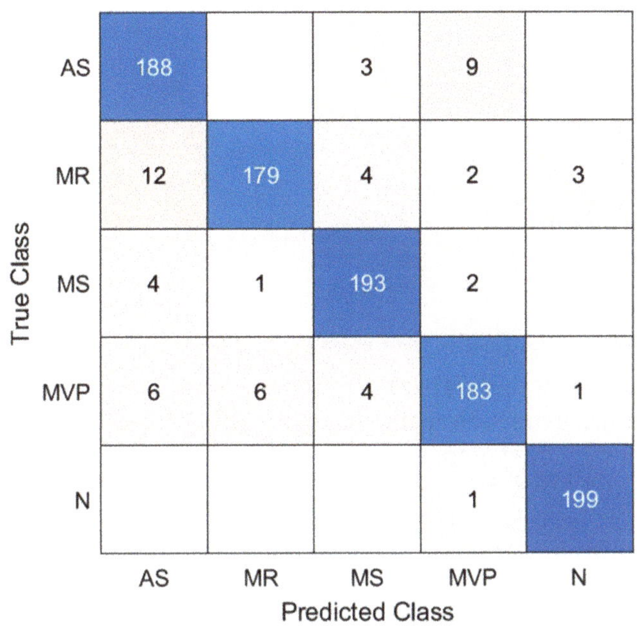

Figure 8.8. Confusion matrix for multiclass classification in PCG signals.

robustness of the performance is ensured by employing 10-fold cross-validation. It is evident from the table that a bagged tree classifier detected all the classes with highest accuracy. The accuracy value is 94.7% which is better than all other ensemble learning classifiers used. The boosted trees and RUS boosted trees provide moderate results. On the other hand, SSD classifier resulted in 67.8% which was the lowest accuracy among all classifiers. Further, the confusion matrix of the results obtained using bagged tree classifier is depicted in figure 8.8. Among all the HVD classes, the bagged tree classifier detects the signals from MS class most accurately with an accuracy of 97%. On the other hand, the classification accuracy is 91.4% for AS class. Moreover, the classifier efficacy is also evident from the ROC curves presented in figure 8.9. The area under curve (AUC) is more than 0.99 for all the classes, which further confirms the robust performance of the proposed method.

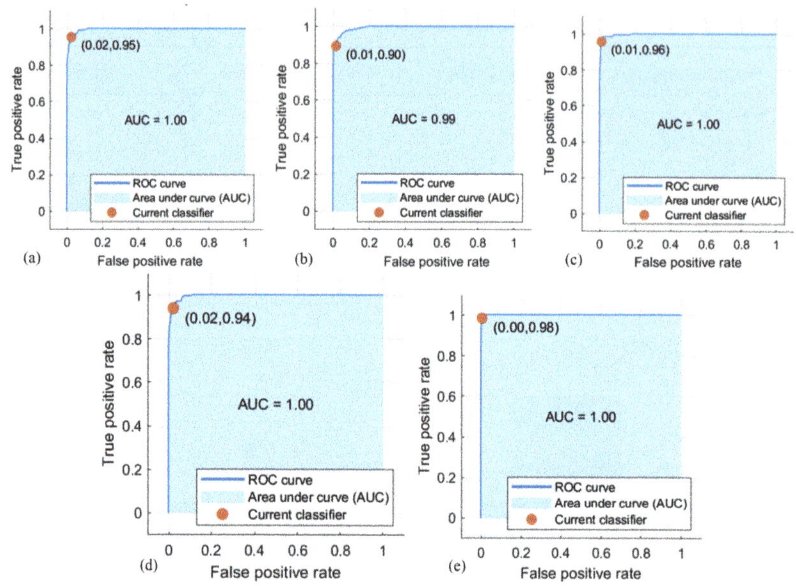

Figure 8.9. The ROC curve for bagged tree ensemble learning classifier to detect HVD in (a) AS, (b) MR, (c) MS, (d) MVP and (e) normal PCG signals.

8.4.3 Comparison of the results with existing methods

The comparison results of the HVD detection by proposed modulating features and the existing feature extraction methods are shown in table 8.5. The SVM and the DNN classifiers were used in the research published in [26] to assess the performance of the MFCC and DWT-based features. Using MFCC and DWT characteristics, they achieved an accuracy of 91.60% and 92.30%, respectively, using the SVM classifier. They further performed the experiment using DNN classifier and achieved accuracy of 86.50% and 87.80% with MFCC and DWT features, respectively. However, when MFCC and DWT features were jointly given as the input to the SVM, the classification accuracy achieved is 97.90%. The proposed technique achieves greater accuracy value by using ensemble learning classifiers as compared to the methods involving separate MFCC and DWT features with SVM [26]. However, the proposed features have a lower accuracy value than that of the combination of both DWT and MFCC features using SVM. Moreover, the proposed method only used 14 features, whereas the method presented in [26] used a total of 43 features, including 24 DWT and 19 MFCC features. The authors of references [8] and [59] used a variety of wavelet domain features to detect HVDs and the reported accuracy values are 91.96% and 85.50%, respectively. The tunable Q-wavelet transform (TQWT) domain sub-bands of PCG signal were used by the authors of [20] to extract various statistical features, and they reported an overall accuracy of 94.01% using a least-square-SVM classifier. Ghosh *et al* [21] used time–frequency magnitude and phase features to improve the accuracy of HVD detection using random forest classifiers, and they obtained a significant improvement in the

Table 8.5. Comparison table for HVD detection.

Author	Features used	Classifier	Accuracy (%)
Yaseen *et al* [26]	MFCC features	SVM	91.60
	DWT features		92.30
	DWT and MFCC features		97.90
Yaseen *et al* [26]	MFCC features	DNN	86.50
	DWT features		87.80
	DWT and MFCC features		92.10
Ari *et al* [8]	Wavelet domain features	Least-square-SVM	91.96
Li *et al* [59]	Wavelet packet norm features	Twin-SVM	85.50
Patidar *et al* [20]	Statistical features using TQWT domain	Least-square-SVM	94.01
Ghosh *et al* [21]	Time–frequency magnitude and phase features	Random forest	95.13
Proposed work	Modulating features	Ensemble learning	94.7

result with an accuracy of 95.13% with fewer features, but they classified the samples into four different classes, excluding MVP. To improve the accuracy of all five classes, the proposed model employs ensemble learning classifiers with modulating features on all five existing classes. The modulating features play a significant role in improving the model's classification and recognition accuracy. For binary class and multiclass classifications, the proposed model has accuracies of 99.5% and 94.7%, respectively. The classification using the proposed method between HVD and normal PCG signals is more accurate. We have also observed some misclassifications in the AR, MS and MVP classes, which may be due to the use of a limited number of features. The classification accuracy of the above classes may increase by including a higher number of modulating features. Overall, the proposed model shows the significance classification accuracy with a smaller number of features (only 14) for PCG classification/HVD detection employing all five classes.

8.5 Conclusion

In this chapter, we have presented a model-based technique utilizing multi-tone AFM signal model and various ensemble learning classifiers for PCG classifications and HVD detection. For the purpose of estimating the parameters of multi-tone AFM signals, the AE and IF functions are extracted from DESA and then individually analyzed. There are a total of 14 modulating features computed and used as feature vector for both binary and multiclass classification using ensemble learning classifiers with 10-fold CV. We performed two experiments on PCG signal classifications using modulating features. The first experiment performed is as binary classifier to detect the HVD patients from normal classes of people. The second experiment is a multiclass classifier which shows the results of five different classes of PCG signals. The experimental results reveal that the proposed method for HVD detection using bagged trees classifier achieved best accuracy. The overall accuracy achieved for the binary classification is 99.5% and for the multiclass classification is 94.7%, outperforming the existing methods.

References

[1] Li S, Xu L D and Zhao S 2015 The Internet of Things: a survey *Inf. Syst. Front.* **17** 243–59

[2] Bandyopadhyay D and Sen J 2011 Internet of Things: applications and challenges in technology and standardization *Wirel. Pers. Commun.* **581** 49–69

[3] Kaur S and Singh I A survey report on internet of things applications *Int. J. Comput. Sci. Trends Technol.* **4** 330–5

[4] Virani S S *et al* 2021 Heart disease and stroke statistics—2021 update *Circulation* **143** E254–743

[5] Chandraratna P A N, Lopez J M and Cohen L S 1975 Echocardiographic observations on the mechanism of production of the second heart sound *Circulation* **51** 292–6

[6] Mondal A, Kumar A K, Bhattacharya P S and Saha G 2013 Boundary estimation of cardiac events S1 and S2 based on Hilbert transform and adaptive thresholding approach *2013 Indian Conf. Med. Informatics Telemedicine, ICMIT (2013)* 43–7

[7] El-Dahshan E-S A, Ali M and Yahiea A 2020 An efficient computational approach for phonocardiogram signals analysis and normal/abnormal heart sounds diagnosis *Arab J. Nucl. Sci. Appl.* **53** 162–77

[8] Ari S, Hembram K and Saha G 2010 Detection of cardiac abnormality from PCG signal using LMS based least square SVM classifier *Expert Syst. Appl.* **37** 8019–26

[9] Sacks M S and Yoganathan A P 2007 Heart valve function: a biomechanical perspective *Phil. Trans. R. Soc.* **B 362** 1369

[10] Hinton R B and Yutzey K E 2011 Heart valve structure and function in development and disease *Annu. Rev. Physiol.* **73** 29

[11] Nivitha Varghees V and Ramachandran K I 2017 Effective heart sound segmentation and murmur classification using empirical wavelet transform and instantaneous phase for electronic stethoscope *IEEE Sens. J.* **17** 3861–72

[12] Mishra M, Banerjee S, Thomas D C, Dutta S and Mukherjee A 2018 Detection of third heart sound using variational mode decomposition *IEEE Trans. Instrum. Meas.* **67** 1713–21

[13] Matulevicius S A, Rohatgi A, Das S R, Price A L, DeLuna A and Reimold S C 2013 Appropriate use and clinical impact of transthoracic echocardiography *JAMA Intern. Med.* **173** 1600–7

[14] Joseph M X, Disney P J S, Da Costa R and Hutchison S J 2004 Transthoracic echocardiography to identify or exclude cardiac cause of shock *Chest* **126** 1592–7

[15] Malik S B, Chen N, Parker R A and Hsu J Y 2017 Transthoracic echocardiography: Pitfalls and limitations as delineated at cardiac CT and MR imaging *Radiographics* **37** 383–406

[16] Reed T R, Reed N E and Fritzson P 2004 Heart sound analysis for symptom detection and computer-aided diagnosis *Simul. Model. Pract. Theory* **12** 129–46

[17] Arora V, Leekha R, Singh R and Chana I 2019 Heart sound classification using machine learning and phonocardiogram *Mod. Phys. Lett.* **33** 1950321

[18] Dwivedi A K, Imtiaz S A and Rodriguez-Villegas E 2019 Algorithms for automatic analysis and classification of heart sounds—a systematic review *IEEE Access* **7** 8316–45

[19] Daniel E, Durga S, Iwin Thanakumar Joseph S, Angelin D and Raj S B E 2022 IoT-based ensemble method on PCG signal classification to predict heart diseases *Secure Communication for 5G and IoT NetworksEAI/Springer Innovations in Communication and Computing* (Cham: Springer) pp 101–16
[20] Patidar S and Pachori R B 2014 Classification of cardiac sound signals using constrained tunable-*Q* wavelet transform *Expert Syst. Appl.* **41** 7161–70
[21] Ghosh S K, Tripathy R K, Ponnalagu R N and Pachori R B 2019 Automated detection of heart valve disorders from the PCG signal using time–frequency magnitude and phase features *IEEE Sensors Lett.* **3** 1–4
[22] Karhade J, Dash S, Ghosh S K, Dash D K and Tripathy R K 2022 Time–frequency-domain deep learning framework for the automated detection of heart valve disorders using PCG signals *IEEE Trans. Instrum. Meas.* **71** 1–11
[23] Her H and Chiu H-W 2016 Using time–frequency features to recognize abnormal heart sounds *2016 Computing in Cardiology Conf. (CinC)* 1145–7
[24] Litvin Y, Cohen I and Chazan D 2010 Monaural speech/music source separation using discrete energy separation algorithm *Signal Process.* **90** 3147–63
[25] Debbal S M and Bereksi-Reguig F 2007 Time–frequency analysis of the first and the second heartbeat sounds *Appl. Math. Comput.* **184** 1041–52
[26] Yaseen S G Y and Kwon S 2018 Classification of heart sound signal using multiple features *Appl. Sci.* **8** 2344–4
[27] Uğuz H 2012 Adaptive neuro-fuzzy inference system for diagnosis of the heart valve diseases using wavelet transform with entropy *Neural Comput. Appl.* **21** 1617–28
[28] Zeng W, Lin Z, Yuan C, Wang Q, Liu F and Wang Y 2021 Detection of heart valve disorders from PCG signals using TQWT, FA-MVEMD, Shannon energy envelope and deterministic learning *Artif. Intell. Rev.* **54** 6063–100
[29] Ismail S, Siddiqi I and Akram U 2018 Localization and classification of heart beats in phonocardiography signals—a comprehensive review *EURASIP J. Adv. Signal Process.* **2018** 26
[30] Debbal S M, Bereksi-Reguig F and Tani A M 2004 The fast Fourier transform and the continuous wavelet transform analysis of the phonocardiogram signal *J. Mech. Med. Biol.* **4** 257–72
[31] Gopika P, Sowmya V, Gopalakrishnan E A and Soman K P 2019 Performance improvement of deep learning architectures for phonocardiogram signal classification using fast Fourier transform *Proc. 2019 9th Int. Conf. Adv. Comput. Commun. ICACC* vol 2019 290–4
[32] Debbal S M and Bereksi-Reguig F 2008 Computerized heart sounds analysis *Comput. Biol. Med.* **38** 263–80
[33] Ghosh S K, Ponnalagu R N, Tripathy R K and Acharya U R 2020 Automated detection of heart valve diseases using chirplet transform and multiclass composite classifier with PCG signals *Comput. Biol. Med.* **118** 103632
[34] Morshed M, Fattah S A and Saquib M 2022 Automated heart valve disorder detection based on PDF modeling of formant variation pattern in PCG signal *IEEE Access* **10** 27330–42
[35] Zeng W, Su B, Yuan C and Chen Y 2022 Automatic detection of heart valve disorders using Teager–Kaiser energy operator, rational-dilation wavelet transform and convolutional neural networks with PCG signals *Artif. Intell. Rev.* **56** 781–806

[36] Beritelli F, Capizzi G, Lo Sciuto G, Napoli C and Scaglione F 2018 Automatic heart activity diagnosis based on Gram polynomials and probabilistic neural networks *Biomed. Eng. Lett.* **8** 77

[37] Maknickas V and Maknickas A 2017 Recognition of normal–abnormal phonocardiographic signals using deep convolutional neural networks and mel-frequency spectral coefficients *Physiol. Meas.* **38** 1671–84

[38] Faust O, Hagiwara Y, Hong T J, Lih O S and Acharya U R 2018 Deep learning for healthcare applications based on physiological signals: a review *Comput. Methods Programs Biomed.* **161** 1–13

[39] Oh S L, Jahmunah V, Ooi C P, Tan R S, Ciaccio E J, Yamakawa T, Tanabe M, Kobayashi M and Rajendra Acharya U 2020 Classification of heart sound signals using a novel deep WaveNet model *Comput. Methods Programs Biomed.* **196** 105604

[40] Shwedyk E, Balasubramanian R and Scott R N 1977 A nonstationary model for the electromyogram *IEEE Trans. Biomed. Eng.* **BME-24** 417–24

[41] Sircar P and Syali M S 1996 Complex AM signal model for non-stationary signals *Signal Process.* **53** 35–45

[42] Sircar P and Sharma S 1997 Complex FM signal model for non-stationary signals *Signal Process.* **57** 283–304

[43] Upadhyay A, Sharma M, Pachori R B and Sharma R 2020 A nonparametric approach for multicomponent AM–FM signal analysis *Circuits Syst. Signal Process* **39** 6316–57

[44] Hood A S, Pachori R B, Reddy V K and Sircar P 2015 Parametric representation of speech employing multi-component AFM signal model *Int. J. Speech Technol.* **18** 287–303

[45] Bansal M and Sircar P 2018 Parametric representation of voiced speech phoneme using multicomponent AM signal model *Proc. 17th IEEE/ACIS Int. Conf. on Computer and Information Science (ICIS 2018)* 128–33

[46] Bansal M and Sircar P 2018 Low bit-rate speech coding based on multicomponent AFM signal model *Int. J. Speech Technol.* **21** 783–95

[47] Bansal M and Sircar P 2019 Phoneme based model for gender identification and adult-child classification *2019 13th Int. Conf. on Signal Processing and Communication Systems (ICSPCS 2019 Proc.)*

[48] Bansal M and Sircar P 2019 A novel AFM signal model for parametric representation of speech phonemes *Circuits Syst. Signal Process* **38** 4079–95

[49] Pachori R B and Sircar P 2010 Analysis of multicomponent AM–FM signals using FB-DESA method *Digit. Signal Process.* **20** 42–62

[50] Bansal M and Sircar P 2021 AFM signal model for digit recognition *2021 Int. Conf. on Wireless Communications, Signal Processing and Networking (WiSPNET 2021)* pp 354–8

[51] Bansal M and Sircar P 2022 Phoneme classification using modulating features *2022 IEEE Region 10 Symp, (TENSYMP) (Mumbai)* pp 1–5

[52] Sharma R, Pachori R B and Upadhyay A 2017 Automatic sleep stages classification based on iterative filtering of electroencephalogram signals *Neural Comput. Appl.* **28** 2959–78

[53] Sagi O and Rokach L 2018 Ensemble learning: a survey *Wiley Interdiscip. Rev. Data Min. Knowl. Discov.* **8** e1249

[54] Cho S H, Hur J and Chung I Y 2014 An applicability of Teager energy operator and energy separation algorithm for waveform distortion analysis: harmonics, inter-harmonics and frequency variation *J. Electr. Eng. Technol* **9** 1210–6

[55] Susmaga R 2004 Confusion matrix visualization *Intelligent Information Processing and Web MiningAdvances in Soft Computing* vol 25 (Berlin: Springer) pp 107–16
[56] Goutte C and Gaussier E 2005 A probabilistic interpretation of precision, recall and *F*-score, with implication for evaluation *Lect. Notes Comput. Sci.* **3408** 345–59
[57] Davis J and Goadrich M 2006 The relationship between precision–recall and ROC curves *ACM Int. Conf. Proc. Ser.* **148** 233–40
[58] McKight P E and Najab J 2010 Kruskal–Wallis test *The Corsini Encyclopedia of Psychology* (New York: Wiley)
[59] Li J, Ke L, Du Q, Li J, Ke L and Du Q 2019 Classification of heart sounds based on the wavelet fractal and twin support vector machine *Entropy (Basel)* **21** 472

IOP Publishing

Internet of Things in Biomedical Sciences
Challenges and applications
Varun Bajaj and Irshad Ahmad Ansari

Chapter 9

Role of Internet of Things, artificial intelligence, and machine learning in biomedical devices: a comprehensive review

Nitesh Singh Bhati, Priya Sharma and Hiba Shakeel

With the advent of Internet of Things (IoT), artificial intelligence (AI), and machine learning (ML), many sectors have seen rapid growth by adopting these technologies and have improved tremendously in terms of efficiency and performance of end products. The benefits of these technologies lie in the fact that they can easily be used in conjunction with multiple other technologies and provide deeper understanding without human intervention. With the help of AI enabled machines and devices, the decision-making of humans can be reduced, and these devices also provide much better predictive abilities. In the current era of technologically advanced medical devices, the use of ML allows devices to learn and recognize patterns in data that humans can miss. When applied to IoT devices specifically designed for medical use, both will enable the development of colossal functional devices. The paradigm is of great interest to researchers and developers worldwide. Using this powerful amalgamation as motivation, this chapter explores the different applications, research scope, gaps, and future possibilities of the said topic in a comprehensive way. This chapter's review study revolves around IoT and AI applications in biomedical systems in biomedical wearables, diagnostic devices, connected hospital machinery/devices, point-of-care technologies, etc. It explores their scalability and transparency issues with highlighted case studies and recent technological novelties.

9.1 Introduction

The introduction of IoT, AI, and ML-based techniques has revolutionized the application delivery of many sectors, including healthcare. A massive number of advancements in the respective fields have led to the evolution of their specific applications and are thus making considerable contributions in many areas they are employed in. This chapter aims to explore the research advancements in the

doi:10.1088/978-0-7503-5311-3ch9

development of biomedical devices concerning the role of IoT, AI, and ML in their development. The chapter also aims to seek out the deficiencies and research gaps in the current processes and propose future research directions. The title should bring new insights into the field and a deeper understanding for readers from distinct backgrounds such as medical, engineering, product development, biomedical, etc. This also fulfills the common social interest of improving healthcare and the quality of life by introducing new diagnostic tools, techniques, and point-of-care devices. The contents on the latest advancements in biomedical device development with the help of IoT, AI, and ML have highlighted these major applications:

- Rapid and improved disease diagnosis;
- Accessible and low-cost healthcare;
- Remote patient monitoring and treatment;
- Improved medical informatics.

New advancements in these techniques have also been discussed with a focus on scalability and transparency. The modern-day clinical scenario is predominantly computerized, with significant data generation daily. This data can be used and converted into useful information for the diagnosis, treatment, and other clinical inferences using ML and AI-based techniques. The most common source of biomedical data are medical images in the form of x-rays, CT (computed tomography) scans, MRI (magnetic resonance imaging), etc, and other forms of health records [1]. It is important to note that procuring all these datasets, even for biomedical analysis, poses several challenges regarding patient data privacy, security, and usage, which are further discussed in this chapter.

9.2 Data workflow in IoT, ML, and AI for biomedical applications

As indicated above, the most common sources of data used in biomedical devices include imaging data, such as x-rays, CT scans, MRI, PET-CT, ultrasonography (USG), etc, and patients' health records. Advanced analysis of the image datasets is required to find crucial elements that can aid in disease diagnosis. This image pattern analysis is also helpful for remote patient monitoring and treatment, allowing physicians to monitor and treat patients without being physically present in the patient's environment. Combined with ML and AI, this facilitates the development of sophisticated biomedical systems capable of combating deadly diseases. The discipline of big data analysis, as shown in figure 9.1, derives from the fact that millions of data are generated every day, which, when combined, form a large amount of information containing many hidden patterns and valuable information that may be exploited using ML-based systems [2].

Kouanou *et al* have conducted an insightful study on the most optimal methods and methodologies for big data analysis for healthcare reasons. In this, the authors suggest a straightforward framework for the collecting, analysis, storage, classification, and diagnosis through medical images [3]. Before, they highlighted that using compressed medical images mentioned as MapReduce in Hadoop and Spark

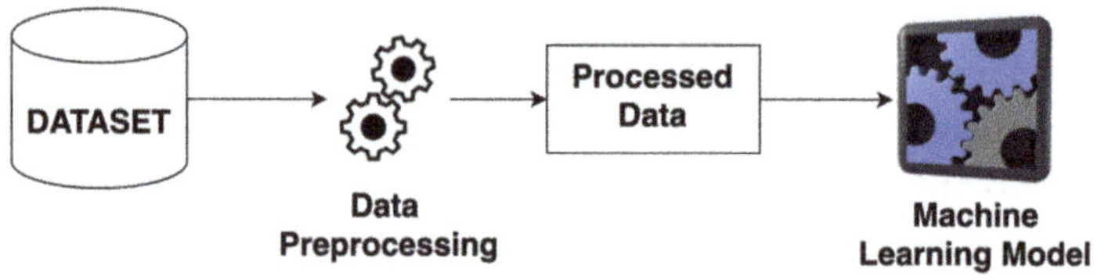

Figure 9.1. Workflow of data in a typical machine learning model.

performs significantly better, with Spark being the most of the Moon algorithm for dealing with large dataset sizes.

In a similar case study, Istephan and Siadat [4] demonstrated that unstructured healthcare datasets for epilepsy disease detection might also be utilized by organized querying using ML methods. The importance of this framework resides in the fact that it can be applied to other unstructured healthcare records outside of the problem statement at hand. Many more researches have been conducted for improved feature extraction and data analysis methods in the medical domain, all focusing on the application of unstructured or structured healthcare records.

In the process of big data development for radiological data, for instance, image acquisition, clarification, novel annotation detection of coma significance, diagnosis, and classification are required. Kansagra *et al* [5] demonstrated a novel implementation sequence that is optimal for analyzing radiological data and its curation. This type of implementation sequence development for different medical data is said to aid in tailoring dataset development in academic departmental laboratories and accelerate the process of employing them in ML and AI-based applications; these approaches would lead to rapid, low-cost, point-of-care treatment.

9.3 Robotic surgeries and telemedicine

When AI and ML technologies are combined with IoT, several convergence issues arise, including the feasibility and viability of communication between the various connected components, the coordination and exchange of information, and privacy and security of the shared data. AI is still in its infancy regarding its applications in healthcare and medical technologies. Its predictive skills have outperformed conventional disease detection and pattern recognition methods in healthcare, but its implementation in conjunction with IoT devices is still being investigated. As shown in figure 9.2, the telemedicine framework is a fairly straightforward model that employs data transmission via telecommunications technology for diagnosis, disease treatments, consulting and education, management, and treatment [6]. There are four forms of telehealthcare communications:

1. Teleconsultation: In this setting, healthcare providers can confer with patients remotely without being physically present.
2. Tele-education: This realm of tele-education includes several well-known websites, such as WebMed [7], where patients can obtain medical information about symptoms and diagnoses via the internet without visiting a doctor or physician.

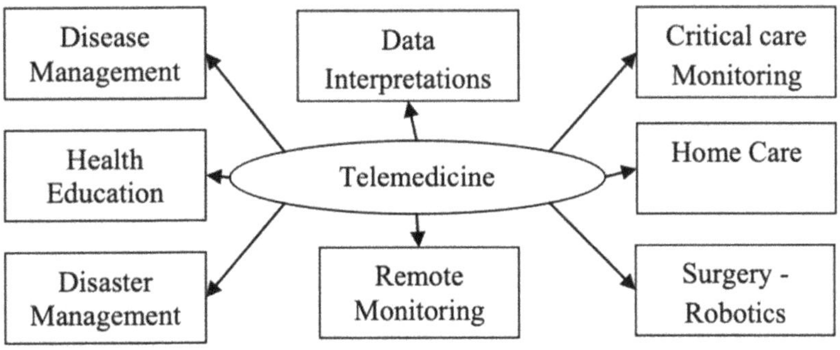

Figure 9.2. Distinct applications of telemedicine in various clinical scenarios.

3. Telemonitoring: Remote patient monitoring is under the ambit of telemonitoring, in which healthcare data can be delivered across a network without the need for physical records.
4. Telesurgery or robotic surgery: It involves using robotic arms to aid in surgical procedures while receiving instructions from a physician remotely or in the vicinity.

Robotic surgery is an interdisciplinary field in medicine, engineering, and healthcare. It is vital to facilitate doctor–patient interaction in surgical settings where the doctor cannot be physically present. Given situations when the doctor is physically present for surgery, robotic surgery helps to ensure the maximum level of precision required in critical microsurgeries. Robotic technology can aid in robotic operational procedures and in maintaining digital health records, medical history, and medical imaging data. It can speed up the disease diagnosis and intervention process. Apart from operational applications, robotics has also been utilized in developing certain assistive technologies, such as the Sister Kenny Home Therapy system (SKOTEE), developed by Lars *et al*, which facilitates the rehabilitation of patients following their doctor's recommendations and medication and check-up regimens. This point-of-care system comprises numerous wearable and wireless sensors for vital sign monitoring. As a result, patients with multiple conditions can be monitored and prescribed medications easily while simultaneously receiving real-time data about their health condition and sharing it with their doctors [8].

A similar study by Anett *et al* [9] focuses on robotics-enabled movement tracking using electroencephalogram signals derived from brain activity (EEG). Yepes *et al* [10], on the other hand, implemented an Android application-controlled KUKA KR6 robotic arm for robot-assisted healthcare.

9.3.1 Brief history

Some fundamental milestones in the history of robotics for healthcare are given in table 9.1.

Table 9.1. Some fundamental milestones in the history of robotics for healthcare [8].

Year	Research Institute/Researcher	Motive/Research
1989	Computer Motion	Robotic surgical methods
1992	Integrated Surgical Systems	Robotic hip surgery
1993	AesopTM 1000	Robotic laparoscopic surgery
1995	FM, RY and JF	Surgical robot to aid doctors
1997	Jacques Himpens and Guy Cardier	Telesurgery
1997	Integrated Surgical Systems Inc.	Neurosurgery via robots
1998	Carpentier *et al*	Mitral valve replacement
1998	Dr Frank Diamiano	Reanastomosis of a fallopian tube utilizing the Zeus method
1999	London Health Sciences Centre	Robotically-assisted closed-chest beating heart cardiac bypass surgery
1999	London Health Sciences Centre	Closed-chest beating heart cardiac hybrid revascularization treatment
1999	Penn State College of Medicine	Robotic aided beating heart bypass
2000	Intuitive Surgical Inc.	Laparoscopic surgical operations
2000	Dr Francois Laborde of L'Institut Mutualiste Montsouris Chiosy	Endoscopic closures of the patent ductus arteriosis utilizing Computer Motion's Zeus robotic aid
2001	ZEUS® Robotic Surgical System	Robotically-assisted laparoscopic and thoracic tools
2001	CyberKnife®	Image-guided robotic system for non-invasive cancer surgery
2000	Intuitive Surgical Inc. and Computer Motion Inc.	Operative surgical robots, telesurgery, and operating room integration.
2004	Intuitive Surgical Inc. and Computer Motion Inc.	Robotic-like equipment to assist in coronary artery bypass surgery
2005	The University of Illinois Clinic	Laparoscopic right hepatectomy
2008	ROBODOC	THA robot
2016	Rockwell Automation, Preferred Networks and Cisco	Field Internet of Robotic Things (IoRT)

9.3.2 Remote patient monitoring and treatment

Remote patient monitoring is one of the most recent developments in the ever-changing field of healthcare. With ever-increasing health complications, this system makes healthcare accessible without graphical limitations. This technology, which began as a simple method of vital signs monitoring alongside hospital beds, has evolved into a home-based assistive system that facilitates real-time patient data exchange and monitoring via sensors. Various biomedical signals, including blood pressure, heart rate, body temperature, glucose level, and respiration rate, are monitored remotely using a variety of sensors. In addition to enhancing the quality of life of chronic patients, remote healthcare technology is also adaptable for monitoring the elderly, neonatal, coma, and chronic to acute patients. These modifications can be made by the patient's health condition, their respective illnesses, or their particular operational circumstances. New technological advances also suggest contactless sensors, which require a patient to be close to the sensor instead of using sensors that are sitting on the surface or are invasive. This type of sensor-enabled technology assists the physician in remote monitoring and can enhance the monitoring process's efficiency. For example, people affected by sleep disorders and their regulations are prone to developing serious and complex health problems, such as cardiovascular disease, diabetes, and other psychotic disorders. Specialized sleep clinics employing nocturnal polysomnography, also known as PSG, have been established to evaluate and study these sleep disorders. This technique again employs multiple biomedical signals generated by sensors, as shown in figure 9.3. In a conventional medical setting, polysomnography is performed by trained medical professionals using standardized screening techniques. This manual examination is essential for identifying a patient's type of sleep-based disorder. Still, it is susceptible to subjective inaccuracies, manual errors, and increased costs. This is where ML and AI come into play. Deep learning and neural network-based systems have outperformed manual inspection techniques by achieving 97% accuracy relative to the gold standard method [9]. This ensures a rapid, accurate, and inexpensive diagnosis of a serious medical condition. With the rising cost of healthcare in the modern era, the transition from bedside treatment to preventive diagnosis bridges a substantial gap in increasing the healthcare condition. Aside from living data exchange regarding a patient's health, remote patient monitoring can also provide potential analysis and data patterns highlighting a hidden issue,

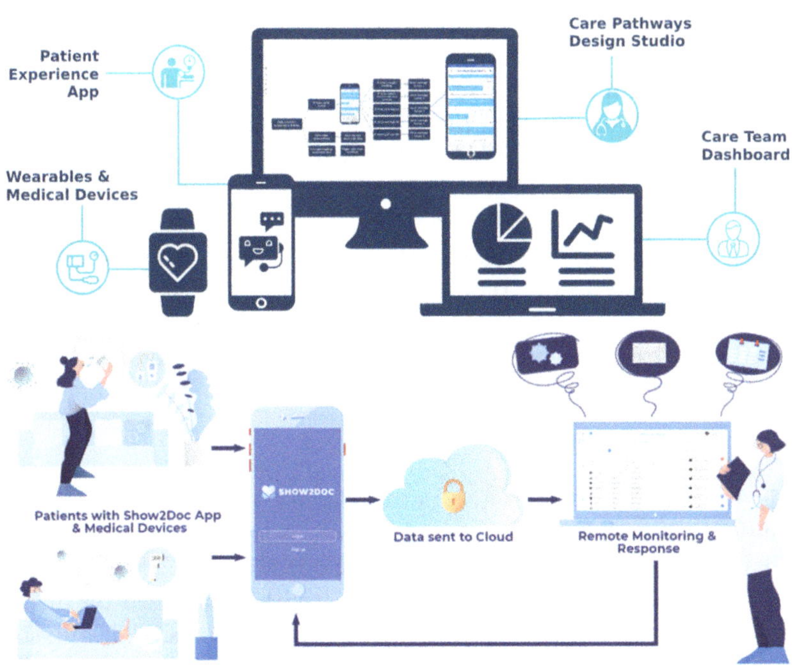

Figure 9.3. Workflow of data in a typical ML model.

such as identifying potential heart and blood pressure anomalies using basic data such as continuous heart rate.

9.3.3 Internet of Robotic Things (IoRT)

Internet of Robotic Things (IoRT) helps with rapid sensing, data collection, analysis, and manipulation and ensures faster decisions and proper data analysis. An ML-integrated IoT system is more intelligent than any conventional IoT system with interconnected robotic components. These systems rely on a WiFi-controlled central processor. Chen *et al* [10] conducted one of the most important studies on the subject. They focus on recognizing patients' emotions and facilitating communication between them via a cloud platform. Using robotics, Al-Taee *et al* [11] conducted a noteworthy study that improved glucose level sensing in diabetic patients. In addition to these major advantages for the IoRT, the incorporation of AI and ML into IoT has also raised concerns about the autonomy of self-enabled robotic systems. There is a severe lack of experimental evidence regarding the accuracy and precision of these systems, and the lack of tactile feedback provided to the medical practitioner is a barrier to their widespread adoption. Conventionally, doctors rely heavily on the tactile feedback they receive during an operation or surgery. However, it enabled robotic approaches to eliminate this feedback system, limiting the healthcare practitioner's decision-making ability. It is necessary to design sophisticated and intelligent systems that can provide either haptic feedback or dimension measurement during surgery to assist surgeons in making crucial decisions.

9.4 Sensors and wearable devices

Biomedical devices and sensors provide a multitude of benefits and potential applications in health monitoring, management, and treatment for stopping heavy equipment in laboratories and hospitals are continuously being replaced with smaller and smaller devices with the help of embedded smart sensors which are revolutionizing the healthcare scenario. Nowadays, the healthcare market has been seeing a massive rise in the development of smart devices such as smart syringes, EpiPens, and even smart pills. Biomedical smart innovations not only help in the rapid diagnosis of diseases but also in disease treatment and management. Some of the notable applications of smart devices and sensors in the biomedical sector are discussed further in this current section.

9.4.1 Biosensors

To enable healthcare providers to control disease treatment, management, and monitoring outside of hospitals and clinics, various sensors that transmit real-time medical data over the internet have been developed. A vast array of sensors, also known as biosensors, can collect vital patient health data based on their sleeping patterns, body movement tracking, physical activities, and overall health status. For example, biosensors can measure vital signs like oxygen saturation, cardiac cycle, hypertension, and glucose levels. In addition, they have a mechanism for informing doctors of any severe abnormalities observed. This contributes to the prevention of disease-related complications and improves the patient's quality of life. This data analysis can also give physicians the same or hidden disease patterns and a clear picture of disease progression.

9.4.2 Wearable sensors

We have investigated the applications of sensor-based activity tracking in healthcare, but numerous devices are not marketed as medical technology on the market. For instance, biomedical devices capable of functioning as smart wearable watches can be used for health monitoring and cosmetic or other purposes. Such devices' (figure 9.4) continuous data collection can be intelligently analyzed to predict potential future outcomes. With the advancements in material science over the past few decades, certain assistive and prospective technologies have also risen in popularity. With the incorporation of robotic technology, sensor-embedded prosthetics can offer patients lacking muscular strength and power greater mobility and flexibility. Applications have been found for both therapeutic and assistive purposes. In simple terms, the primary purpose of these wearable sensor devices is to identify and record our activities with geographical annotations [12, 13].

Depending on the use scenario and requirements, wearable devices can be utilized with or without expert intervention. For instance, medical-grade smart pills or ingestible sensors, in addition to invasive wearables, necessitated valid medical prescriptions for determining the dosage. On the other hand, some wearable devices, such as blood pressure monitoring patches and wearable ECG sensors, can be purchased by patients for proper disease understanding and education. A survey conducted by Seneviratne *et al* sheds light on the subject by categorizing wearable devices into smartwatch-based, head-mounted, jewelry-embedded, e-textile/patches, and sports and fitness-based devices [14].

9.4.3 IoT-based communication technology for wearable devices

The distance at which data can be transmitted is limited by all devices' power consumption constraints. Although most biomedical devices use small systems powered by small batteries to maintain minimal power consumption, they still have their own power constraints based on the amount of storage and processing power required and the distance they can travel. Very brief range communications such as near field communication (NFC) require extremely low power consumption. But they can only transfer a small amount of data internally and require contact transmission within a range of approximately 4–5 cm. Figure 9.5 describes the architecture of IoT devices in wearables. The contactless card payment system is a very common example of this type of data transmission.

Slightly larger data transfer range is possible with Bluetooth technology. It is a low-cost and energy-efficient technology that enables data transfer up to a hundred meters away. Typically, devices powered by a small coin cell battery employ Bluetooth technology. A maximum of eight devices can form a network, with one master node and the others functioning as auxiliary slave notes. Due to its limited

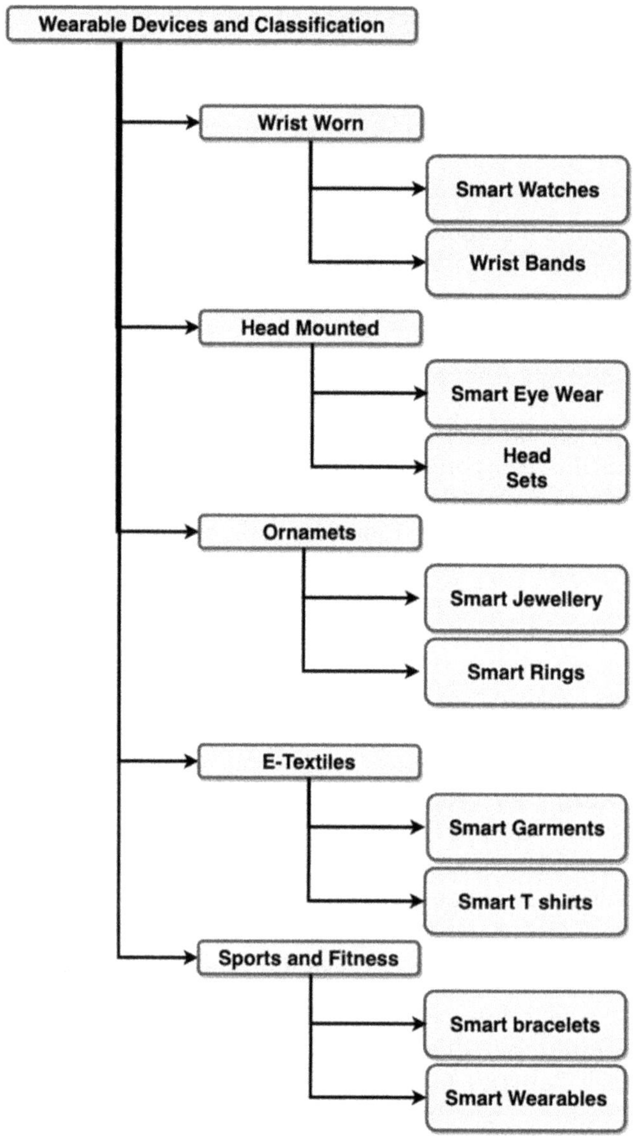

Figure 9.4. Types of wearable devices.

data transfer capacity, it is unsuitable for transferring large files for multimedia communications. Most modern mobile phones are equipped with Bluetooth technology, which is still utilized in Bluetooth-based headphones. ANT is a lesser-known short-distance data transfer protocol widely used in the sports industry and equipped with fitness and heart-monitoring devices (figure 9.6). SensRcore is a typical example of this device. The survey paper by Seneviratne *et al*, referenced in the preceding section, can provide a deeper understanding of the operation of such devices [14].

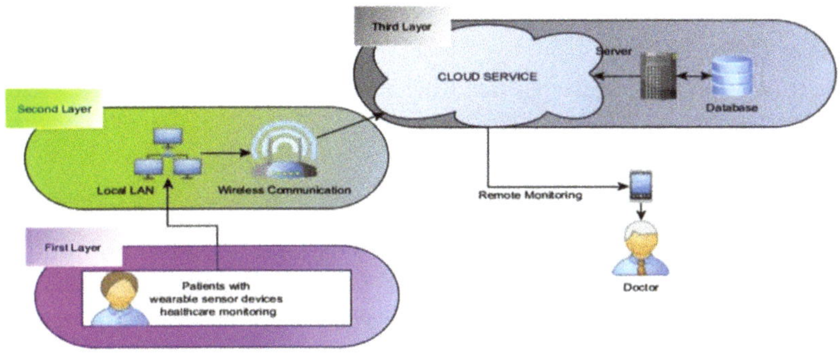

Figure 9.5. IoT architecture in wearable devices.

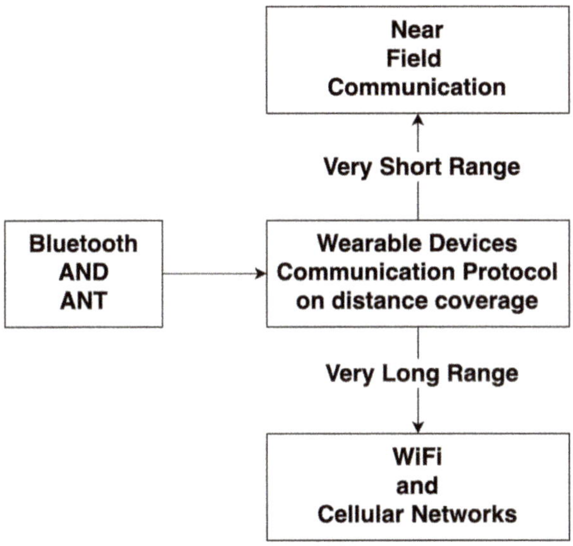

Figure 9.6. IoT-based communication technologies in wearable devices.

Lastly, utilizing WiFi and cellular networks is the best option for long-distance data transfer. this kind of data transfer process can be utilized for large-size multimedia transfers such as video and voice data.

Some key applications of IoT-based wearable sensors are outlined below:

- Variable easy sensors for detecting driver drowsiness while driving to prevent road accidents [15].
- Wearable IoT-based sensors for patient identification and monitoring in heterogeneous healthcare environments [16].
- Machine learning-based wearable sensors for detecting post-traumatic stress disorders [17].
- Non-invasive blood pressure measurement using wearable sensors [18].
- Blood sugar measurement for remote patient monitoring and insulin dosage prediction using wearable sensors.

- Intelligent sports and fitness systems for monitoring activity and calorie intake [19].
- Wearable navigation assistance devices for visually impaired patients [20].

9.5 Diagnostic technologies

Using technology, multiple diagnostic technologies have been formed which have helped people with diseases such as Parkinson's disease, acquired immunodeficiency disease (AIDS), and diabetic retinopathy etc. Figure 9.7 mentions how a healthcare diagnostic chain with information input, recommendations, and outcomes is formed.

9.5.1 Parkinson's disease diagnosis

Parkinson's disease falls under neurodegenerative disorders that affect the patient's motor function. It is a disease with a slow progression whose symptoms include tremors, dysphonia, general slowness, and mental or behavioral changes in some cases, shown in figure 9.8. Parkinson's disease is typically caused by genetic inheritance or environmental triggers [21]. The conventional methods for diagnosing Parkinson's include a thorough medical examination and neurological evaluation. Reaching autopsy provides the most conclusive diagnosis due to the presence of Lewy bodies in the midbrain region [22]. A conclusion during clinical examination requires multiple follow-up assessments. Due to the factors above, the clinical diagnosis of this disease is not always accurate, given that the patient is aware of the gradual onset of these symptoms. Several efforts have been made to improve the

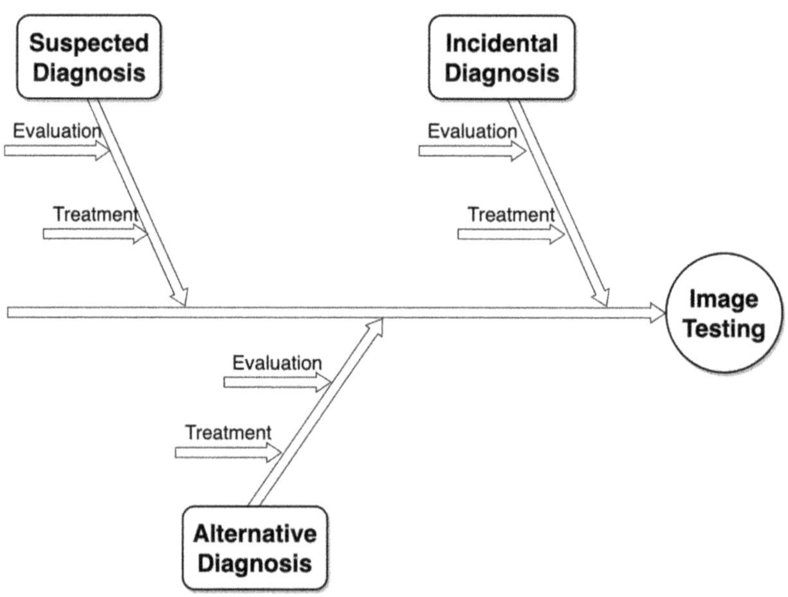

Figure 9.7. Typical example of a healthcare diagnostic chain with information input, recommendations, and outcomes.

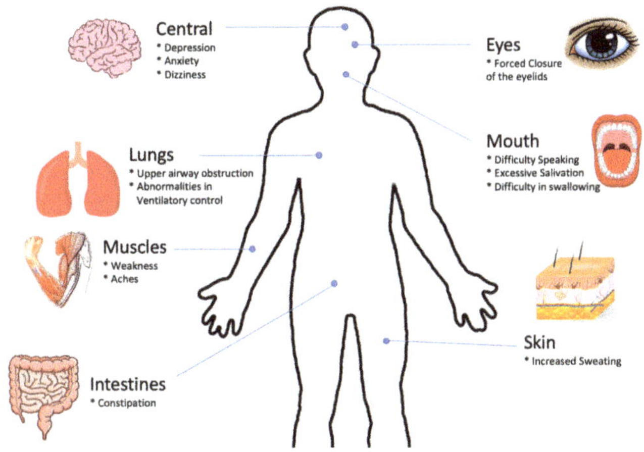

Figure 9.8. Symptoms of Parkinson's disease in terms of motor impairment and reduced systemic activity [27].

diagnostic accuracy of this disease. In contrast, others have focused on improving patients' quality of life through using technologies for rehabilitation. A standardized screening method is also being made to develop diagnostic criteria for early disease detection to ensure proper disease management. the most dependable and prevalent standard in use is a set of criteria for the UK Queen Square Brain Bank that uses bradykinesia, postural anomalies, and rigidity as determining factors [23].

Several AI-based techniques have been instrumental in developing computer-assisted Parkinson's disease diagnosis for the past decade. Utilizing classification algorithms such as regression, decision trees, the Bayes algorithm, and multi-layer perceptron (MLP), post-operative machine learning has played a crucial role in assisting doctors with the diagnosis decision-making process. Several techniques, including support vector machines (SVMs), artificial neural networks (ANNs), linear discriminant analysis (LDA), and fuzzy networks, aid in voice analysis-based disease diagnosis. These techniques have already been applied to medical image analysis and the analysis of biosensor signals, such as EEG and ECG, for Parkinson's disease diagnosis [24].

Literature review suggests using triaxial gyroscopic sensors for activity tracking and recording and the region of interest isolation using spectral analysis based on the sensors and symptoms being monitored. Numerous studies have employed inertial sensors, accelerometers, and electromyogram-based motor analysis to detect tremors. Using the appropriate sensors, other motor symptoms such as dyskinesia or bradykinesia can also be used to diagnose Parkinson's disease.

As previously stated, there is currently no cure for Parkinson's disease and no diagnostic method demonstrating a very high degree of accuracy. Several image processing techniques have also gained prominence in Parkinson's disease diagnosis. Nevertheless, detecting the disease area can improve the patient's quality of life and potentially save their life. This disease requires years of experience and expertise, and very few doctors have this kind of exposure; therefore, they require assistance in making diagnostic decisions. In addition to different ML-based techniques, certain parametric models can be used during medical image processing and analysis to analyze the structural changes in the collected dataset. To achieve optimum predictive performance.

9.5.2 Acquired immunodeficiency disease (AIDS)

Human immunodeficiency virus (HIV) infection causes acquired immunodeficiency disease or AIDS, which results in various medical complications. This disease primarily affects the body's immune response and ability to detect or fight incoming infections. As a result, all opportunistic infections and rapidly growing cancers can take over the body's machinery without interference from immune cells.

This makes diagnosing and treating this disease a priority since early detection of the virus will aid in planning treatments to enhance the immune response. Very recently, ML has been used to combat HIV by identifying and monitoring the spread of new infections using distinct patterns of immediate body reactions and behaviors. HIV can also be diagnosed based on behavioral patterns and biological database monitoring. SVM, logistic regression (LR), and decision trees/random forests are the most prevalent ML-based methods utilized in diagnosing the disease. Most of these models are used to accurately diagnose diseases based on similarities between the patterns of HIV-positive patients and those being examined for the disease.

9.5.3 Diabetic retinopathy

The persistent presence of high blood sugar levels in a patient is classified as diabetes or diabetes mellitus. This disorder is typically caused by either a lack of insulin hormone production by the body or an inability to utilize the hormone produced by the pancreas. The treatment of this condition is of the utmost importance because it has the potential to evolve into multiple other acute and chronic conditions, such as ketoacidosis, cardiovascular disorders, stroke, foot ulcers, and other kidney-related problems [25].

Diabetic retinopathy is a diabetic complication that affects the eyes and can result in visual impairment if not controlled or treated promptly. Patients with long-term diabetes are highly likely to develop diabetic retinopathy, which can even result in total blindness. Due to changes in the body's glucose levels, the retinal blood vessels undergo abnormal changes such as swelling or leakage, causing irreversible damage to the eyesight.

Fundus or retinal images analyzed for microaneurysms and other changes in the form of hemorrhages, exudates, or morphological changes are essential in diagnosing diabetic retinopathy. Medical professionals search for such indicators and conclude after weighing all symptoms in conventional settings. This process is very time-consuming and prone to human error unless years of experience are combined, necessitating the development of more reliable pattern recognition techniques to aid in disease diagnosis. Numerous AI-based systems utilizing well-established pattern recognition techniques, such as SVM, CNNS (convolutional neural networks), and k-Nearest Neighbors, have been utilized for this purpose and have proven to be highly effective and reliable [26].

9.6 Conclusion

IoT has no unified standard and is not yet integrated. Every day, a new wearable device is added to the IoT applications, making integrating heterogeneous devices complex in terms of scalability and adaptability. Furthermore, when scaling in the domain of naming and addressing, it is challenging to identify devices in the application and real-time environment. The transition from IPv4 to IPv6 is proving extremely difficult due to the 100 billion devices currently in use. Working with IoT devices generates massive amounts of data at gigabits per second; therefore, controlling this data is critical. Furthermore, because the server always receives data, identifying sensor data in a healthcare application is challenging. Confidential health information is gathered and distributed without the individual's knowledge. It is difficult to validate data obtained from healthcare and other applications. The ever-increasing patient privacy concerns also add to the challenge and demand more transparency in the AI-based systems employed in healthcare. The reliability of these IoT, ML, and AI-based systems when making decisions about life and death is also always cross-examined in terms of replacing conventional techniques. For example, robotic surgeries have proven to be more precise and efficient in the application. But the lack of haptic response from the doctor poses a hindrance to its widespread adoption in real-life operational scenarios. Thus, to increase the scalability and feasibility of these technologies, more efforts have to be made to make their decisions transparent, subjective, and precise.

References

[1] Oussous A, Benjelloun F-Z, Ait Lahcen A and Belfkih S 2018 Big Data technologies: a survey *J. King Saud Univ. - Comput. Inf. Sci.* **30** 431–48

[2] Xing E P, Ho Q, Xie P and Wei D 2016 Strategies and principles of distributed machine learning on big data *Engineering* **2** 179–95

[3] Kouanou A T, Tchiotsop D, Kengne R, Zephirin D T, Armele N M A and Tchinda R 2018 An optimal big data workflow for biomedical image analysis *Inform. Med. Unlocked* **11** 68–74

[4] Istephan S and Siadat M-R 2016 Unstructured medical image query using big data—an epilepsy case study *J. Biomed. Inform.* **59** 218–26

[5] Kansagra A P *et al* 2016 Big data and the future of radiology informatics *Acad. Radiol.* **23** 30–42

[6] Chakraborty C, Gupta B and Ghosh S K 2013 A review on telemedicine-based WBAN framework for patient monitoring *Telemed. E-Health* **19** 619–26

[7] Folio L R, Yancy W and Yancy R 1999 Internet-based continuing medical education in remote areas of China: WebMEd: economical PC-based tele-education and telemedicine *SAE Technical Paper*

[8] Mishra D R K History of Robotic Surgery. https://laparoscopyhospital.com/history_of_robotic_surgery.htm (accessed 5 August 2022)

[9] Stephansen J *et al* 2017 The use of neural networks in the analysis of sleep stages and the diagnosis of narcolepsy (unpublished)

[10] Chen M *et al* 2016 CP-Robot: Cloud-assisted pillow robot for emotion sensing and interaction *Industrial IoT Technologies and Applications* (Cham: Springer) pp 81–93

[11] Al-Taee M A, Al-Nuaimy W, Muhsin Z J and Al-Ataby A 2017 Robot assistant in management of diabetes in children based on the Internet of Things *IEEE Internet Things J.* **4** 437–45
[12] Martin T and Healey J 2007 2006's Wearable computing advances and fashions *IEEE Pervasive Comput.* **6** 14–6
[13] Avila L and Bailey M 2015 The wearable revolution *IEEE Comput. Graph. Appl.* **35** 104
[14] Seneviratne S *et al* 2017 A survey of wearable devices and challenges *IEEE Commun. Surv. Tutor.* **19** 2573–620
[15] Li G, Lee B-L and Chung W-Y 2015 Smartwatch-based wearable EEG system for driver drowsiness detection *IEEE Sens. J.* **15** 7169–80
[16] Lomotey R K, Pry J and Sriramoju S 2017 Wearable IoT data stream traceability in a distributed health information system *Pervasive Mob. Comput.* **40** 692–707
[17] McWhorter J, Brown L and Khansa L 2017 A wearable health monitoring system for posttraumatic stress disorder *Biol. Inspired Cogn. Archit.* **22** 44–50
[18] Xin Q and Wu J 2017 A novel wearable device for continuous, non-invasion blood pressure measurement *Comput. Biol. Chem.* **69** 134–7
[19] Yong B *et al* 2018 IoT-based intelligent fitness system *J. Parallel Distrib. Comput.* **118** 14–21
[20] Bai J, Lian S, Liu Z, Wang K and Liu D 2018 Virtual-blind-road following-based wearable navigation device for blind people *IEEE Trans. Consum. Electron.* **64** 136–43
[21] Kalia L V and Lang A E 2015 Parkinson's disease *Lancet* **386** 896–912
[22] Gibb W R and Lees A J 1988 The relevance of the Lewy body to the pathogenesis of idiopathic Parkinson's disease *J. Neurol. Neurosurg. Psychiatry* **51** 745–52
[23] Salarian A *et al* 2003 An ambulatory system to quantify bradykinesia and tremor in Parkinson's disease *4th Int. IEEE EMBS Special Topic Conf. on Information Technology Applications in Biomedicine, 2003* 35–8
[24] Valli A and Jiji G W 2014 Parkinsons disease diagnosis using image processing techniques a survey *Int. J. Comput. Sci. Appl.* **4** 57–67
[25] WHO | Diabetes Web.archive.org. https://web.archive.org/web/20130826174444/ (accessed 6 August 2022)
[26] Mansour R F 2017 Deep-learning-based automatic computer-aided diagnosis system for diabetic retinopathy *Biomed. Eng. Lett.* **8** 41–57
[27] Parkinson's Care & Support UK 2019 Symptoms and diagnosis *Parkinson's Care and Support UK* https://parkinsonscare.org.uk/symptoms-and-diagnosis/ (accssed 30 December 2020)

IOP Publishing

Internet of Things in Biomedical Sciences
Challenges and applications
Varun Bajaj and Irshad Ahmad Ansari

Chapter 10

Internet of Medical Things-based wearable medical devices

Ruby Jain and Bhoumik Mahajan

Health is one of the most important aspects of life. Therefore, the last decade has witnessed extensive research in the field of healthcare services and their technological upgradation. As the Internet of Things (IoT) becomes a hot and trending topic nowadays, with the help of biomedical IoT it has become the Internet of Medical Things (IoMT). IoMT has various applications like medical devices, wearable sensors, communication systems, and mobile user interfaces. As a part of IoT, wearable devices have been developed to help people get the right treatment for themselves. The reliable and valid system, easily carried, helps the doctor to monitor patients from a far distance expectantly to overcome problems. The main aim of this chapter is to comprehensively discuss the role of IoT in wearable medical devices.

10.1 Introduction

The IoT plays an important role in healthcare monitoring using wearable devices. As the name suggests, IoT is a network of physical objects equipped with sensors and software that can communicate and exchange data over the internet. Nowadays, wearables are becoming an important part of IoT technology. IoT enables our medical wearable devices to provide individuals with the information needed to achieve better health outcomes. In today's market, wearable systems are available in a wide variety of forms, including tiny sensors integrated into textiles, consumer electronics embedded in fashionable clothing, computerized watches, belt-worn PCs with head-mounted displays, and glasses, which can all be worn on a variety of parts of the body [1]. As the smart wearable uses other devices for computing and communication, such as smartphones [2], it can integrate with other devices as well. Smart wearable devices are becoming increasingly significant as a result of the mobility of both humans and animals since they can collect and transmit data while on the move and consequently receive information from the internet, which can be

doi:10.1088/978-0-7503-5311-3ch10

used to make smarter decisions. The use of smart wearables can bring efficiency and optimization to the applications, enhance the quality of life, and increase productivity or safety. The sports and healthcare industries benefit from wearable healthcare devices [3]. A wearable healthcare technology device may improve the accuracy of health data, encourage healthier behavior in individuals, and reduce healthcare costs by improving their health.

We have witnessed a rapid development of smart wearable products adapted for various applications during the past few years. Here are some examples of wearable smart devices: smartwatches, wristbands, eyewear, headsets, earbuds, and warning devices, etc [2] (figure 10.1).

The power consumption of wearable IoT devices is considered a vital outline factor since they are battery-operated. While a wearable device cannot execute multiplex processing or retransmit a large amount of data, it is limited by the considerable amount of power that will be consumed in these situations. It is generally necessary to charge the battery of wearable IoT devices more frequently if they perform a great deal of processing and transmit large amounts of data. In many applications and usage scenarios, this is quite possible. For instance, in a situation where the wearable IoT device is used to detect falls, the device might be worn during the time that the wearer is not asleep and can be charged during his/her sleep time. Additionally, wearable IoT devices used during sports activities can drain the battery during the duration of the activity, which usually lasts a few hours, and can be recharged afterward. Using an IoT device to determine the trajectory of a bird within a year will not only require limiting the processing and data transmission but also energy harvesting methods to prolong battery life.

This chapter aims to evaluate the wearable healthcare devices both in scientific papers and commercial efforts. In this study, we focus on the most important wearable devices, which directly compute the health position parameters. Readers can find comprehensive and useful information about the most reliable current devices and concepts in this area.

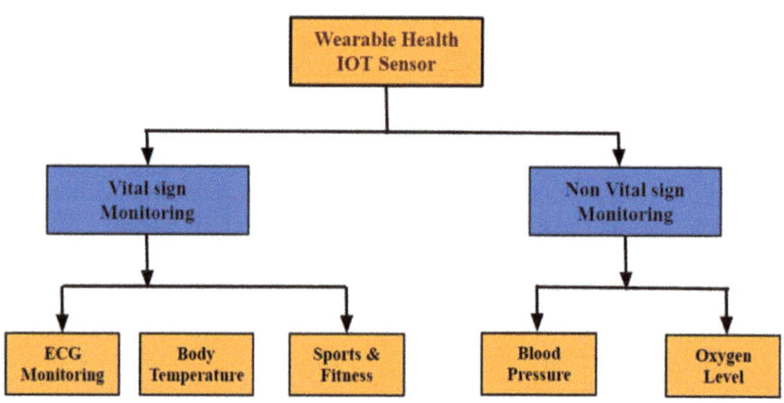

Figure 10.1. Types of IoT sensors.

Below is a concise summary of the rest of this evaluation chapter. Section 10.2 covers health monitoring under changing eco-friendly situations and while in motion. Section 10.3 presents a review of recent studies on wearable devices, beginning with a discussion of motion tracking and the research perspective and implementations in this field, followed by a comparison of some of the most recent commercial devices. In section 10.4 we discuss wearing devices to monitor environmental conditions and vital signs. Section 10.5 discusses the challenges that may be faced by potentially available devices. A summary of the conclusions is presented along with suggestions for further research

10.2 Smart wearables

Today, in a time-constrained world, people, especially the working class, often neglect their health and fitness [4]. Visiting a doctor in a clinic can take several hours, as a variety of tests are carried out for diagnosis, prescriptions, and finally treatment. That is why many patients go to the hospital when they are seriously ill. For this reason, many people are searching for a replacement, for example, a wearable device that monitors the user's health continuously in real time and gives timely insight on various health parameters to both the user and the physician [4] (figure 10.2).

10.3 Architectural aspects

In most cases, wearable devices are connected to the internet by connecting to a smartphone. Consequently, if the gateway battery is empty or the connection options are inadequate, the gateway's operational efficiency may be limited. Currently, some wearable devices have an infrared radio that can transmit a long distance. However, the continuous use of wearable devices is not recommended because of the high-power consumption [11]. Prior to e-health systems, patients wore specialized devices, such as biomedical sensors, to monitor their health like smartwatches. A storage and computation facility was used to access these devices. This facility was either local or remotely located on the internet [12]—the first architecture of wearable devices is a separate device. Wearables are capable of

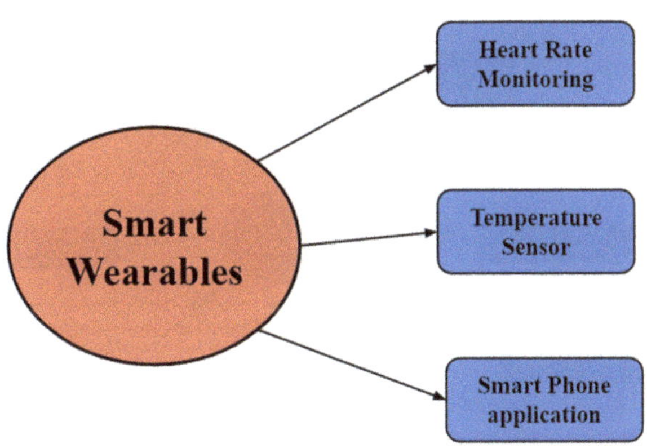

Figure 10.2. Some functions of smart wearable.

monitoring a user's status by collecting information ranging from physiological signals (e.g., heart rate, body temperature, and physical activities) and interactions with the surrounding environment.

Wired links connected wearables to more powerful external devices during the next phase of architecture evolution. The form factor limitation of wearables prevents them from performing certain data processing tasks. As a result of these architectures, mainly found in healthcare-related applications, users' mobility was restricted, which was seen as a barrier to the expansion of wearable technologies. Healthcare services needed to provide real-time alerts in critical situations to be considered smart, which means tracking patients' health conditions without frequent visits to medical centers or hospitals [13]. This has led to the replacement of traditional wired health monitors with wireless wearable ones.

Consumer wearables are becoming more and more integrated into an individual ecosystem, rather than standalone devices, as smartphones become part of the personal wearable cloud. In the end, the system was redesigned where smartphones act as gateways for transmitting data to the cloud, either directly or after being processed by custom applications. In addition, IoT technologies enable users to connect with a multitude of general-purpose smart devices, allowing them to be within proximity of the device they need. The IoT devices provide additional details about the environment surrounding the user, which can be adapted to meet their specific requirements.

IoT gateways are also called monitoring stations in the IoT architecture described in [14] for people with disabilities, and are part of their perception layer. It makes sense that a star-shaped topology is supposed to be used for communications with the development of wearable clouds. Wearable devices began communicating purely centrally, with gateway devices acting as masters, after Bluetooth became a leading technology for connecting devices. The fourth evolution step in figure 10.3 can be seen in fitness, sports, and healthcare products that exchange data with smartphone applications. To comply with the growing demand for wearable devices, device manufacturers consider equipping wearables with short-range and long-range connectivity chip sets in several scenarios where a wearable cannot connect to the

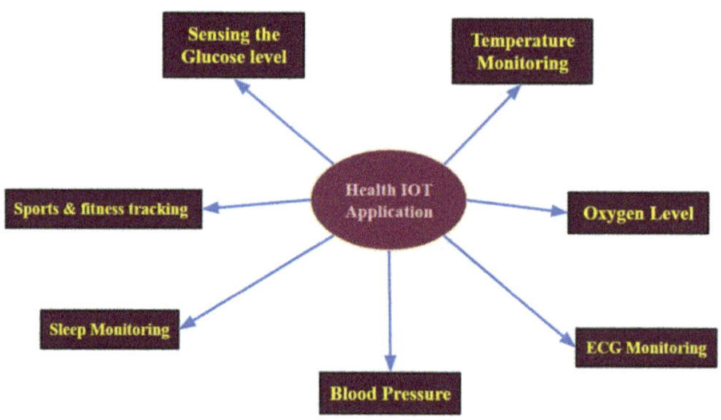

Figure 10.3. Applications of IoT.

network, such as the absence of a nearby smartphone, non-installed applications, or outdated phone software [15]. These independently functioning wearables are independent of other devices, so they can function independently.

There are currently at least two wireless interfaces on board most wearable devices today. In the future, vendors will likely add more wireless modules in response to the trend of unifying operations. Technological selection mechanisms will be intelligently selected based on improved situational awareness as a result of the trend.

While this standalone wearable-based architecture allows for the separation of wearables from other personal devices and permits direct cloud access, it poses some network design and sizing challenges. Specifically, the absence of pre-processing, normally handled by gateway devices, will place additional demands on wireless networks. Additionally, battery life and device complexity are reduced due to the implementation of low-power communication technologies.

There are currently two or more wireless networks on most wearable devices today. Retailers will be able to add more networking modules as a result of the trend toward simplifying operations. Using improved situational awareness to select technology could result in intelligent technology selection mechanisms.

10.4 Some applications of smart wearables

A variety of IoT-based applications are developed using IoT services/concepts. Several concepts have been suggested to the service of mankind by researchers working in these areas. The conceptual model is more developer-centric, and the application model is more user-centric. Wearable sensors, portable gadgets, and medical devices have become more affordable and user-friendly thanks to the rapid development of IoT technology. Information about patients can be collected, diseases detected, health monitored, and alerts generated in case of medical emergencies can be sent out through these systems. Here are some recent commercially available devices discussed in the following subsections. Furthermore, numerous IoT-based applications have been investigated, including those addressing both single and multiple conditions.

10.4.1 Electrocardiogram (ECG) monitoring

An electrocardiogram (ECG) shows the electrical activity of the heart's ventricles atria as a result of depolarization and repolarization. An ECG provides information about the basic rhythms of the heart muscles and acts as an indicator for various cardiac abnormalities. This population can identify several abnormalities, including arrhythmias, prolonged QT intervals, and myocardial ischemia. An abnormal heart rhythm can be detected early through the monitoring of an ECG using IoT technology. There have been many studies in the past that have used IoT to monitor ECGs [5–10]. In [10], an IoT-based ECG monitoring system is proposed that consists of a wireless data acquisition system and a receiver. Real-time cardiac abnormalities were detected by using a search automation method.

10.4.2 Oxygen saturation monitoring

Oxygen saturation measurement can be done non-invasively through pulse oximetry, which is a critical parameter in healthcare research. Compared to conventional methods, the non-invasive method allows for real-time monitoring and eliminates the associated issues. As IoT-based technology is being integrated into pulse oximetry, it shows potential applications in the healthcare field. The non-invasive tissue oximeter proposed in [16] measures several parameters, including oxygen saturation in the blood, heart rate, and pulse rate. Zigbee and Wi-Fi are both feasible communication technologies for transmitting recorded information to the server. Based on recorded data, it was able to decide whether medical supervision was necessary. In another study [17], to detect a critical oxygen saturation level, an alarm system is used to determine the oxygen saturation level of a patient. In addition to the pulse oximeter, the Blynk server was used to connect the pulse oximeter to the WLAN router. Furthermore, one of the first multispectral sensors has been proposed by Von Chong *et al* [18]. It has been proposed in [19] that remote patient monitoring systems can be low-power and cost-effective. Monitoring in real time can be effectively accomplished with this device.

10.4.3 Temperature monitoring

A person's body temperature contributes significantly to many diagnostic processes because it indicates the body's homeostasis. In addition, a change in body temperature could indicate an underlying illness such as trauma or sepsis. In many diseases, doctors can determine a patient's health condition by tracking changes in temperature over time. An attached mouth, ear, or rectum temperature thermometer is the traditional way to measure temperature. These methods are always ineffective due to patient discomfort and the high possibility of getting infected. As a result of recent advances in IoT-based technologies, a variety of solutions have been proposed to this problem. Wearable 3D printed devices for the ears were proposed in [20]. Through the use of an infrared sensor, this device measures the body's core temperature. The device was integrated with a wireless sensor module and a data processing unit. Environments and other physical activities do not affect the measured temperature here. Utilizing IoT technologies such as Arduino and Raspberry Pi, Gunawan developed a temperature monitoring system. An online web page presented temperature data stored in the database that was accessible from a desktop or mobile device [21]. Real-time body temperature measurements were performed on infants using wearable and lightweight sensors in another study [22]. As soon as the temperature rises above a critical value, it can also alert parents.

10.4.4 Blood pressure monitoring

The measurement of blood pressure (BP) is an essential part of any diagnostic process. At least one person is required to take BP measurements using the most common method. The IoT and other sensing technologies have revolutionized how BP can be measured. In [23], an implantable cuffless device was proposed that measures both systolic and diastolic pressure. As well as storing recorded information in the cloud, users can access the information at any time.

Validation of accuracy and efficiency was also performed on this device. An IoT-based BP measurement system developed by Guntha employs cloud and fog computing [24]. This preparation helps prepare the system to be monitored in real time over a long period. Additionally, the device can record and store data for later use. Systolic and diastolic BP were evaluated by a convolutional neural network model for deep learning [25]. Categories of IoT applications: monitoring of BP using the ECG signal and telephotography (PPG), recorded from the fingertip, have been used for rehabilitation of patients with hypertension and the treatment of asthma and depression. Other various applications include checking of ECG, BP, temperature, mood, medication, wheelchairs, glucose level, and oxygen saturation [26]. In this application, BP was computed and stored in the cloud using the attached microcontroller module.

10.4.5 Sports and fitness tracking

Sports wearables enable users/athletes to record metrics as they exercise to improve their performance. This category is for applications that use wearables during sports activities. Applications in this bunch consider gathering data regarding the recognition of human and animal daily activities. Various metrics of a user's/athlete's activity are recorded during sports activities to improve performance. The applications in this cluster are not limited to the medical diagnostics or out-of-hospital healthcare categories, though they can have some applications in these areas. Two related activities are discussed in this section. Physical activities are recognized as part of the first set of activities [27] and sports-related activities are recognized as part of the second set [28]. Walking, walking backward, jogging, sleeping, running, lifting one's arms, raising one's knees, and jumping are some of the routines and movements that can be tracked when tracking daily physical activities. The concept also encompasses static postures, such as sitting, sitting and relaxing, standing, lying down, or transferring from one posture to another, like going from standing to sitting.

A measure or estimate of sports performance and feedback related to parameters such as timing, angle, amount, or angle at which force is applied or released can help increase performance accuracy. They help players improve their performance by providing them with real-time feedback on their performance. It has been suggested that wearable devices can improve the quality of sports activities or even enable wearers to do things they wouldn't be able to do otherwise. An indication of the quality of performance or tips on how to proceed is usually given to the wearer via a message. It is possible to view these messages on a wearable device or another place. In addition to receiving messages, the wearer may also receive audio or haptic indications of messages. In addition to badminton [29, 30] basketball [31, 32], rowing [33, 34], swimming [35, 36], hockey [37], skiing [38, 39], martial arts [40], weightlifting [41], tennis [42], baseball [43] and golf [44, 45], researchers have searched for the effects of different sports on performance.

10.5 Challenge and future scope

IoT-based wearable devices must provide easy-to-use access to IoT devices through powerful applications. Using technology to solve healthcare-related problems has become increasingly common in the last few years. Healthcare services are now at the fingertips of everyone, which has contributed to a significant improvement in healthcare services. Using smart sensors, cloud computing, and automation, IoT has effectively restructured healthcare. Research in IoT may be able to fill a gap in future technology development due to certain challenges and issues. A major portion of this section discusses wearable data processing, privacy, security, and transmission issues. The adoption, hardware constraints, interoperability, and scalability points are then drawn, followed by localization and communication challenges. The challenges are discussed below.

10.5.1 Power consumption

It is generally the case that the execution of complex operations involves an additional utilization of energy and resources, thereby reducing the battery's lifespan. However, these drawbacks suggest that it would still be a worthwhile starting point in reducing the potential risk of future attacks, despite the mitigation strategies discussed already. It is quite challenging to implement these concepts on wearable devices. In today's technological age, wearable technology's security aspects are being explored by developers and researchers, particularly in fields such as medicine and industry. As part of a study published in [46], the authors investigated the executability of symmetric and asymmetric cryptography primitives, block ciphers, and elliptic curve cryptography primitives, as well as conventional hash functions. Wearable devices experience higher computational loads when using widely used methods than smartphones, for example. To design efficient devices with limited resources, this study highlights the need for the development of lightweight primitives while considering the trade-off between energy consumption and safety.

10.5.2 Security and data privacy

Monitoring in real time has become increasingly feasible thanks to the integration of cloud computing. As a result, healthcare networks have become more vulnerable to cyber-attacks, allowing patients' valuable private information to be mishandled and potentially affecting patient treatment. Several preventive measures can be taken when designing an IoT system to protect it from such malicious attack. Detecting and stopping attacks on medical and sensing devices embedded in the IoT requires evaluating and implementing identity authentication, secure booting, fault tolerance, authorization management, whitelisting password encryption, and reliable pairing protocols. It is also imperative to integrate routing mechanisms and message integrity verification practices into network protocols such as Wi-Fi, Bluetooth, Zigbee, etc. Considering that the IoT is a network where each user is connected to a server, any flaw in the IoT's security services may compromise the privacy of the user. With the combination of advanced algorithms and cryptography, this could be fixed by creating a more secure environment.

10.5.3 Conduction by sweat

In wearables, charging takes a bit less time since it can be done anywhere. Many IoT devices take a few minutes to power up, but wearables can be recharged on their hands at any time. For people to charge their wearable devices, sweat will be collected from their hands and sweat contains sodium chloride.

10.5.4 Wearability

Wearable IoT devices must be comfortable when they are used by the user. It is imperative that they are lightweight and designed so they don't interfere with the user's normal activities. One major challenge is the trade-off between computation complexity and wearable weight. Chen *et al* [47] introduce the idea of smart wearables that integrate the human body with the cloud, solving the discomfort caused by wearing multiple sensors on different parts of the body.

10.5.5 Environmental impact

Integrating biomedical sensors with semiconductor-rich devices is necessary to develop an IoT system. Earth metals and other toxic chemicals are primarily used in manufacturing and fabrication. It may have a negative impact on the environment. To regulate and control the production of sensors, a proper regulatory system must be developed. Furthermore, biodegradable materials must be utilized more frequently in the development of sensors (figure 10.4).

10.5.6 Conclusion

Adding wearable IoT to real-life applications can open up a wide variety of possibilities. Wearables and the IoT research community efforts were reviewed in

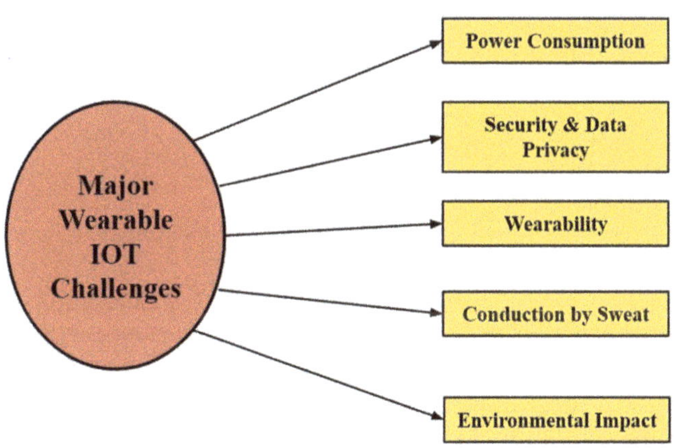

Figure 10.4. Major challenges IoT devices.

this chapter. When integrated IoT systems are available for wearables, they have significant potential. Because of this, wearables and IoT are not taken advantage of to their full potential. Providing a comprehensive overview of this field of research was the main purpose of this work. As well as reporting on all wearable health monitoring devices, it provides an overview of the complete range of tools. Performance, efficiency, and power consumption are considered the most relevant factors in this study. We conclude by discussing some of the biggest challenges facing the IoT and some of the most promising prospects. The challenges described above will serve as a basis for future research and development. As a result, readers who are planning to initiate their research in the field of IoT devices have been provided with comprehensive up-to-date knowledge of the devices.

References

[1] Haghi M, Thurow K and Stoll R 2017 Wearable devices in the medical internet of things: scientific research and commercially available devices *Healthc. Inform. Res.* **23** 4–15

[2] Dian F J, Vahidnia R and Rahmati A 2020 Wearable and the internet of things application opportunities and challenges: a survey *IEEE Access* **8** 69200–11

[3] Cheung M L, Chau K Y, Lam M H S, Tse G, Ho K Y, Flint S W, Broom D R, Tso E K H and Lee K Y 2019 Examining consumers' adoption of wearable healthcare technology: the role of health attributes *Int. J. Environ. Res. Public Health* **16** 2257

[4] Xu S, Zhang Y, Jia L, Mathewson K E, Jang K I and Kim J *et al* 2014 Soft microfluidic assemblies of sensors, circuits, and radios for skin science *Science* **344** 70–4

[5] Tekeste T 2018 Ultra-low power QRS detection and ECG compression architecture for IoT healthcare devices *IEEE Trans. Circuits Syst.* I **66** 669–79

[6] Bathilde J B 2018 Continuous heart rate monitoring system as an IoT edge device *Proc. of 2018 IEEE Sensors Applications Symp. (SAS) (Seoul, Korea, March 2018)* 1–6

[7] Drew B J, Califf R M and Funk M *et al* 2004 Practice standards for electrocardiographic monitoring in hospital settings *Circulation* **110** 2721–46

[8] Dash P 2002 Electrocardiogram monitoring *Indian J. Anaesth.* **46** 251–60

[9] Agu E 2013 The smartphone as a medical device: assessing enablers, benefits and challenges *Proc. of the 2013 IEEE Int. Workshop of Internet-of-Things Networking and Control (IoT-NC) (New Orleans, LA, June 2013)* 48–52

[10] Liu M-L 2012 Internet of the things-based electrocardiogram monitoring system *Chinese Patent* **102** 118

[11] Qaim W B, Ometov A, Molinaro A, Lener I, Campolo C, Lohan E S and Nurmi J 2020 Towards energy efficiency in the internet of wearable things: a systematic review *IEEE Access* **8** 175412–35

[12] Carroll R, Cnossen R, Schnell M and Simons D 2007 Continua: an interoperable personal healthcare ecosystem *IEEE Pervasive Comput.* **6** 90–4

[13] Magno M, Benini L, Spagnol C and Popovici E 2013 Wearable low power dry surface wireless sensor node for healthcare monitoring application *Proc. IEEE 9th Int. Conf. on Wireless and Mobile Computing, Networking and Communications (WiMob)* (Piscataway, NJ: IEEE), 189–95

[14] Domingo M C 2012 An overview of the Internet of Things for people with disabilities *J. Netw. Comput. Appl.* **35** 584–96

[15] Djapic R, Vivier G, Zhen B, Wang J, Lee J and Haiming W 2018 *Wearables White Paper, TNO, etc*

[16] Fu Y and Liu J 2015 System design for wearable blood oxygen saturation and pulse measurement device *Procedia Manuf.* **3** 1187–94

[17] Agustine L 2018 Heart rate monitoring device for arrhythmia using pulse oximeter sensor based on android *Proc. of the 2018 Int. Conf. on Computer Engineering, Network and Intelligent Multimedia (CENIM) (Surabaya, Indonesia, November 2018)* 106–11

[18] Von Chong A, Terosiet M, Histace A and Romain O 2019 Towards a novel single-LED pulse oximeter based on a multispectral sensor for IoT applications *Microelectron. J.* **88** 128–36

[19] Larson E C 2012 SpiroSmart: using a microphone to measure lung function on a mobile phone *Proc. 2012 ACM Conf. on Ubiquitous Computing (New York, September 2012)* 280–9

[20] Ota H, Chao M and Gao Y *et al* 2017 3D printed 'earable' smart devices for real-time detection of core body temperature, ACS *Sens.* **2** 990–7

[21] Gunawan I 2020 Design and development of telemedicine-based heartbeat and body temperature monitoring tools *Proc. of the IOP Conf. Series: Materials Science and Engineering, (Gambang, Malaysia, November 2020)* 012018

[22] Zakaria N A 2018 IoT (Internet of Things) based infant body temperature monitoring *Proc. 2018 2nd Int. Conf. on Biosignal Analysis, Processing and Systems (ICBAPS) (Kuching, Malaysia, July 2018)* 148–53

[23] Xin Q and Wu J 2017 A novel wearable device for continuous, non-invasion blood pressure measurement *Comput. Biol. Chem.* **69** 134–7

[24] Guntha R 2019 IoT architectures for noninvasive blood glucose and blood pressure monitoring *Proc. 2019 9th Int. Symp. on Embedded Computing and System Design (ISED) (Kollam, India, December 2019)* 1–5

[25] Chao P C-P and Tu T-Y 2017 Using the time-domain characterization for estimation continuous blood pressure via neural network method *Proc. of the Information Storage and Processing Systems(August 2017) (San Francisco, CA)*

[26] Dinh A 2017 Blood pressure measurement using finger ECG and photoplethysmogram for IoT *Int. Conf. on the Development of Biomedical Engineering in Vietnam* (Berlin: Springer), pp 83–9

[27] Qi J, Yang P, Hanneghan M, Tang S and Zhou B 2019 A hybrid hierarchical framework for gym physical activity recognition and measurement using wearable sensors *IEEE Internet Things J.* **6** 1384–93

[28] Mencarini E, Rapp A, Tirabeni L and Zancanaro M 2019 Designing wearable systems for sports: a review of trends and opportunities in human–computer interaction *IEEE Trans. Hum. Mach. Syst.* **49** 314–25

[29] Wang Z, Guo M and Zhao C 2016 Badminton stroke recognition based on body sensor networks *IEEE Trans. Hum. Mach. Syst.* **46** 769–75

[30] Raina A, Lakshmi T G and Murthy S 2017 CoMBaT: wearable technology-based training system for novice badminton players *IEEE 17th Int. Conf. Advanced Learning Technology* 153–7

[31] Maglott J C, Xu J and Shull P B 2017 Differences in arm motion timing characteristics for basketball free throw and jump shooting via a body-worn sensorized sleeve *IEEE 14th Int. Conf. Wearable Implantable Body Sensor Networks* 31–4

[32] Bogers S and Megens C 2017 Design for balanced engagement in mixed level sports teams *SIGCHI Conf. Extended Abstracts of Human Factors in Computing Systems* 994–1002
[33] Wang Z, Zhao H, Qiu S and Gao Q 2018 Stance phase-detection for ZUPT-aided foot-mounted pedestrian navigation system *IEEE/ASME Trans. Mechatronics* **20** 3170–81
[34] Wang Z, Wang J, Zhao H, Yang N and Fortino G 2016 CanoeSense: monitoring canoe sprint motion using wearable sensors *IEEE Int. Conf. on Systems, Man, and Cybernetics (Budapest)* 644–9
[35] Pansiot J, Lo B and Yang G Z 2010 Swimming stroke kinematic analysis with BSN *Int. Conf. Body Sensor Networks (Singapore)* 153–8
[36] Bächlin M, Förster K and Tröster G 2009 SwimMaster: a wearable assistant for swimmer *UbiComp '09: Proceedings of the 11th international conference on Ubiquitous computing* 215–24
[37] Häkkilä J, Alhonsuo M, Virtanen L, Rantakari J, Colley A and Koivumäki T 2016 MyData approach for personal health—a service design case for young athletes *49th Int. Conf. Syst. Sci. (Hawaii)* 3493–502
[38] Haladjan J, Reif M and Brügge B 2017 VIHapp: a wearable system to support blind skiing *ACM Int. Joint Conf. Pervasive Ubiquitous Computing/ACM Int. Symp. on Wearable Computing* 1033–7
[39] Niforatos E, Fedosov A, Elhart I and Langheinrich M 2017 Augmenting skiers' peripheral perception *ACM Int. Symp. on Wearable Computing* 114–21
[40] Chi E H, Song J and Corbin G 2004 Killer App' of wearable computing: wireless force sensing body protectors for martial arts *17th Annual ACM Symp. on User Interface Software and Technology* 277–85
[41] Pan M, Salvi S and Brady E 2018 Designing auditory feedback from wearable weightlifting devices *Extended Abstr. Hum. Factors Comput. Syst.* paper LBW561
[42] Havlucu H, Bostan I, Coskun A and Özcan Ö 2017 Understanding the lonesome tennis players: insights for future wearables *Extended Abstracts on Human Factors in Computing Systems* 1678–85
[43] Lapinski M, Berkson E, Gill T, Reinold M and Paradiso J A 2009 A distributed wearable, wireless sensor system for evaluating professional baseball pitchers and batters *2009 Int. Symp. on Wearable Computers* (Linz, Austria) pp 131–8
[44] Arvind D K and Bates A 2008 The speckled golfer *3rd Int. Conf. on Body Area Networks*
[45] Ghasemzadeh H and Jafari R 2009 Sports training using body sensor networks: a statistical approach to measure wrist rotation for golf swing *4th Int. Conf. on Body Area Networks (BodyNets'09) (Los Angeles, CA, April 1–3 2009)*
[46] Ometov A, Masek P, Malina L, Florea R, Hosek J, Andreev S, Hajny J, Niutanen J and Koucheryavy Y 2016 Feasibility characterization of cryptographic primitives for constrained (wearable) IoT devices *Proc. of Int. Conf. on Pervasive Computing and Communication Workshops (PerCom Workshops)* (Piscataway, NJ: IEEE) 1–6
[47] Chen M, Ma Y, Li Y, Wu D, Zhang Y and Youn C 2017 Wearable 2.0: enabling human–cloud integration in next-generation healthcare systems *IEEE Commun. Mag.* **55** 54–61

IOP Publishing

Internet of Things in Biomedical Sciences
Challenges and applications
Varun Bajaj and Irshad Ahmad Ansari

Chapter 11

Low-cost solutions for cardiac care services based on IoT capabilities

Rene Ivan Gonzalez-Fernandez, Margarita Mulet-Cartaya, Gisela Montesde Oca-Colina, Alejandro Lopez-Reyes, Daniel Jimenez-Gonzalez and Jose L Caceres-Hernandez

The Internet of Things (IoT) has emerged as a rapidly developing field in recent years, having a significant impact on all fields of human activity, including health services. Heart disease is the worldwide leading cause of death according to the World Health Organization reports. To face this situation, IoT-based systems provide the required tools to guarantee ubiquitous care services available for the majority. The authors present their experiences in the care of cardiac patients through three specific examples: a cardiac event recorder derived from a Holter system, a device to follow-up cardiac arrhythmias and an assistive device for elderly patients who remain alone in their homes much of the time. In all cases, emphasis is placed on minimizing the cost of the proposal and providing a comfortable and reliable health service. In the experimental implementations, basic services of public data networks have been used and thus operational costs have been minimized.

11.1 Introduction

The vertiginous development and spread of the internet have had a dramatic impact on the life of today's societies. There is no sphere of modern life that has not received its positive influence, although new risks have also been created that must be faced continuously to ensure the proper functioning of systems based on this technology. The high speed of data transmission, the high reliability of all processes and the ease of connecting to the worldwide web in much of the planet have been basic elements for the birth of services that could have been unthinkable a few decades ago and have also allowed the improvement of traditional services that have greatly increased their productivity and customer satisfaction.

doi:10.1088/978-0-7503-5311-3ch11

The accelerated development of communications has been combined with the technological advances of electronics and thus IoT has emerged as a response to the dreams of researchers and entrepreneurs who more than a century ago took the first steps in this endeavour. Suffice it to point out that there is evidence that at the end of the 19th century, more exactly in 1874, a group of French researchers installed a group of devices for measuring meteorological variables in Mont Blanc and the data acquired was transmitted to Paris through radio link. This rudimentary implementation is considered as the most distant predecessor of the IoT [1]. The evolution of communication technologies allowed the development and extensive use of telemetry in the 20th century. However, the term IoT was first used in 1999 by the British Kevin Ashton to describe a system in which objects in the physical world could connect to the internet and communicate with each other regardless of their geographic location [2, 3]. It should not go unmentioned that Nikola Tesla, an eminent Serbian scientist and inventor, predicted in 1926 the growth of global connectivity and technological miniaturization until achieving what he defined as a 'big brain' [4].

To get an idea of the impact of the IoT in today's society, it suffices to point out that many analysts agree that by 2025 there will be around one hundred billion devices connected to the IoT and its impact on the world economy will be in the order of trillions of USD [5, 6]. However, the IoT also generates great challenges in terms of privacy, information security and system stability. The attacks generated against these IoT systems by ill-intentioned specialists are becoming more frequent and sophisticated; this reality leads to the creation of increasingly complex security and protection tools.

Health services from industrialized countries, backgrounded by great financial resources, have not been immune to this technological revolution and thus the IoT has led to the IoMT (Internet of Medical Things). This new concept is associated with the use of internet technologies in the field of medicine to integrate smart devices, software and protocols into services that contribute to continuously improving the health services provided while expanding their reach to remote regions with difficult access [6]. The last features cited make the IoMT an attractive option for low-income countries, characterized by big population and weak health systems, unable to satisfy all the people.

The aim of this chapter is to emphasize some characteristics of IoMT and describe the main characteristics of three systems implemented within this area of knowledge. In the examples cited, emphasis is placed on minimizing costs because they were designed for use in public health systems in low-income countries. The proposals shown are focused on caring for heart diseases and the elderly.

The complexity and potential of IoT-based systems largely depends on the communications infrastructure. Currently there are great differences between the communications networks of highly developed countries and those with low resources, so the systems that use these public data networks must take into account the platform on which they will be mounted. The examples shown only use basic features implemented in any public data network supporting internet protocols.

11.2 Internet of Medical Things

An impressive technological revolution has occurred in recent years in the fields of computing, communications and electronics; this process has provided new health services based on sophisticated technologies that allow increasingly effective diagnoses and medical treatments. Artificial intelligence, virtual reality, big data and IoT techniques are combined achieving surprising results in this sector. This is how the approach known as IoMT has emerged as a powerful and unlimited tool.

The combination of public data networks and current medical devices, characterized by being increasingly reliable and stable in their operation, have allowed many health services to be implemented outside hospitals, bringing services closer to the homes of people requiring medical attention. With this approach, commonly called telemedicine, hospital costs are reduced and the comfort of sick people is increased since they receive different medical services without the traditional movement from their homes to a health center. Visits to the hospital are minimized using modern medical devices connected to the internet that communicate between physicians and patients ubiquitously. This includes IoMT integrated intelligent medical devices, internet services and cloud-based software.

Medical technology companies manufacture a wide variety of medical devices, about half a million, such as electrocardiographs, pacemakers, blood glucose monitor meters and many others. As an example of the importance given to IoMT today, it stands out that designers of medical equipment and devices consider the ability to connect to the internet and send information in real time to health professionals to be an essential feature.

The main benefits provided by the IoMT technology are the following:

- Real-time acquisition of signals and variables that allow characterizing the health status of the subjects analyzed regardless of their geographical location.
- Follow-up of the long-term evolution of patients. The storage of large amounts of information allows the implementation of very precise prediction methods to intervene therapeutically before a dangerous health event occurs.
- Reduction of hospital costs. The implementation of remote monitoring systems, with the study subjects remaining in their respective homes, contributes to the reduction of hospital costs.
- Decrease in diagnostic errors and application of treatments. The combination of artificial intelligence and big data techniques has emerged as a powerful tool for diagnosis and prediction of dangerous disturbances in chronic diseases. The highly specialized medical knowledge can be modelled to be applied in a ubiquitous approach where geographic location of patients and physicians is unimportant. By automating diagnostic methods, errors due to specialist burnout, distractions, and visual impairments due to aging are eliminated.
- It improves the patient experience in the health center, with personalized appointments and better optimization of the care space.

The variety of medical devices considered within the IoMT is very large and can be classified in different ways. Taking into account the technology and how it is used, they can be classified as:

- Devices for telemedicine: Telemedicine is responsible for providing medical and health services remotely, without the need for patients to travel or serving as support for their transfer to hospital centers. In this way it is possible to provide health care in remote regions with difficult access or where the required technology or specialists are not available.
- Wearables: Wearables are medical devices that patients carry, such as watches, vests and bracelets, to measure their vital data. All this information is uploaded to the cloud where applications are in charge of storing and automatic processing to create the proper working scenario for physicians in charge of medical interpretation.
- Aerial devices: Drones are used in the health sector to speed up the delivery of medical supplies and products such as medicines, samples (blood, urine, or skin, for example), and other medical supplies. These communication-enabled devices are capable of reporting where they are and how long it takes to deliver supplies. Time in medicine is essential to be able to make timely diagnoses and to be able to apply the appropriate treatments as soon as possible. Helicopters and small planes are also used to transport patients in situations of natural disasters, major accidents and other catastrophic events. These means of air transport are equipped with medical devices for the acquisition and transmission in real time of the vital signs of people who are being transferred to a medical care center.
- Augmented reality: This technique combines elements of virtual reality with real environments to help improve patient safety and enable the performance of important operations. It has a great application in the training of specialists. They allow simulations of certain situations to train doctors and educate patients. It is also very useful in rehabilitation and in creating relaxing environments to reduce the stress level of patients suffering from painful diseases, amputations, etc.
- Artificial intelligence and big data: Medical devices connected through IoMT allow the collection of large volumes of information on the subjects studied. These data can be intelligently organized (big data) so that different artificial intelligence methods can be applied, thus obtaining new knowledge that contributes to knowing the health status of the subjects studied and predicting future dangerous situations. Currently, these techniques are widely used in the early detection of diseases, increased productivity in making diagnoses and other processes that require highly specialized or experience-based knowledge.

The classification of devices used in IoMT can also be based on who uses them, medical professionals or patients. Those for exclusive use by health professionals are devices that connect to the internet to select the appropriate treatments and provide punctual and timely help, in addition to preventing chronic diseases. They can also be devices in charge of processing the information transmitted by the sensors connected to the subjects studied. The devices used by the patients are also equipped with sensors that provide signals, values of variables or relevant images for the analysis of the health status of the person studied; its objective is to capture this information with the highest possible quality and transmit it reliably and securely.

From the operational point of view, it is essential to take into account how the devices created for the IoT will be connected and communicate, that is, the communication model to be used must be set from the beginning because it will be decisive in the selection of the necessary electronic components. In March 2015, the Internet Architecture Board (IAB) released a document to guide the creation of smart object networks (RFC 7452), which describes a framework of four common communication models used by IoT devices. The defined models are listed below:

1. Device to device.
2. Device to the cloud.
3. Device to gateway.
4. Data exchange model through a back-end.

The IoMT examples that will be discussed in this chapter are based on models 1 and 2 mainly. These approaches are characterized by their low complexity and cost, so they fit well for our purpose. The device-to-device communication model represents two or more devices communicating directly with each other and not through an intermediary application server. These devices communicate over many types of networks, including IP networks or the internet. However, to establish direct device-to-device communications, protocols such as Bluetooth and ZigBee are often used. These device-to-device networks are used in systems with low data transfer rates and with a small number of devices connected to each other. Frequently, there are interoperability problems with other systems using standard protocols that are more complex and expensive. A way to solve this weakness is to create an optional layer, focused on compatibility with other systems, to translate internal protocols to international standards such as JPEG, PDF, DICOM and so on.

In a device-to-cloud communication model, the IoT device connects directly to a cloud service, such as an application service provider, to exchange data and handle message traffic. This approach often takes advantage of existing communication mechanisms such as Wi-Fi connections or traditional ethernet to establish a connection between the device and the IP network, which then connects to the cloud service. This communication model is widely used in devices for domestic use since they are massive and with this approach costs are reduced for remote detection of faults, devices updating and the creation of new services that increase the value added to extend the capabilities of the device beyond its native features. However, interoperability issues can arise when trying to integrate devices from different manufacturers, so many times the device and the cloud service are from the same technology provider.

11.3 Case 1: a cardiac event recorder derived from a Holter system

Holter systems are focused on the ambulatory study of cardiac activity from the acquisition and storage of several electrocardiographic leads, typically two or three, which are analyzed offline by specialized software to detect heart rhythm disorders, fundamentally, although they can also be used for studies of cardiac ischemia based on ST segment analysis. These systems are also capable of performing other studies from the ECG such as heart rate variability and analysis of the temporal or spatial dispersion of the QT interval in dependence of the used lead system; some of these techniques study spatial phenomena and others are focused on cardiac rhythm. The authors of this chapter participated in the development of a Holter system, called Excorde, which had significant success in health systems in several Latin American countries. This device is capable of recording three ECG leads for a maximum of 72 s and is combined with a PC software for storing, displaying and analyzing these signals. A front view of the device is shown in figure 11.1.

Holter systems are unable to record only ECG segments corresponding with what is suspected provoked by the symptoms related by the patient, so the ECG review is a heavy and slow process, requiring much time from specialists. Also, cardiac rhythm disorders are prone to appear and disappear depending on many factors, so a 24 h Holter test could be insufficient to record an arrhythmia event, even a 72 h test could fail. When this situation appears, it is necessary to record more time minimizing the patient's discomfort. Another aspect to analyze is the device autonomy, Holter systems are designed to store 72 h as a standard because of the relation between the battery and device power consumption.

In response to the situation described above, cardiac event recorders emerged, devices able to monitoring heart rhythm in real time and storing in an internal memory only the signals corresponding to the detected arrhythmic events [7, 8].

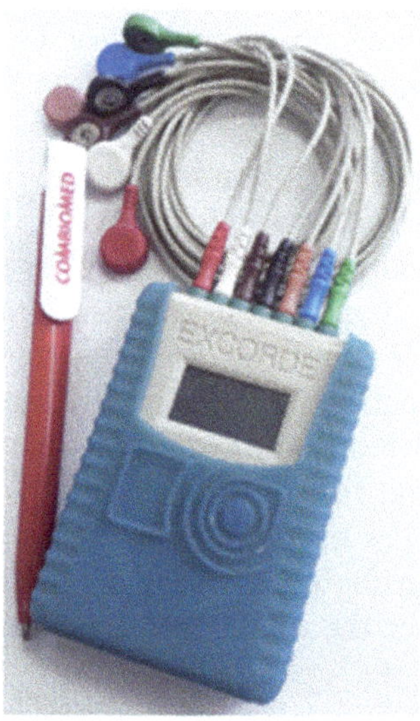

Figure 11.1. The Excorder recorder, a three-channel ECG Holter logger designed by the authors.

With this approach, greater autonomy and greater comfort are achieved for the patient since they can connect and disconnect whichever device they want.

Initially, event recorders were limited to real-time ECG analysis and storage of the signal associated with detected arrhythmic events [8–10]. With the development of the IoMT, these devices evolved to other alternatives capable of transmitting the signals to a server so that they can be analyzed in real time or not, depending on the kind of implemented health service. Nowadays, the following types of cardiac event recorders are available [9]:

1. Patch recorder: This approach is good for two weeks and has everything contained in one unit (patch) attached to the patient's chest.
2. Symptom event monitor: The patient puts the sensors on and turns the device on when they have symptoms.
3. Loop memory monitor: The patient keeps the sensors on and starts the device when they have any symptom. It can record the ECG while symptoms are happening, but also a minute or two before and after they start.
4. Implanted loop recorders: These are implanted under the skin. This approach is more comfortable, but surgery risk must be evaluated.

The authors of this chapter designed an event recorder based on the initial Holter system recorder created by them [11]. The proposed solution adds the automatic detection of events to the traditional signaling of these by the patient. That feature is not common in this kind of device. Also, a second version of the same device is introduced to upload the ECG segments to the cloud.

11.3.1 First approach to the cardiac event recorder

The first developed alternative was based on a hardware simplification of the Excorde recorder; the three-channel amplifier was reduced to two channels because it is enough for arrhythmia analysis and the second is a backup to guarantee a good signal-to-noise ratio. Also, firmware for real-time ECG processing was implemented. Regarding the software, a reduced version of the Excorde ECG analysis software was developed.

The electronic design of the Excorde logger is based on the MSP430F118 microcontroller and all its circuits have been optimized so that it can be powered by a 900 mAh NiMH technology AAA battery; these criteria also contributed to decreasing the device dimensions. It should be remembered that the Excorde device is capable of acquiring three ECG channels and storing all the samples in an SD memory for 72 h, using a sampling rate of 250 Hz. Simultaneously, it stores information in the same memory about the pacemaker spikes it detects.

In the redesign for the event recorder, one channel was removed from the ECG amplifier to reduce power consumption and simplify the design. It should be remembered that for the analysis of cardiac arrhythmias, which is the device's intended use, one ECG channel is sufficient. However, two ECG channels are preserved because this decision contributes to have a channel with a good signal-to-noise ratio most of the time, although the signal is acquired while the studied subject makes their daily activities.

The plastic case and keyboard are the same as those created for the Excorde recorder, thus reducing the cost and time needed to obtain the final product (time to market). Using the same AAA NiMH battery, a much greater autonomy is achieved since one channel of the amplifier was eliminated and only 2 min of ECG prior to the detected event and a minute after it are recorded in the memory, while in the case of the Holter test the signal is recorded continuously. It is true that the energy consumption associated with the microcontroller is increased because of the real-time ECG processing, but the MSP430F168 microcontroller is a very low-consumption component, so the device autonomy is not affected. The block division of the proposed device can be appreciated in figure 11.2.

The ECG acquisition starts by pressing the two keys of the device simultaneously for more than three seconds and stops in the same way. The connection of the electrodes with the skin of the studied subject is continuously evaluated and when a failure is detected, a message is shown on the device display to alert the user. The pacemaker spikes are detected if the studied subject uses this implanted therapeutic device. When the studied subject feels some discomfort, they must press one of the keys. This action is considered as an electrocardiographic event and the device stores the signal corresponding to the period elapsed between two minutes before pressing the key and a minute after; it would be three minutes of ECG for each event suggested by the studied subject, the same happens when the ECG processing algorithm detects an arrhythmic event. In this way, it is possible to store signal segments associated with all the events. Memory capacity dedicated to signal storage allows storage of more than 5000 three-minute ECG strips, allowing recording over long-term periods.

The electrical safety of the Excorde recorder is endorsed by international technical laboratories, so its electronic design is considered safe for patients. It was considered that this security level can be extended to the proposed designs

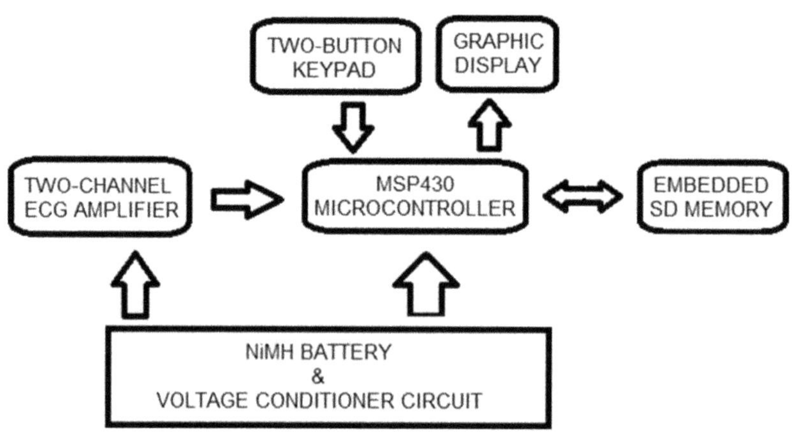

Figure 11.2. Block structure of the proposed device.

because the electronic changes to create the new proposed device do not affect the safety implemented in the original electronic design. The usability of this new recorder was evaluated through the experiences of five adult volunteers aged between 22 and 66 years, whose data is shown in table 11.1.

Usability was quantified through the formulary shown in figure 11.3; this was filled out by the five volunteers who participated in the trial carried out. The average values for each of the evaluated parameters are shown in table 11.2. As can be seen, all the results are favorable and show that the recorder is comfortable and easy to use for patients. At the same time, the cardiologists who participated in the design of this sample were unanimously satisfied with the results.

Table 11.1. Subjects studied with variant 1 of the cardiac event recorder.

Volunteer	Age	Sex	ECG segments acquired	Months using the device	Suffering arrhythmia?
V1	22	M	110	3	No
V2	62	M	446	5	Yes
V3	66	M	1,044	6	Yes
V4	54	F	220	4	No
V5	51	F	244	4	No

	Usability Scale Questionnaires	Strongly Disagree 1	2	⟺ 3	4	Strongly Agree 5
1	I think I would like to use this product frequently					
2	I found this product unnecessary complex					
3	I though the product was easy to use					
4	The support of a technical person is mandatory to use this product daily					
5	I though the functions in the product are well integrated					
6	There was too much inconsistency in this product					
7	I imagine that most people would learn to use this product very quickly					
8	I found the product very awkward to use					
9	I felt very confident using this product					
10	I needed to learn a lot of things before I could get going with this product					

Figure 11.3. Usability formulary to evaluate the proposed cardiac event recorder.

Table 11.2. Summary of the criteria of volunteers regarding the proposed device.

	Usability scale	V1	V2	V3	V4	V5	Average
1	I think I would like to use this product frequently	2	5	5	4	4	4.00
2	I found this product unnecessarily complex	1	1	1	1	1	1.00
3	I thought the product was easy to use	5	5	5	5	5	5.00
4	The support of a technical person is mandatory to use this product daily	1	1	1	3	1	1.40
5	I though the functions in the product are well integrated	5	5	5	5	5	5.00
6	There was too much inconsistency in this product	1	1	1	1	1	1.00
7	I imagine that most people would learn to use this product very quickly	1	5	5	4	4	3.80
8	I found the product very awkward to use	1	1	1	1	1	1.00
9	I felt very confident using this product	5	5	5	5	5	5.00
10	I needed to learn a lot of things before I could get going with this product	1	1	1	1	1	1.00

Table 11.2 summarizes the survey results. The full coincidence of the volunteers in their favorable criteria about the proposed cardiac event recorder after having used it for at least three months is demonstrated. Healthy persons were combined with persons suffering cardiac arrhythmias and everybody learned to use the device quickly and understand the importance of the proposed approach and the role of the sick person in the system functioning. Another important fact is that no device was broken during the trial, technical support was always available, and the volunteers never reported unexpected functioning events.

The ECG processing will be explained later as it is common to the solutions proposed for the care of arrhythmic patients. To review the ECG segments stored by the event recorders, a Windows application was developed that inherited many of the tools developed for the Holter system from which the described recorders were derived. The main features of this application are the following:

- ECG display in several formats using a millimetric grid background similar to the traditional ECG thermal recording paper.
- An SQL database to manage all the system data, including physician comments about the patient evolution and treatment changes.
- Trend graphics.
- Reports in PDF format.
- Cloud-based storage to implement a second opinion mechanism.

This alternative for recording and analyzing cardiac events is simple and easy to implement, requiring few resources for its use.

11.3.2 Cardiac event recorder based on IoMT

An internet-connected cardiac event recorder is more powerful for patient care. Internet connection makes it possible for a dangerous event to be attended to in real time and also allows this device to be integrated with more complex systems such as those combining the geographical location of the patient and the closest ambulance to guarantee a quick patient transfer to a hospital facility. The solution described above is feasible because the detected cardiac events can receive immediate attention if the proper system is implemented. To develop the cardiac event recorder as a device for IoMT, greater hardware changes were required than those made in the first described variant. In the firmware, the fundamental change was associated with managing an embedded modem to implement a TCP/IP stack and thus upload the desired signals to an internet server.

The redesign of the hardware, based on the mentioned Excorde recorder, was more expensive than in the previous case because the changes introduced were greater. To the changes already explained in the previous case, the original NiMH battery was substituted by a 3500 mAh lithium polymer battery in order to guarantee the energy required by the embedded GSM/GPRS/GPS modem included as part of the proposed device. These changes resulted in the need for a bigger plastic box, approximately 20% bigger. Electromagnetic shields were also incorporated to protect the ECG amplifier from high-level frequencies. Based on the changes described before, a block diagram of the proposed solution is shown in figure 11.4.

ECG acquisition begins when both keys of the recorder are pressed simultaneously during more than three seconds; the same action stops this process. The quality connection of the electrodes with the skin of the subject studied is continuously tested and when it fails, a message is displayed on the device to alert the user. When the studied subject feels some discomfort, suspecting a cardiac disturbance, he must press one of the keys to record this situation; the signal corresponding to the period elapsed between two minutes before pressing the key and a minute later will be stored in an embedded SD memory. It would be three minutes of ECG recorded for each discomfort indicated by the subject studied; the same period recorded when an arrhythmic event is detected automatically. The same information stored in the device's memory is uploaded to an internet server using the HTTPs protocol; a cloud-based application (Arrhythmia Station) poll where the server is periodically looking for new uploaded ECG segments. Each segment is

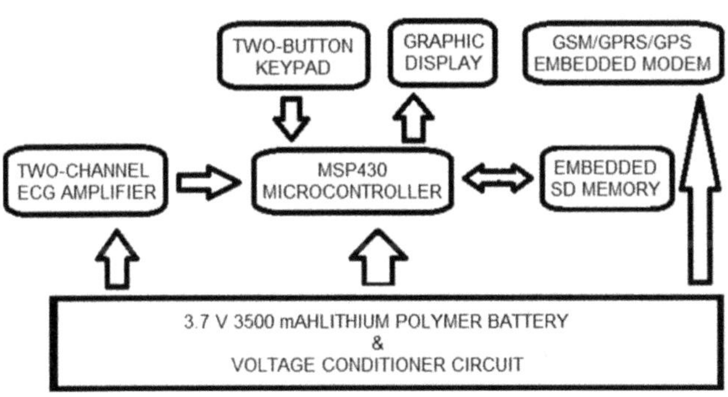

Figure 11.4. Cardiac event recorder block structure for IoMT.

stored in the database to be analyze by the cardiologist any time. Two approaches were conceived for the ECG analysis, which are explained below:

- Offline: This approach is similar to the one explained in the section dedicated to the first alternative of the cardiac event logger. Actions are not taken in real time, but the recorded ECG segments are stored to be analyzed by a cardiologist any time. This specialist logs into the Arrhythmia Station to access the whole information associated with the patients linked to him. Multiple algorithms and software tools are integrated in this software to facilitate signals interpretation.
- Online: This approach is more complex and powerful because of the real-time implementation. Also, it needs more resources and is more expensive. The Arrhythmia Station has to work in a 24/7 scheme, so when the signal corresponding to a detected cardiac event is uploaded to the cloud, it can be immediately analyzed by a specialist who decides the actions to execute (address an ambulance to rescue the patient, send a message to the device asking for a new ECG segment, consider the event as irrelevant or as a false positive, etc). In fact, this approach is very attractive and more powerful, but it also requires procedures, infrastructure and procedures that imply significant operational costs. This proposal also requires a detailed evaluation to improve the response to unforeseen events that usually occur in real-time systems.

As in the previous variant, this cardiac event recorder proposal is capable of storing more than 5000 three-minute ECG segments. Also, the stored data can be used to restore the system database, managed at the cloud level, in case of catastrophic system data loss. When internet connectivity is not available, the ECG segments stored in the recorder can be discharged into a PC to be analyzed using a desktop application designed for this purpose. This is an extreme situation, but it is possible, mainly in low-resource countries.

In this variant of cardiac event recorder, it is impossible to discuss results obtained from trials with volunteers. At the time of writing this document, the prototype's manufacturing process is in progress but it has not been completed. However, the authors consider that the patients' acceptance will be similar to the results reported by the volunteers who used the previous variant. The affirmation is based on how the patient intervention in the system is functioning, it is the same for both proposals of the developed devices. The performance of the ECG segments interpretation service in real time remains unknown because the prototypes are not ready yet and the system implementation will request more resources such as ambulances, offices and so on.

11.4 Case 2: following-up cardiac arrhythmias

In this case, the intended use is different from that explained before. While the cardiac event recorders try to record signals to confirm the suspicions of existing cardiac arrhythmia based on what was referred to by the studied subject, in this case the intended use is focused on the study of persons suffering from cardiac arrhythmia. The aim is to study their evolution to adjust the medical treatment dynamically in order to get a better patient response. It is a process to be followed for the entire life of the patient in order to continuously optimize their medical treatment based on the evidence provided by the ECG acquired periodically. The real-time transmission of signals is never necessary, but the signal is acquired periodically, according to the specialist planning.

The traditional treatment of chronic diseases is based on the periodic visit of patients to the specialist who cares for them so that he or she can evaluate their health state and the effectiveness of the applied medical treatment. In each visit to the health care center, medical tests are performed to get important physiological variables values to characterize the health condition of the studied patient. Cardiac arrhythmias are classified as a chronic cardiac disorder and are treated according to the described procedure. The patient visits the arrhythmia specialist periodically, it could be every three months, a Holter system could be planned to get more information because it is a long-term cardiac test. The great weakness of this traditional approach is the absence of cardiac evidence, such as ECG signals, between consecutive visits to the specialist. It may happen that a sudden and silent deterioration process starts and no therapeutical treatments are indicated because the specialists ignore the new condition. The described situation can be solved with an approach based on IoMT as explained below: for the study of the heart rhythm, the acquisition of one ECG lead is sufficient, being a simple process if the appropriate device is available. If the patient had such a device to acquire a one-lead ECG and upload this signal to an internet server where it is properly stored, a specialist could review the signals and evaluate the patient's progress in detail using specific software for these tasks. If the patient is instructed to acquire three 3-minute ECGs daily, the specialist would be able to see these signals and the variables associated with them (heart rate, number of premature beats, etc) any time. After several days they would have a significant amount of electrocardiographic data available, the same result would be impossible following the traditional approach of medical treatment of chronic diseases. The authors' proposal is focused on creating the necessary tools to implement the monitoring, day after day, of the evolution of the arrhythmic patients studied.

11.4.1 How to solve the described weakness?

The design of the proposed system is based on the requirements set by specialists in cardiology and by patients who have suffered from cardiac arrhythmias for ten years or more. The most important requirements were the following:

- The designed device must be simple, robust, with the greatest possible autonomy and safe. Its use should not imply stress for the patient.
- Specialists need graphical and tabular tools to analyze the ECGs and measurements stored. Trend graphs are required to study the progression of different parameters. Each specialist should only have access to the data of

the patients with them; although tools for medical criteria sharing should be available.

- There should be no additional costs for patients or specialists. The system should be designed for public health systems and its operating costs must be minimal.

The proposed system is composed of three fundamental parts that are shown in figure 11.5 and are explained below.

- The ECG logger: A portable device was designed, powered by NiMH technology batteries, able to acquire a bipolar ECG channel, preferably lead II of the standard ECG because it is accepted as the best lead for heart rhythm analysis. Unlike the cardiac event recorders discussed above, a single bipolar channel ECG amplifier is preferred instead of the two channels used in previous designs. This decision is closely related to the intended use of the designed device; the cost of the device by eliminating one channel of the amplifier and electrodes placement was simplified for better patient comfort. The intended use is the offline evaluation of arrhythmic process across the time based on ECG segments acquired periodically. In the case of event recorders, it is intended to acquire an ECG segment that reflects a cardiac arrhythmia event. If the contact of the electrodes fails or the signal is not of the appropriate quality, the opportunity to record the event will be lost and all you can think about is creating the best conditions to record the signal corresponding to the next one. This is why having two ECG channels was preferred, thus reducing the possibility of not being able to record an ECG signal that has the appropriate signal-to-noise ratio for the intended use. The ECG logger was designed as a low-cost solution, so commercial electronic components were used instead of expensive components such as ASIC, FPGA and so on.

  A low-noise and low-power consumption one-channel ECG amplifier was designed to digitize a bipolar ECG. The amplifier design is based on the OPA4236 operational amplifier and the micro power single-supply INA826 instrumentation amplifier to obtain a power consumption below 10 μA.

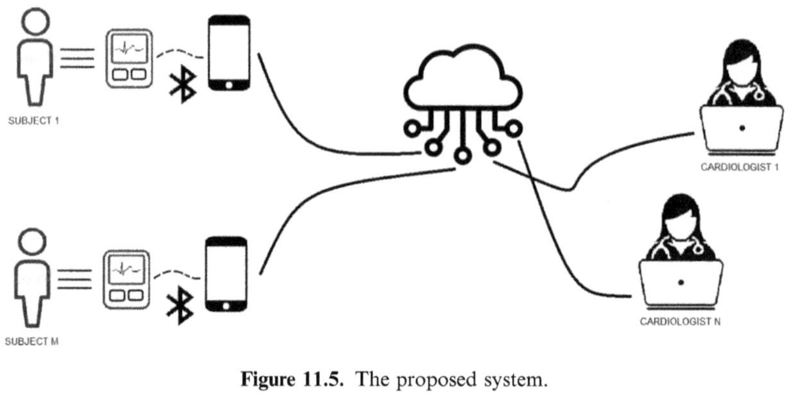

Figure 11.5. The proposed system.

The bandwidth is limited between 0.5 Hz and 40 Hz to improve the signal quality and to keep the main ECG frequency components.

The MSP430F5529 microcontroller from Texas Instruments was selected as the processing unit of the ECG logger; it was programmed in C language and is in charge of all the implemented features. An ultralow-power consumption and a 16-bit RISC architecture with a high-level integration are the main features of this microcontroller. Multiple peripherals such as interrupt controller, timers, serial ports, a twelve-bit A/D converter and memory for data and programs are integrated in a single chip.

The LMX9838 Bluetooth Serial port module was the first option selected because this component was a quality and performance reference in the Bluetooth embedded components market. However, it was replaced because of its cost; do not forget the authors were focused on a solution with a minimal cost. The definitive selection was the RN4678 module. This component provides a friendly and reliable solution for Bluetooth communication; the host communicates with the RN4678 sending commands interpreted and executed by a Bluetooth stack in charge of wireless bidirectional communication.

Two AAA NiMH batteries supply the required isolated voltage for the intended autonomy. An internal battery charger circuit was not implemented in order to simplify the device and reduce its dimension, so batteries should be charged in any commercial charging station which are available at very low prices. A lithium polymer battery could be a better solution, but this technology was expensive and little used in the market when the device design was developed.

The ECG logger design had as one of its main premises to minimize energy consumption, so the firmware was programmed to make intensive use of the MSP430F5529 microcontroller low-power states, that is, whenever the microcontroller is idle it is brought to its 'sleep mode' to minimize power consumption. It only awakes because of a time event occurrence or an interruption event attention request, returning to 'sleep mode' after the event request is attended.

- The mobile collector: It is a mobile-based application to receive the digital ECG transmitted from the ECG logger, store in an intermediate database and upload to the Arrhythmia Station when connectivity is available. It was developed for Android devices, but it can be expanded to other mobile operating systems with minimal changes. The application was programmed in Java language, using Android Studio framework, but several other options are available nowadays. The best choice of these tools will strongly depend of the programmer's skills and will be a determinant to shorten or delay the time to get the final solution.

  The pairing process is mandatory to set the Bluetooth link between the ECG logger and the mobile running the mobile collector. It is set for one time, unless there are hardware changes or failure, and is started from a mobile phone. The embedded Bluetooth hardware selected is fully compatible with this wireless communication standard, so a reliable channel is implemented. A user-level protocol was defined by the authors to guarantee a continuous data and commands flow. ECG samples are transferred by blocks and information about electrode-skin contact quality pacemaker spikes detection is added. Control commands are included as head and tail for each block, contributing to an easy synchronization.

A MySQL database engine was used to implement simple data storage with the basic database operations. The engine selection is based on how simple and standardized SQL technology is today. This database could be very useful if a data restoring process is necessary because of a catastrophic data loss in the cloud application. Also, it is useful when connectivity is not available and the ECG segments recorder should be studied.

The main purpose of the mobile collector is to upload the ECG segments acquired by the ECG logger. This feature was designed considering connectivity failures as a frequent status because designers were focused on solutions for poor countries conditions, where public communication networks are not as stable as the same service in high-income countries. ECGs received from the recorder are stored in the mobile collector's database as a backup and are uploaded when connectivity is available using a secure HTTP protocol. The uploading process includes an encryption algorithm to avoid unauthorized personal data publication, since it is mandatory in IoMT systems [12, 13].

- The Arrhythmia Station: This was designed as a web application to store, analyze and display the ECGs; providing tools for an ECG disturbance predictive. Each cardiologist enrolled in the system can login in to check the information corresponding to any of their patients at any time. The user-password mechanism guarantees secure data access.

The Arrhythmia Station is 'the heart' of the proposed solution; it is able to collect all the ECG information acquired by the ECG loggers and provide tools to make an interactive analysis of this information using tables, graphics and parameters computed by modern methods. A highly detailed analysis is possible because daily information about the cardiovascular functioning is available; it is impossible with the traditional approaches based on periodic visits to health centers and ECG printed in the standard millimetric thermal paper.

A reliable SQL database was implemented to store all general data, ECGs and parameters. Tables and graphics are available to analyze the evolution of any patient, so cardiologists can evaluate the effectiveness of the drug treatment and make any necessary change. Cardiologists' comments and treatment changes are stored in the database too.

Data security is implemented with a user-password mechanism and a database relationship where a cardiologist is linked to several patients, but the patients only are linked to a cardiologist. However, tools are provided to satisfy any cardiologist who wants to get a second qualified opinion about any patients.

Trend charts of different electrocardiographic parameters allow predicting future disturbances. Also, they are a valuable tool to evaluate the treatment effectiveness and introduce changes when necessary.

Classic informatics features such as PDF reports, color and display resolution setup, periodic database saving and so on are available too. Interoperability with other digital systems is guarantee using standard formats to export information.

A simple way to appreciate the advantages of the proposed solution is the following example: a cardiologist instructs a patient to capture three ECGs daily with the ECG recorder (morning, afternoon and night). After a month, the cardiologist has ninety ECGs of the specific patient and he/she can analyze in detail how it is influencing medical treatment in the disease studied. Following the traditional method of visits to the specialist, the cardiologist would take years to accumulate that number of ECGs and would not have the tools to analyze this 'growing big data' in a simple way. Difference will grow exponentially as time goes by. It is possible to affirm that the proposed solution provides a much closer and stronger doctor–patient relationship. Figure 11.6 shows a real ECG segment displayed to be analyzed by the corresponding cardiologist.

The proposed solution was designed as a three-layer system; this concept facilitated the development of the layers simultaneously to reduce the time to market. Digital ECGs are processed at the Arrhythmia Station to facilitate future signal processing software updating tasks at the cloud level only instead of the updating all the ECG loggers. On the other hand, different versions of ECG logger and mobile collector can be used in the same system whenever the data exchange protocols remain unchanged.

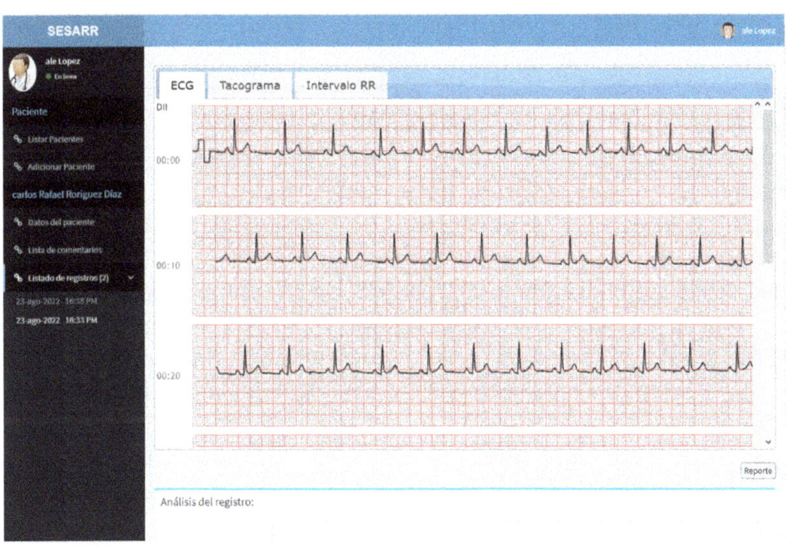

Figure 11.6. Displaying an ECG segment at the Arrhythmia Station.

11.4.2 Overall system functioning

Cardiologists are enrolled in the system by the system administrator while patients are enrolled by the corresponding cardiologist or the system administrator.

When the patient visits the cardiologist for the first time, after their enrolling, they are trained to use the ECG logger and the mobile collector and the latter is installed in the patient's mobile phone. A patient training session is carried out and the necessary elements are delivered to begin the acquisition of ECG segments at home on a regular basis.

Every time a patient uses their ECG logger, the electrocardiographic signal is acquired during the time configured in the device when it was initialized at the patient's training to start the use of the device. ECG samples are acquired and wirelessly transmitted automatically when the ECG recorder is turned on and the mobile collector must synchronize with the incoming data flow; sampling frequency is always set to 250 Hz. If the electrode connection quality is poor, the mobile collector beeps and displays a message to alert the patient and he should correct the electrode's contacts. If this problem cannot be solved, the ECG acquisition is aborted and the acquisition session is reported as aborted due to technical problems Signal quality is very important for the system's intended use because ulterior ECG analysis reliability strongly depends on the primary information, the digital electrocardiographic samples.

The ECG is transmitted in real time to the mobile collector, which is in charge of storing the information in a database and uploading the information to a server whose internet address was written previously in the mobile collector setup. If connectivity fails, no ECG segments are lost because they are stored in the mobile collector database and uploaded to the server when the internet connection is restored.

In the cloud, the Arrhythmia Station periodically polls the server and when it detects that a new ECG segment has been uploaded, it reads all the associated information and stores it in the system database. Every time a cardiologist logs into the system, they have access to all the information of their patients. It is impossible for access to the information of patients to be associated with another cardiologist unless a cardiologist requests a second opinion about a patient. Also, information is always encrypted for transmission from one part of the system to another. The confidentiality and privacy of information is vital in any IoMT-based system and every precaution to combat possible cyber-attacks is useful.

The system administrator is in charge of database saving periodically to guarantee data restoration after catastrophic data loss; they must set a procedure for these processes. Other functions of the system administrator are the new cardiologists' inscription and deregistration when a specialist is out of the system. It is very important because when a cardiologist is permanently out of the system a reliable patient reassignment process is required. On the other hand, cardiologists are responsible for enrolling new patients and for deregistering patients.

11.5 Results and discussion

As explained above, the design of the proposed devices for ECG acquisition takes as starting point the electronic design of the Excorde recorder, a medical device endorsed by international technical laboratories, so its electronic design is considered safe for patients. The changes introduced to obtain the proposed solutions have been aimed at reducing the number of ECG amplifier channels, changing the type of battery and including a GSM/GPRS/GPS modem. The authors consider that the degree of patient safety demonstrated by the Excorde logger can be extended to the proposed designs.

Five prototypes were manufactured and tested by the authors following the IEC 60601-1 medical technology safety standard as a prerequisite for testing with volunteers. The successful results confirm the criterion on the extension of the safety properties of the Excorde recorder to the new proposed devices. The ECG logger usability was tested with five adult volunteers for 60 days, who had suffered from arrhythmia for more than five years. Three ECG segments three times a day obtained 180 segments of signal from each one. Table 11.3 shows age and gender of studied subjects; the type of rhythm disturbance suffered by each is specified in the answer of the subjects to the formulated questions.

Usability was quantified through a survey based on a simple form shown in figure 11.3, while the results obtained are shown in table 11.4. It can be seen that the results for each of the evaluated criteria are favorable, demonstrating that the volunteers were able to use the ECG logger and the mobile collector without difficulty.

Attention should be paid to criterion 5. Two of the volunteers rated it a value of three because they felt that it would be better if there was no need to use a phone and the ECG logger could perform all the tasks associated with the patient. An integrated solution like the one proposed by these patients would be more compact, but could also be more expensive. However, the authors are already working on the analysis of this proposal, which was based on practical experience. The same patients described the solution as slightly annoying, although they recognized its value for monitoring the disease they suffer from.

Three experienced cardiologists with more than 15 years in the specialty used the Arrhythmia Station to review acquired ECG signal segments and agreed that the

Table 11.3. Subjects studied with the proposed solution.

Volunteer	Age	Sex	Rhythm disturbance
V1	58	M	Paroxysmal tachycardia
V2	62	M	Isolated VPC
V3	66	M	Supraventricular tachycardia
V4	74	M	Atrial fibrillation
V5	71	F	Atrial fibrillation

Table 11.4. Summary of the survey applied to the volunteers.

	Usability Scale Questionnaires	V1	V2	V3	V4	V5	Average
1	I think I would like to use this product frequently	5	5	5	4	4	4.60
2	I found this product unnecessarily complex	1	1	1	1	1	1.00
3	I though the product was easy to use	5	5	5	5	5	5.00
4	The support of a technical person is mandatory to use this product daily	1	1	1	1	1	1.00
5	I think the functions in the product are well integrated	5	5	3	3	5	4.20
6	There was too much inconsistency in this product	1	1	1	1	1	1.00
7	I imagine that most people would learn to use this product very quickly	5	5	5	5	5	5.00
8	I found the product very awkward to use	1	1	1	2	3	1.60
9	I felt very confident using this product	5	5	5	5	5	5.00
10	I needed to learn a lot of things before I could get going with this product	1	1	1	1	1	1.00

solution is very useful and easy to use. The main merits that they enunciated were the following:

1. It is possible to simultaneously analyze a number of signals that are almost never available to them.
2. The signals acquired daily allow clearly defining the isolated changes of those that are a trend.
3. It is a friendly and powerful tool for evaluating medical treatments and new drugs.

In summary, the criteria offered by patients and cardiologists support that the proposed system is a powerful, sustainable and useful tool for cardiac arrhythmias follow-up.

11.6 ECG processing

The algorithms used for ECG processing in the proposed systems are very similar, so they will be explained in a single section. The big difference is the implementation, real-time or offline approach. The first one combines thread-based programming with the use of data queues. It always is more complex and prone to unexpected events. Reference will be made to these aspects when necessary.

The ECG processing begins with its own acquisition since an analog signal is converted into a digital one that tries to be faithful enough to the original. A sampling rate of 250 Hz is used, which is sufficient according to the sampling theorem [14] and provides a small digitization error compared to the duration of the events to be measured. Also, sampling rate represents a compromise between data to be managed and the computing power available; it is very important for real-time applications.

Digital filtering is the next step; the goal is to maximize the signal-to-noise ratio minimizing the presence of noise and baseline wandering in the acquired signal. A FIR (finite impulse response) moving average filter proposed by Ligtenberg and Murat [15] was implemented. It was used by the authors in previous projects with good results; an attractive characteristic is that the filter is based on integer arithmetic only; although a detailed interpretation of the expression is needed before programming. The mathematical expression of the implemented digital filter is as follows:

$$y(k) = \frac{1}{K^2} \sum_{m=k-K+1}^{k} \sum_{n=m-K+1}^{m} x(n) - \frac{1}{L^2} \sum_{m=k-L+1}^{k} \sum_{n=m-L+1}^{m} x(n) \tag{11.1}$$

where:

$x(n)$: input signal.
$y(k)$: output filtered signal.
K, L: filter constants strongly associated with cut-off frequencies.

The expression seems complex, but when analyzing the limits of the four sums, it is observed that by means of recursive techniques is possible to simplify the computational processing. This analysis combined with the strict use of integer arithmetic, make possible a real-time implementation.

The authors have implemented a QRS complex detection based on an energy collector and two thresholds; it is a simplified approach to the Pan and Tompkins algorithm [11]. The energy function is easy to implement in real time because it is based on integer arithmetic.

The energy function is defined as the sum of the squared differences of the samples corresponding to a pre-established time window previous to the studied sample. The windows width is set to 150 ms taking into account the width of ventricular beats which are prone to durations over 120 ms. Expression (11.2) corresponds to the described energy collector.

$$y(k) = \frac{1}{N} \sum_{n=k-N+1}^{k} [x(n) - x(n-1)]^2 \tag{11.2}$$

where:

$x(n)$: input signal
$y(k)$: energy function.

This energy collector approach can be affected by signals contaminated with high frequency noise and QRS detection could be affected. A better approach tested by the authors is the Teager energy operator [18–20], defined as shown in expression (11.3).

$$\mathrm{TEO}(x[n]) = x^2[n] - (x[n-1] * x[n+1]) \tag{11.3}$$

where:

$\mathrm{TEO}(n)$: Teager energy operator for each sample.
$x(n)$: ECG samples.

Replacing the subtraction operation contained in expression (11.2) by the expression corresponding to the Teager operator, see expression (11.3), we obtain a new energy collector which is able to increase differences among the ECG segments associated with the QRS complexes and the rest of the signal.

The energy function is combined with two thresholds. The first one is used to detect high-energy peaks and the second threshold is applied to a rough onset and offset identification for each QRS complex. R waves are identified as the wave including the most positive peaks within each QRS complex, so a peak detection algorithm is applied after the onset and offset events were detected.

RR intervals are computed after the identification of all R wave's peaks as the difference between two consecutive peaks. It is a previous step to compute heart rate taken in the RR interval as the period of the cardiac rhythm. Each cardiac beat is classified as premature or not premature according to their previous RR interval duration. This classification process is very important for any arrhythmia analysis; the main goal is a good classification of premature beats to help cardiologists in their analysis. An ECG segment is classified as 'arrhythmic' if more than 10% of the detected QRS complexes meet this criterion. This percentage should be set at the Arrhythmia Station setup and cardiologists can modify according to the patients.

After a QRS complex has been detected, it should be classified. The main goal of the classification process is a reliable identification of premature beats in order to compute the premature beat ratio. The increase in this parameter can be the prelude to such dangerous events as ventricular tachycardia and ventricular fibrillation and the last one is non compatible with life.

Detected QRS complexes are classified as normal (NB), premature (PB) and unclassified (UB). To facilitate the execution of the process, simple and effective rules must be defined without losing effectiveness. The defined criteria were the following:

- A normal beat must be preceded by an RR interval whose duration is greater than 80% of the average duration of previously measured intervals of this type and less than 110% of it.
- The width of a normal QRS complex has to be greater than 85% of the average value of this variable for the previously detected complexes and less than 110% of it.
- A premature beat must be aberrant and its duration must be greater than 120% of the average value of this parameter for the previously detected QRS complexes.
- The RR interval preceding a premature beat (PB) must be short and this concept is expressed as 80% of the average duration of the previously measured RR intervals.
- The duration of an RR interval previous to a PB must be less than 80% of the average duration of this interval.

When the previous rules are analyzed, it stands out that all of them can be implemented making exclusive use of computational operations of integer arithmetic, something that greatly reduces the execution time and facilitates the real-time implementation. The criteria used in these rules are based on the authors' experience developing other medical devices such as bedside monitors and others used in the study of cardiac arrhythmias [17, 18].

The premature beats rate is easy to calculate when QRS complexes are classified. Typically, this parameter is updated each 15 or 20 s. Unclassified beats are not studied.

Table 11.5 shows results when the QRS complex detector was tested with the MIT-BIH database, considered as a gold standard for this purpose [19, 20]. A high sensitivity value was obtained, so the QRS complex detection algorithm is enough for the intended use. This was verified when the proposed solutions were evaluated with volunteers under real conditions of use, that is, the volunteers using the ECG acquisition devices by themselves, without the help of specialized personnel.

Throughout the explanation of the ECG processing algorithms, the authors have insisted on the use of integer arithmetic to minimize the consumption of time dedicated to processing. This is vital because it is impossible to simulate all the situations that will arise when the proposed solution is working under real

Table 11.5. Results with 30 min ECG strips from MIT-BIH database.

Record	QRS per strip	QRS detected	Sensitivity	Record	QRS per strip	QRS detected	Sensitivity
100	2273	2273	100.00%	201	1963	1960	99.85%
101	1863	1861	99.89%	202	2136	2127	99.58%
103	2084	2084	100.00%	205	2656	2624	98.80%
104	2229	2220	99.60%	207	1860	1833	98.55%
105	2572	2549	99.11%	208	2955	2933	99.26%
106	2027	2007	99.01%	209	3005	2996	99.70%
107	2137	2120	99.20%	210	2650	2631	99.28%
108	1762	1741	98.81%	212	2748	2746	99.93%
109	2532	2507	99.01%	213	3251	3220	99.05%
111	2124	2111	99.39%	214	2262	2241	99.07%
112	2539	2538	99.96%	215	3363	3360	99.91%
113	1795	1794	99.94%	217	2208	2177	98.60%
114	1877	1860	99.09%	219	2154	2136	99.16%
115	1953	1951	99.90%	220	2048	2046	99.90%
116	2412	2398	99.42%	221	2427	2407	99,18%
117	1535	1520	99.02%	222	2483	2466	99.32%
118	2278	2253	98.90%	223	2605	2581	99.08%
119	1987	1981	99.70%	228	2053	2018	98.30%
121	1863	1861	99.89%	230	2256	2253	99.87%
122	2476	2475	99.96%	231	1571	1568	99.81%
123	1518	1516	99.87%	232	1780	1772	99.55%
124	1619	1592	98.33%	233	3079	3036	98.60%
200	2601	2576	99.04%	234	2753	2750	99.89%

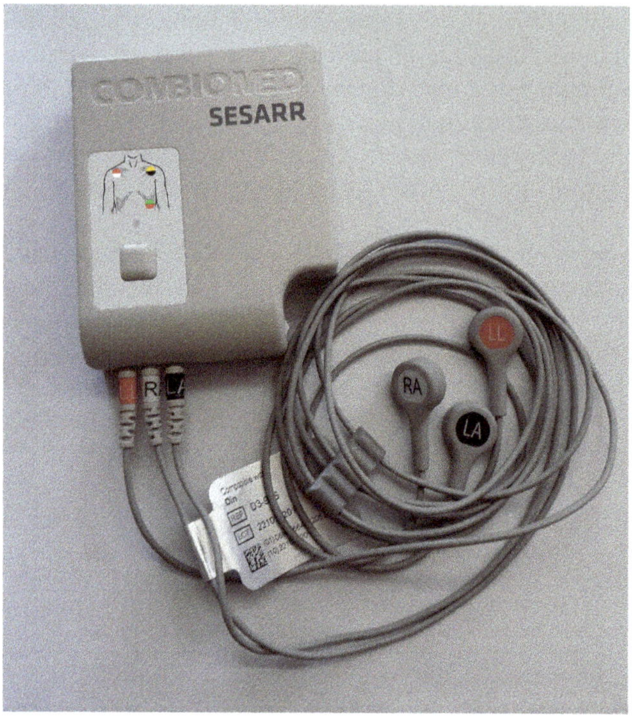

Figure 11.7. Top view of the ECG logger.

conditions. Real-time applications are characterized by the unexpected appearance of events that can be catastrophic if no measures have been taken to mitigate their effects. One of these measures is that the processor always has idle times reserved to respond to the unforeseen delays provoked by unexpected events. Also, this approach based on integer arithmetic operations contributes to reduce the energy consumption of the proposed solutions, increasing their autonomy and the patient's comfort.

11.7 Case 4: assistant device for the eldery

In recent years, there has been a marked growth in the elderly population worldwide [21, 22]. Initially, the growth of this population sector was exclusive to highly developed countries, but in the last two decades a similar situation has arisen in middle- and low-income countries with a growth trend. This is a new problem to be faced by the health systems of these poor countries, which were no longer capable of successfully dealing with public health problems with the financial and human resources available to them [23, 24]. Another aspect that makes the situation more complex is that many elderly people are forced to live alone, mainly due to the exodus or death of their closest relatives, or to stay alone for much of the day because the people living with them have to work long hours in order to satisfy the domestic economy requirements. Under these conditions, these elderly people can suffer a sudden illness or a significant fall while alone, so they need some easy-to-use means to request immediate help or the consequences can be serious, even fatal.

To respond to the situation described, the authors of this chapter developed a device that could be classified as what is currently known as an SOS button, an emergency button or a panic button because it allows the wearer to request help by pressing only one key. Although it has been designed for the elderly, it can also be useful for pregnant women, people recovering from illnesses and people with some mobility disabilities. The proposed design is represented in figure 11.8.

The electronic design of the proposed device is as simple as possible. A display was not included to simplify the user interface and to reduce cost; the user interface is reduced to pressing or not pressing a key. A microcontroller of the MSP430 family controls the operation of the device, which is based on managing the embedded GSM/GPRS/GPS modem when one of the keys, A or B, generates an interruption attention request when pressed by the elderly person. Attention to the event generated by the pressed key consists of generating an SMS to each of the telephones previously configured in the device and unanswered calls, only set communication until ringing status, to send notifications to the emergency care system, the family doctor and the closest relatives. Up to five phone numbers are configured, so the probability that the elderly person will quickly receive help is very high.

The device setup is very simple and fully-automatic. Every time the device is turned on, it automatically connects to an HTTP server to read a file containing the phone numbers to call for help. The server address is recorded on the device through a USB connection with a PC running a Windows application for this purpose. Phones numbers linked to each device are stored in the cloud and can be updated by a cloud-based application developed for this purpose.

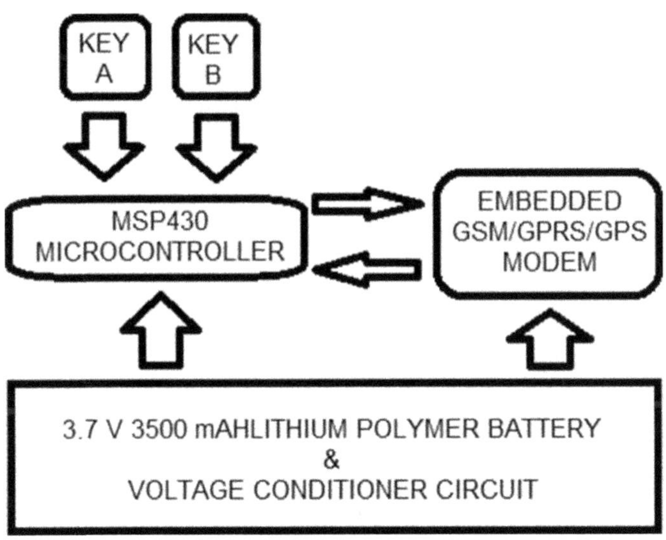

Figure 11.8. Block diagram of the proposed design.

Two keys are included in the device design to request help as easily as possible. If the elderly person is very nervous, it is easier for them to press any of two keys, or both, than to press a single available key. If the device suffers damage, it is more robust to duplicate the keys than have a solution based on only one key.

The same microcontroller and modem used in the solutions described above are used to lower component acquisition costs and reuse purchased development tools.

The product design has two variants, one to hang around the neck and one to use as a wrist bracelet. Three prototypes of the first alternative were made and used by three volunteers whose data is shown in table 11.6. The volunteers were instructed, as it was a trial, to use the device whenever they wanted and write the time and date in a diary.

The obtained results can be summarized as follows:

- Prototypes were tested for three months and no breakage or unexpected functioning was reported, this is an indication that the proposed solution is robust.
- The volunteers requested help 581 times according to what they wrote in their diaries. All requests were received.
- The weight of the device hanging around the neck did not bother any of the volunteers. All agreed that the bracelet variant will be more exposed to mechanical impacts increasing device damage.
- The volunteers agreed that the device is very useful. They told neighbors and relatives in their age range, over 70 years old, about this device and they were all enthusiastic because they considered it a great help.
- One of the volunteers suggested that key combinations could be used to encode the type of help required. This suggestion increases the complexity of the device, but it is being tested for certain users.

The implementation of the full system, supporting patient requests, is beyond the scope of the authors of this solution, but it is not something that is difficult to implement. The SMS service is available on all cell phone networks, it is cheap and very little used nowadays, so it is a very cheap and safe option. The selected embedded modem offers the possibility of transmitting the GPS coordinates, making it feasible to locate the elderly person. Based on the proposed device, other warning services could be implemented to detect when a person with cognitive disorders leaves their home or is approaching the limits of the area where they can be safe.

Table 11.6. Age and sex of volunteers.

Volunteer	Age	Sex	Cognitive disorders
V1	80	M	No
V2	76	F	No
V3	84	M	No

11.8 Data security

Ensuring the security, reliability, resilience, and stability of IoMT applications and services is critical to building trust in their use. If users do not believe in the devices they are using and their advantages for the effective treatment of the disease they suffer from, they will not make stable and efficient use of this technology [24].

As more devices are connected to IoMT, the potential for new security vulnerabilities increases. Poorly secured IoT devices serve as a gateway to cyber-attacks that can jeopardize the stability of the system under attack and can even affect the health of patients using the services under attack [24, 25]. Creating cost and performance competitive solutions minimizing the costs associated with security is a major challenge for IoMT designers. Every poorly secured device connected online potentially affects the security and resiliency of the internet globally, not just locally, and this is very dangerous in the field of health. On the other hand, an expensive and secure device could fail in the market where customers look for a good cost–benefit relationship.

Human beings are increasing their dependence on internet services while more and more devices are connected to the World Wide Web—nowadays it is difficult to imagine life without this interconnection. In the same proportion that these services grow, more vulnerabilities are available for malicious people with computer skills focused on cyber-attacks to put out of order this kind of service and system. In the case of health services, people's lives could be compromised by the failure of one of these IoMT-based systems. Imagine a successful cyber-attack on a telesurgery system while a patient is undergoing surgery, it would be a lethal danger [26].

It is imperative that everyone who interacts with IoMT-based systems be aware of the importance of security and protection against cyber-attacks. Many times, the device designers for IoMT systems come from previous design schemes in which the device was totally closed and intended to perform a repetitive function with high reliability, that is, their design concepts did not take into account the possibility of cyber-attacks because they just didn't exist. By connecting the same device to a phone, a computer, or directly to the internet, the whole scenario changes and unexpected events can occur that cause a serious failure. That is why, from the design stage, when designers are thinking about risks and how to mitigate them, measures must be considered to protect data, secure communication protocols must be implemented and periodic checks of the operation of the critical parts must be designed. Of course, all these measures will increase the cost of the device, but they will guarantee its operation and therefore reduce operating costs.

Based on the foregoing, the following recommendations are made:

1. Any new design or modernization of a device for IoMT systems must thoroughly analyze the risks that the essential connection to the internet implies and define what measures can mitigate these risks.
2. Any new tool or platform that is developed for IoMT has to include protocols, solutions and tools to combat the risks of cyber-attacks.
3. The deployment of many IoMT systems will consist of the connection of identical devices, an example could be an intensive care monitoring room in

which all vital parameter monitors are connected to each other and to a superior system. This homogeneity amplifies the potential impact of any security vulnerability simply because of the large number of devices that have the same characteristics. It is necessary to analyze how to combat cyber-attacks in this scenario, which may be the most common.

4. Long-term management of the devices for IoMT is vital. Many of them have a longer useful life than the computers to which they are connected because computers are prone to obsolescence provoked by new versions of operating systems emerging continuously and the electronics market dynamic.
5. Updated policies must be issued for IoMT medical devices. When a flaw in a model is detected, the update process should be mandatory because the security of many updated devices can be compromised because others were not updated and remain vulnerable.

11.9 Conclusions

The solutions explained in this chapter are examples of low-cost systems to provide effective tools for cardiac rhythm disturbance analysis and follow-up. The proposed solutions were designed to minimize costs because the goal is their implementation in low-income countries. IoMT could be a good approach to solve many health problems affecting people in poor countries, highly specialized medical knowledge could be applied to cure or diagnose big populations without resources to access the health centers located in big cities.

Several theatrical concepts were mentioned to emphasize their importance. Frequently, data security is forgotten for some device designers and it is a dramatic error. Any new design for IoMT must take care about connectivity vulnerabilities and cyber-attack risks from the initial stages.

The authors would like to combine their practical experiences with theoretical topics to share the cumulative knowledge in several years of developing medical devices. We hope this chapter will be instructive for young biomedical engineers and a motivation to improve the solutions exposed and create new ones.

Acknowledgments

The authors would like to acknowledge the collaboration of colleagues from hospitals and technical testing laboratories who supported the development of the proposed systems. Without them it would have been impossible to get these results. The financial support of the Ministry of Science of the Republic of Cuba for the execution of the projects associated with the presented systems is also appreciated.

Conflict of interest

The authors guarantee that there is no conflict of interest with the information published in this document.

References

[1] Tschofenig H 2015 Architectural considerations in smart object networking *Tech. No. RFC7452. IAB* https://www.rfc-editor.org/rfc/rfc7452.txt

[2] Atzori L, Iera A, Morabito G and Nitti M 2012 The social Internet of Things (sIoT)–when social networks meet the internetofthings: concept, architecture and network characterization *Comput. Netw.* **56** 3594–608

[3] Karkouch A, Mousannif H, Moatassime A and Noel T 2016 Data quality in Internet of Things: a state-of-the-art survey *J. Netw. Comput. Appl.* **73** 57–81

[4] Seifer M J 1998 *Wizard: The Life and Times of Nikola Tesla: Biography of a Genius* (New York: Citadel Press/Kensington Publishing)

[5] Holler J, Tsiatsis V, Mulligan C, Avesand S, Karnouskos S and Boyle S 2015 *From Machine-to-Machine to the Internet of Things* (Amsterdam: Elsevier)

[6] Hui G 2014 How the Internet of Things changes business models *Harv. Bus. Rev.* **92** 1–5

[7] [15]; Pradhan B, Bhattacharyya S and Pal K 2021 IoMT-based applications in health care devices *J. Healthc. Eng.* **2021** 6632599

[8] Miorandi D, Sicari S, De Pellegrini F and Chlamtac I 2012 Internet of things: vision, applications and research challenges *Ad Hoc Networks* **10** 1497–516

[9] Scalvini S, Zanelli E, Martinelli G, Baratti D, Giordano A and Glisenti F 2005 Cardiacevent recording yieldsmore diagnoses than 24-hour Holter monitoring in patients with palpitations *J. Telemed. Telecare* **11** 14–6

[10] Kwok C S, Darlington D, Mayer J, Panchal G, Walker V, Zachariah D, Phan T, Mallen C D, Barker D and Patwala. A 2022 A review of the wide range of indications and uses of implantable loop recorders: a review of the literature *Hearts* **3** 45–53

[11] Rodríguez A R, Rodríguez G, Almeida R, Pina N, Montes de Oca G and González R 2010 Design and evaluation of an ECG Holter analysis system *Comput. Cardiol.* **37** 521–3

[12] Fleisch E, Weinberger M and Wortmann F 2015 Business models and the Internet of Things *Interoperability and Open-Source Solutions for the Internet of Things* (Cham: Springer), pp 6–10

[13] Sethi P and Sarangi S 2017 Internet of Things: architectures, protocols, and applications *J. Electr. Comput. Eng.* **2017** 9324035

[14] Lai E 2003 Converting analog to digital signals and viceversa *Practical Digital Signal Processing* (Boston, MA: Newnes) pp 14–49

[15] Ligtenberg A and Kunt M 1983 A robust-digital QRS-detection algorithm for arrhythmia monitoring *Comput. Biomed. Res.* **16** 273–86

[16] Pan J and Tompkins W J 1985 A real-time QRS detection algorithm *IEEE Trans. Biomed. Eng.* **BME-32** 230–6

[17] Gonzalez-Fernandez R *et al* 2020 Combining ECG and pulse oximetry for newborn cardiovascular screening *Acta Sci. Med. Sci.* **4** 49–54

[18] Gonzalez-Fernandez R, Mulet-Cartaya M, Lopez-Cardona J D and Lopez-Rodriguez L 2015 A mobile application for cardiac rhythm study *Computing in Cardiology Conf. (CinC)* 393–6

[19] Kakria P, Tripathi N K and Kitipawang P 2015 A real-time health monitoring system for remote cardiac patientsusing smartphone and wearable sensors *Int. J. Telemed. Appl.* **2015** 373474

[20] Beyramienanlou H and Lotfivand N 2018 An efficient teager energy operator-based automated QRS complex detection *J. Healthc. Eng.* **2018** 8360475

[21] Tison G H, Zhang J, Delling F and Deo R C 2019 Automated and interpretable patient ECG profiles for disease detection, tracking, and discovery *Circ.: Cardiovasc. Qual. Outcomes* **12** e005289
[22] Moraes E, Barros L P, Rodrigues A E, Pagliara A T and Carvalho A C 2012 Pre hospital electrocardiography: prevalence of clinically important ECG findings of a public health system in a developing country *2nd Int. Conf. on Global Tele Health (26–28 November, Sydney)* (Australian Tele Health Society)
[23] Silva B N, Khan M and Han K 2018 Towards sustainable smart cities: a review of trends, architectures, components, and open challenges in smart cities *Sustain. Cities Soc.* **38** 697–713
[24] Dijkman R M, Sprenkels B, Peeters T and Janssen A 2015 Business models for the Internet of Things *Int. J. Inf. Manage.* **35** 672–8
[25] Minh D, Piran J, Han D, Min K and Moon H 2019 A survey on Internet of Things and cloud computing for health care *Electronics* **8** 768–72
[26] Constantiou I D and Kallinikos J 2015 New games, new rules: big data and the changing context of strategy *J. Inf. Technol.* **30** 44–57

IOP Publishing

Internet of Things in Biomedical Sciences
Challenges and applications
Varun Bajaj and Irshad Ahmad Ansari

Chapter 12

Patient empowerment with direct insights from healthcare professionals questionnaires

Antonio Pesqueira and Sama Bolog

The dissemination of clinical research findings and medical evidence through electronic medical records, direct insights, and virtual clinical trial datasets is viewed as a major driver for delivering valuable scientific findings to patients and clinicians.

Different viewpoints on patient data differ, and the use of different datasets in research, and clinical studies, as well as for generating value for patient communities, is strongly criticized, and evaluated.

A survey sent to 278 primary care health professionals asked which information sources they thought were relevant and which datasets and data correlated points they considered most important, for enhancing the value of an overall benefit to patients in terms of different clinical areas.

The purpose of conducting a variety of comparisons with a variety of research assumptions and research questions in this paper was to gain insight into the complexity of the datasets analyzed and evaluate the overall value of the patients' empowerment and increase in information.

The findings of this study and comparable studies indicate the importance of combining new technologies and better clinical, patient-reported, and mobile health data to enhance patient and primary care healthcare professionals' ability to make more effective diagnoses, perform better medical procedures, and access relevant patient information.

12.1 Introduction

Despite being a new topic in the healthcare context, digital/electronic data can bring benefits to different stakeholders in the healthcare field, but not everyone benefits directly from it. Having access to accurate and reliable data is an advantage of an advanced healthcare system and ecosystem. To optimize healthcare business processes, health data must be characterized by large, complex, and sensitive datasets [30].

doi:10.1088/978-0-7503-5311-3ch12

The health industry is constantly creating new applications for analyzing and displaying big data available to all stakeholders in the health system in a powerful way. These applications, however, can be a driving force of change in the sector, particularly with the use of digital mobile data [11].

Different stakeholders are responsible for different data components, such as healthcare providers related to providing better healthcare services, researchers and developers of new products aimed at improving quality of life as well as other stakeholders involved in health-related processes and sharing digital healthcare data (DHD). Despite the potential benefits and more tailored responses they can provide with a better quality of life, privacy and ethics are central concerns with big data-related ventures. Personal health data are sensitive, therefore ethical, and legal questions must be considered when analyzing this data [22].

A global value chain in the health sector (pharma, healthcare providers, citizens, and all other stakeholders) can be enhanced by defining specific policies and technologies that enable big data analysis of healthcare data for the European Union, as well as contributing to the creation of a digital single market [32].

By using digital health data, the healthcare sector will be more efficient, costs will be reduced, and patients will become more empowered with self-data-accessible options. As a new way to take a clearer look at data about clinical research, medical evidence, electronic medical records, direct insights, virtual trial datasets, and mobile health data, as well as diving into the industry to gain insight into the data strategies employed by different companies to guide future developments [9].

Thus, this study introduces the rule that well-being computerized information strategies are certainly central to making information for better dynamic cycles associated with patients and the general business. Utilizing brain network systems, information researchers can further develop consideration, learning, and navigation, upheld by applications that help them in their undertakings. The reason for this examination, which recognizes the requirement for information models to foster explicit value chains for patients, is likewise to empower associations' execution of information methodologies and models to be economically and precisely upheld straight by patients and the whole business.

12.2 Literature review

12.2.1 Real-world data (RWD), electronic medical records (EMRs), electronic health records (EHRs), and health data

Real-world data (RWD) refers to information obtained from a variety of daily activities that cannot be included in highly controlled randomized trials (RCTs). As an example of RWD, we can look at the large quantities of data collected from the use of a variety of medical devices by different users, such as self-checked glucose meters and sphygmomanometers. The actual, practical data obtained from RWD cannot be synthesized in a clinical trial. As part of RWD, a variety of previously collected data is also included, including information from hospitals' electronic medical records (EMRs), National Health and Nutrition Examination Surveys,

Adverse Event Reporting Systems (AERS) or Health Insurance Review and Assessment Service [21].

Using electronic health records (EHRs), healthcare providers and patients can enhance patient care, embed performance measures into clinical practices, and improve the identification of eligible patients and their recruitment for clinical research. As a macroeconomic tool, EHRs (by facilitating pragmatic clinical trials) may be used for assessing whether new treatments or innovations will improve outcomes or reduce healthcare costs [10].

There are many concerns about the current state of different clinical research: a shortage of recruits, a burdensome data collection process, and uncertainty about generalizability to clinical practice. In addition to these factors, declining investment in clinical research can be attributed to the increasing costs of clinical research [26].

From another point of view, EHRs are a major tool that can be used to decrease the costs and timelines of clinical trial research, provide better evidence for clinical decision-making, and advance healthcare. Clinical research has become increasingly efficient, streamlined, and enhanced as EHRs have become available over the past decade. During clinical trials, electronic health records and data handling devices are used for many purposes, from feasibility assessments to data collection during care delivery. For healthcare stakeholders to take advantage of these opportunities, they must work together to address critical challenges associated with EHR data leveraging, including data quality and completeness, information security, stakeholder engagement, and expanding the research infrastructure and governance. Clinical data accumulated by EMR are increasingly used for medical research and are reported to improve research quality and clinician satisfaction around the world. EMR-based clinical research has been shown to increase the quality of research and clinician satisfaction worldwide. Study designs and objectives may allow for the use of various types of data in EMR research, such as medication prescriptions, treatment decisions, and clinical research data. EMR data, therefore, are considered the most reliable RWD, due to their definitive nature. The analysis of RWD yields real-world evidence (RWE), and scholars are concentrating their efforts on RWE research with broad collections of RWD as well as issues of big data. Clinical research has been expanded to broaden the range of relevant studies [20].

There is a fundamental reason for maximizing the mutual complementarity between the new format of research, RWE, and the traditional research format, RCT. The tendency among scholars to mistrust the results of RWE, despite comprehensive reports on the benefits of RWE, persists despite the extensive reports on its importance. It requires trial and error for many researchers to overcome an array of biases that can arise in EMR-based RWE research. A past study of the use of EMRs and DHDs focused on the availability and accommodation of these records. As EMR frameworks aggregate broad information, it is possible to utilize this information during clinical examinations. RWE based on EMRs tends to suffer from the same shortcomings as partner studies (e.g., follow-up costs, long review periods, and consistent support throughout the review period) and RCTs (e.g., loss of members at follow-up, changes in treatment, long review periods, and costs). By testing related factors from the EMR framework, the specialist can rapidly confirm speculation in EMR-based clinical exploration [14].

12.2.2 Prediction data models based on artificial intelligence

With profound changes resulting from the COVID-19 pandemic crisis, emerrging and becoming prevalent lately, individuals are turning out to be progressively keen on computerized reasoning that uses profound learning. Profound learning-based man-made reasoning eventually needs the usage of a broad scope of aggregated information. As EMRs have been executed generally in emergency clinics, there is expected to be an uncommon expansion in the examination of gathered EMR information. To get clinically huge information from enormous emergency clinics, a clinical information stockroom can be a significant device, while EMR will possibly prompt differently sorts of clinical examinations. Notwithstanding, most genuine EMR-based profound learning projects have neglected to arrive at the level first expected. At the core of the disappointment is information assortment [6].

Different calculations created utilizing natural information have now and again neglected to proceed as expected. It is preposterous to expect to sum up and find results with the outcomes obtained from natural and inferior quality information. Consequently, emergency clinics have as of late initiated further developing admittance to orderly decontamination of information [19].

The present world is associated remotely. This is reflected by the way that the quantity of cell phone memberships has overwhelmed the number of individuals like healthcare consumers in the world, a peculiarity that is joined by an expansion in broadband associations for these telephones, which makes a pervasive portable framework. This opportunity has been held onto by a large number of organizations, engineers, confidential businesspeople, and new companies, which have made a torrential slide of portable applications with administrations centered around diversion, infotainment, and the simplicity of day-to-day existence methods. Strangely, the improvement of medical services-related applications and gadgets addresses the quickest developing region inside the data and correspondence DHD innovation area. This offers colossal open doors for worldwide medical services frameworks confronting the test of working on understanding consideration by making it more exact, proficient, and practical while further developing availability, particularly for far-off regions. Until now, the greater part of the advancement in the versatile DHD area has been driven by privately owned businesses, yet focal designs to guarantee the nature of existing and new items have not yet been laid out. This critical need has been perceived by the World Health Organization (WHO), the European Union, public states, and a large number of clinical affiliations [12].

As a great many patients have unfavorable experiences, susceptible illnesses might profit from DHD developments, the European Union made a team to evaluate the best in class as well as the future capability of DHD in the field of clinical and medical practices. Not very many DHD applications had been clinically approved and many were not subject to rules or clinical proof. From that point forward, different examinations have assessed the benefits, ease of use, productivity, and dangers of versatile DHD advancements in unfavorably susceptible disease areas [33].

12.2.3 Data privacy law, data regulations, data security

The collection of the enormous scope of patient information and clinical preliminaries utilizing such information raises the significant issue of the insurance of individual data. Security concerns should be referenced while considering different DHD and RWD datasets [27].

DHD should incorporate the way the collected information, and data are straightforwardly connected with protection, for example, a location, phone number, and email will be eliminated. Any blend that can prompt the ID of an individual, for example, clinic enlistment number and date of birth, should be eliminated quickly preceding the phase of the investigation. The process of de-identification should also be sufficiently robust to ensure that combining anonymized data points does not lead to the identification of the data subjects [1].

Further, all records on the removed data should be scrambled and afterward filed in an encoded DHD, open just to the assigned scientist. Moreover, the items in propositions should not manage the individual data of patients; scientists ought to accentuate that the examination has no chance of inflicting any kind of damage at all on the subjects [31].

At last, it should be determined that the development assent of the patient isn't required given the namelessness of the subjects through encryption of information and that there is no impact on the privileges and government assistance of the subjects since past information, gathered in the wake of having finished treatment, is utilized [29].

To get to business sectors, limit dangers, and gain importance by giving a vital degree of trust, DHD administrations should meet the prerequisites of various lawful spaces. Tragically, a considerable number of these need worldwide harmonization. For example, clinical responsibility and distant treatment are not covered by global arrangements or acts and vary across Europe. Consequently, a worldwide standard covering all legitimate parts of DHD exhaustively is not feasible. Notwithstanding, certain lawful regions offer instruments for making worldwide guidelines. The European Union has long been a leader in the field of data privacy with the General Data Protection Regulation (GDPR) being regarded as a global standard for data protection. Personal health data are considered sensitive data under the GDPR, requiring data subjects to explicitly consent to the processing [13].

In practice, this means that data subjects need to give an additional confirmation which in the digital environment could be provided through an electronic form. Particularly important in the healthcare sector is the patient's consent to both the medical intervention and the treatment-related processing of the health data. The processing of DHD for clinical trial purposes, however, goes beyond the original consent given for treatment purposes and is often referred to as secondary use of data [18].

In the case of encrypted data, the GDPR allows this further processing without requiring additional consent thus showing the importance of the encryption process.

In a lack of efficient processes, patients might lose their ability to control the usage of their health data, in particular, if they are not able to consent to the secondary use due to the lack of oversight [8].

The GDPR sets out to ensure that this lack of control does not occur by requiring controllers to disclose their practices, define the purposes and base the data processing on legitimate grounds, such as consent. While this has certainly increased the level of privacy, the Regulation has a complex and open language that leaves significant room for interpretation and has made it increasingly difficult for businesses to pursue their activities as they strive to ensure compliance [34].

In the healthcare sector, in particular, professionals have voiced their concern that the GDPR impedes research activities and the global sharing of health data. Furthermore, with the appearance of new technologies the GDPR alone may not be able to address patients' risk of losing control over their health data, especially where data is stored digitally in more than one location [1].

In response to these challenges, the European Union has released its first proposal (the Proposal) on the European Health Data Space (EHDS). The Proposal aims to create a privacy-preserving space where healthcare professionals and researchers can access DHD and EHR both for primary and secondary use. At the same time, it seeks to ensure that individuals have more control over their data by establishing the right to access and the right to receive an electronic copy of the EHR, among others. Additionally, the Proposal might provide a solution for the above-mentioned reluctance in creating technical solutions for managing DHD and EHR. Under future regulations, EHR systems would have to comply with the requirements laid down in Annex II before being placed on the market, including safety, security, and interoperability requirements. These requirements also aim to facilitate the interoperability of wellness applications with EHR systems [28].

Furthermore, the RWD gathered from medical devices, wellness applications and other digital health applications can also be processed for secondary use, thus enabling RWE research. While this may lead to ground-breaking discoveries and possibly improve global health, the secondary use of such data may also negatively impact the individuals' right to privacy [17].

The European Data Protection Board (EDPB) and the European Data Protection Supervisor (EDPS) have both expressed their concern and recommended the secondary use of such data be excluded from the Proposal. The reason for this reluctance is due to the applications' features that monitor every single movement made by the individual. The information indeed includes valuable medical information that enables innovative research, but it may exceed what is necessary for the research and even make wrong health assumptions based on data related to the data subject's private life [16].

At this point, it is unclear whether the Proposal will be amended to exclude this type of secondary use. The other option, again provided by the EDPB and the EDPS, would be to ensure that data subjects can make informed decisions about whether this RWD shall be shared and which categories of it should be processed for secondary use [5].

From a data privacy perspective, both recommendations would effectively protect data subjects from possibly invasive processing. From a healthcare perspective, its implementation might lead to the same issues faced now with the GDPR, namely the hindrance of innovative research [25].

12.2.4 Health data future challenges, research analysis barriers

Contrasted and RCT, an EMR-based RWE concentrate on presenting challenges in controlling for predispositions that might influence the review results. Research projects should be started with a conclusive plan to limit such predispositions. Data quality management (DQM) is the main piece of the removed information in RWE. As separated information could be considered side-effects of the most common way of treating patients, as opposed to information extravagantly coordinated and organized as per the reasons for the exploration, and the nature of the information. There might be numerous errors or wrong contributions over their assortment. Through DQM, examination with unique information can be affirmed, including the blended utilization of numbers and letters, mistaken portrayals, and genuine errors. This stage might be tedious, contingent upon the number or limit of information. The most genuine inclination regularly happens at this stage [15].

As referenced above, it is critical to get a bigger example size to raise generally the dependability of RWE. Albeit bigger amounts of information are not guaranteed to raise precision and dependability, utilizing the equivalent would assist with limiting the predisposition that happens in the most modest number. Indeed, even with a lot of really separated information, a specialist might wind up barring an enormous number once the information is arranged as per the reason for the exploration [35].

For instance, there are many cases in which the fundamental benchmark results, like level/weight and circulatory strain, end up overlooked. Without pattern values, there can be no development, and changes in clinical lab information cannot be analyzed. There likewise are continuous cases in which the genuine by and a large number of exploration subjects is decreased by the greater part, for example, when patients for whom follow-up is beyond the realm of possibilities or patients who moved to one more emergency clinic in the examination are avoided. The prohibition of countless examples is in itself a critical predisposition, and it is the part of EMR-based clinical exploration brought up most often by diary commentators as a hard limit [2].

Surely, not all information is accessible in EMR or DHD-related systems. For one, it is challenging to affirm the consistency of the subjects utilizing EMR, including whether they consumed medications as trained in drug-related research. Subsequently, appraisal of the viability or adequacy of medications will in general be troublesome in RWE research [12].

Disappointment of the clinical staff to make passages in the clinical graph is likewise an issue. The legitimate examination would be conceivable on the off chance that the clinical staff depicts the condition of patients precisely and exhaustively. Further, although patient circumstances and medicines can be depicted, EMR cannot be utilized to clarify experimentally causal connections [33].

The area of RWE notwithstanding, EMR information referenced in this work is very expansive. It tends to be gathered straightforwardly from the patient through a different scope of clinical gadgets and by using a wide scope of information. In like manner, RWD is expanding in volume, though RWE is slowly extended, with the nonstop progression of their particular logical capacities and conventions [2].

Notwithstanding the significance of the amount of information, it is important to focus on the method for appropriately organizing and using quickly amassed clinical information. RWE and RCT research are not in a commonly cutthroat relationship. As of now, RWE research cannot substitute RCT research. Nonetheless, RCT research gave the most noteworthy unwavering quality, and RWE research seen to mirror the genuine clinical viewpoint, can be demonstrated to share a commonly strengthening relationship to turn into the most remarkable asset in proof-based medication [22].

12.3 Empirical methodological approach

To cover all topics proposed, we developed a survey. For enhancing the value of an overall benefit to patients in a variety of clinical areas, 278 primary care health professionals (HCPs) were asked which information sources they thought were relevant and which datasets and data correlated points they thought were most important. This quantitative study analyzed the collected questionnaire data to better understand and summarize dependent and independent variables, key statistics parameters, correlations, associations, and principal components of data associations. Additionally, measurement instruments like the questionnaire can be used to define study objectives with measurable variables in addition to the COVID-19 lockdown restrictions preventing face-to-face interviews [7].

In using this sampling technique, we were able to select a representative sample of the population and divide them into subgroups with the right expertise and experience for the study objectives. Several criteria elements were required for inclusion in this sample [4].

A combination of proximity and expertise from the researchers made the population eligible for inclusion. Hence, in this paper we investigated the complexity of the datasets analyzed and the overall value of patients' empowerment and knowledge increase by conducting a variety of comparisons based on a range of assumptions and questions. To answer the research question identified, we used quantitative methods to assess the differences between organizations with and without a DHD strategy. We developed a structured questionnaire for gathering information based on an in-depth literature review. In non-probabilistic sampling procedures, convenience samples can be used whenever it is difficult to obtain a complete sample. Our method of selecting individuals in corporations across the world with a confidence level of 95% (and $p = q = 0.5$). Table 12.1 provides detailed information about how the data was collected and analyzed.

Following the descriptive analysis, we can understand that all the consulted HCPs have significant experience working in the connected themes as well as holding senior positions within the affiliated companies. As seen in figure 12.1, the sample

Table 12.1. Fact sheet.

Fieldwork	February 2022 to March 2022
Sample size	278 surveyed
Sample type	Convenience and geographic quota sampling
Survey type	Structured online questionnaire
Geographical area	177 Europe, 79 North America, 7 China, 7 APAC, and 9 others

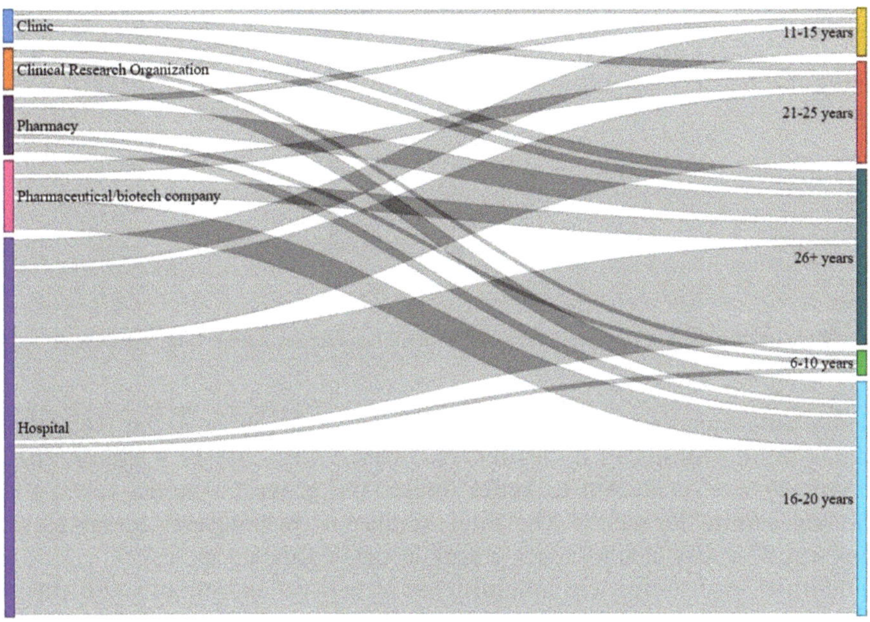

Figure 12.1. Working and affiliated organizations and years of experience.

includes HCPs working mainly in hospitals representing 74%, where 11% work in pharmaceutical or biotechnology companies, 7% correspond to HCPs working in pharmacies, 5% in clinical research organizations, and 3% in clinics.

With a total percentage of 22%, respondents to the questionnaire were from oncology, followed by 17% from vaccines, then 14% from endocrinology, followed by rare diseases at 13%, and cardiology at 13%, with the other distributions of the therapeutic areas in which the HCPs were connected shown below (figure 12.2).

12.3.1 Questionnaire design and variable selection

Using the methodology approach process described previously, we formulated a structured questionnaire based on the results of the literature review. The changes affect healthcare organizations (HCOs) regardless of whether they utilize DHD. The research, which is based on a survey to analyze the current adoption and application

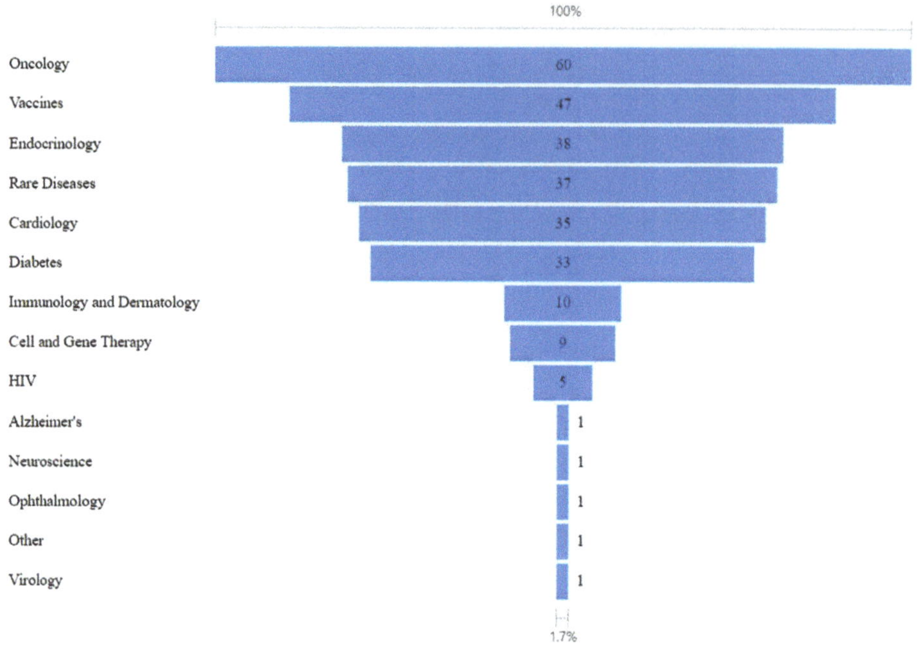

Figure 12.2. Therapeutic areas connected with affiliated organizations from respondents.

of health data technology, is proposed to shed light on how the technology is becoming more widespread in healthcare. From 8 February to 4 March 2022, an online survey was conducted to better understand general attitudes toward DHD technology within the sector. The total number of respondents across all global regions was 278, of which all are working in the healthcare sector.

In addition, one survey was administered to external consultants and experts to gauge their views on DHD technologies. Based on previous studies that were translated and validated by an expert committee consisting of two specialists, a statistician, and the authors, the study used a self-administered survey developed by the authors using Google Forms. The questionnaire was administered in English and included demographic questions like gender and age. Respondents were asked to complete an anonymous questionnaire to respect their right to privacy and to not identify their affiliated organizations in the database. An open-ended and closed-ended questionnaire was used, and the questions were mostly designed to complement closed questions in cases when one or more possible answers did not fit respondents. To validate the consistency of the questionnaire, ten respondents, a representative sample of the study population, were analyzed before the distribution of the survey [23].

As part of the questionnaire invitation email, digital health data was defined as a new emerging technology having significant implications for healthcare, medical direct insights, EMRs, EHRs, and virtual clinical trial data management, among other relevant areas.

12.3.2 Results and statistical analysis

According to the questionnaire results, this section summarizes the most important topics. This study's data analysis was carried out using SPSS and Microsoft Excel. There will be some statistical hypotheses presented in this section, and some correlations and connections analyzed, with special attention paid to many key variables, data management components, and security issues regarding DHD processes, technologies, and programs being discussed. Moreover, we conducted statistical and descriptive analyses of the sample of industry professionals and decision-makers to determine whether it was representative of the entire population. In terms of categorical and numerical variables, understanding which tests were preferred required close attention during data classification activities. The differences between organizations that use DHD and those that do not were analyzed using an analysis of covariance (ANCOVA). A Shapiro–Wilk test was conducted to determine whether the null hypothesis of normality was rejected. With a multivariate design with covariates, other covariate variables, such as psychological variables, can be reduced, which can reduce damage. Using this method, individual differences in variance were estimated through a regression between the dependent variable and the covariable. ANOVA was then performed on these adjusted scores after statistically adjusting the dependent variable for the covariable variable.

To eliminate variation due to the mismatch of the ANOVA error, the analysis controls the effect of the covariable variable. To investigate technological and related DHD differences, the following hypotheses were examined, and in table 12.2 the adjusted mean for each group is presented [24].

Table 12.2 shows the adjusted means, *F*-statistics, and *p*-values, demonstrating that not all variables related to the presence of DHD show statistically significant differences, with the variables, present showing with DHD a higher score in organizations, indicating that a high statistical significance is associated with this variable. The factors identified from this analysis were then subjected to an

Table 12.2. Adjusted means, *F*-statistics, and *p*-values.

Variables	With DHD	No DHD	F	p
Digital data volume	161 128	59 153	58 385	0.071**
Data quality	161 101	59 631	44 633	0.000***
Availability of data	161 367	59 614	7234	0.12*
Data ownership	161 377	59 571	93 375	0.000***
Cost of data	161 278	59 568	61 542	0.000***
Lack of technology	161 119	59 861	63 377	0.012**
Shortage of talent/skills	161 035	59 738	71 934	0.005***
Privacy concerns	161 231	59 912	85 069	0.0653**
Data security	161 288	59 837	98 908	0.135*

*$p < 0.1$;
**$p < 0.05$;
***$p < 0.01$.

exploratory factorial analysis to further understand the connections and relationships between the variables [24].

A factor that has nine items and is referred to as the DHD dimension can explain 83.93% of the variance of the matrix of challenges, as determined by the extraction method. Using Varimax as the rotation procedure, a second factor explaining 50.908% of the variance, along with the DHD security dimension, was identified. 84.874% of the variance can be explained by these two extracted factors (table 12.3), and a Kaiser–Meyer–Olkin index larger than 0.7 is supported by a Bartlett test of sphericity of 4633.704 (p-value <0.000).

A Cronbach's alpha of 0.7 or greater is recognized for this study, as is a composite reliability index of 0.7 or greater, and average variance extracted of more than 0.5 is noted for this study. Validity measures are also adequate, such as higher coefficients of standard loadings, more than 0.7 means, a lower confidence interval of correlations, and higher coefficients of standardized loadings [3].

On the main analysis axis, we have validated the scales for data management and data security with five indicators each, with technology deficiencies and talent shortages carrying the highest loads and in connection with the organizations with DHD presence. As we proceeded with our analysis (table 12.4), we analyzed globally the differences that may exist between organizations with DHD-related processes and strategies in terms of both data management and data security.

According to table 12.4, DHD-oriented organizations perform better both in management and data security. In terms of practical business implications, an organization with DHD-related skills will be able to make better business decisions since accurate and valuable data are used to make the decision.

Table 12.3. Exploratory factor analysis.

			Components	
Item	Skewness	Kurtosis	1	
Digital data volume	−0.739	0.147	0.841	
Data quality	0.253	−1.057	0.691	
Availability of data	−0.048	−1.625	0.763	
Data ownership	−0.501	−0.370	0.912	
Cost of data	−0.150	−1.444	0.840	
Lack of technology	−0.203	−1.262	0.829	
Shortage of talent/skills	−0.131	−1.517	0.637	
Privacy concerns	−0.966	−0.207	0.627	
Data security	−0.174	−1.645		0.728
% Variance explained				50.908%
Kaiser–Meyer–Olkin index			0.762	
Bartlett's test of sphericity			Chi-square = 4633.704; sig <0.000	

Table 12.4. ANCOVA. Data management and data security. Adjusted means, *F* statistics, and *p*-values.

Dimensions	DHD	No DHD	*F*	*p*
Data management	161 255	59 570	71 016	0.000***
Data security	161 197	59 792	24 735	0.000***

*$p < 0.1$;
**$p < 0.05$;
***$p < 0.01$.

Table 12.5. Evaluation of the structural relationship.

	DHD		No DHD	
Structural relationship	Coef.	Value *t**	Coef.	Value *t**
DS → DM	0.884 35	48.31***	0.1403	0.97

*$p < 0.1$;
**$p < 0.05$;
***$p < 0.01$.

As soon as the measurement model was validated, an exploratory analysis was necessary to find out if there is a relationship between data security and data management and if the organization has a data science strategy. According to table 12.5, we used the maximum likelihood analysis for structural equation models because it is robust to non-normal data, whereas we used the standardized coefficients for this structural relationship analysis.

This analysis suggests that there exists an empirically supported positive association between data security and data management within organizations implementing DHD-related technologies and processes. Alpha coefficients of each of the selected scales were computed to measure the scales' internal reliability.

12.4 Conclusions

Using a survey of 278 healthcare professionals, this study explores DHD's application to the healthcare industry, where they were asked which information sources, they considered relevant and which datasets and data correlation points they deemed important. As part of Patient Empowerment with Electronic Medical Records, Direct Insights, and Virtual Trial Datasets, we aim to enhance the value of an overall benefit to patients in terms of different clinical areas. In this study and comparative studies, the importance of combining new technologies with better clinical, patient-reported, and mobile health data is illustrated. For the industry to be able to implement the described techniques and models effectively for the management of DHD, there is a need to develop a strong organizational culture and a strong practical capacity.

As part of our analysis of DHD strategies, we consider key dimensions such as RWD, EMRs, EHRs, and health data, prediction models powered by artificial intelligence, data privacy law, data regulations, data security, and future challenges in health data analysis. We can conclude from our chosen methodology that companies should enhance their data security to achieve better results in DHD, a concern with data management that most companies see as a growing concern. Based on the results of the literature review, we devised a structured questionnaire based on the methodology approach, and a few statistical hypotheses were formulated based on these findings. A special focus was placed on understanding key variables, data management components, and security issues relating to DHD processes, technologies, and programs, as well as some correlations and connections. Regardless of whether an HCO uses DHD, the changes affect them, where the research is based on a survey that analyses the current adoption and application of DHD technology to shed light on how the technology is becoming more prevalent in healthcare. In addition, we can conclude that DHD needs to consider how the collected data, information, and phone numbers are directly connected to protection, for example, eliminating the location, phone number, and email.

Elimination of any DHD-connected risks that may reveal an individual's identity, such as a clinic's enrolment number and date of birth, should be done immediately before the screening phase, and the de-identification process should be robust enough to ensure that the combination of anonymized data points does not identify subjects. From the conclusions presented, whether DHD-related projects are amended to include more security and data regulation protocols and ensure that data subjects can make informed choices about whether to share RWD and which categories of it should be processed for secondary use, from a data protection perspective, both recommendations would effectively protect data subjects from potentially invasive processing.

References

[1] Appenzeller A, Hornung M, Kadow T, Krempel E and Beyerer J 2022 Sovereign digital consent through privacy impact quantification and dynamic consent *Technologies* **101** 35

[2] Archer N, Fevrier-Thomas U, Lokker C, McKibbon K A and Straus S E 2011 Personal health records: a scoping review *J. Am. Med. Inform. Assoc.* **184** 515–22

[3] Barati M, Taheri-Kharameh Z, Farghadani Z and Rásky É 2019 Validity and reliability evaluation of the Persian version of the heart failure-specific health literacy scale *Int. J. Community Based Nurs. Midwifery* **73** 222

[4] Bhardwaj P 2019 Types of sampling in research *J. Pract. Cardiovasc. Sci.* **53** 157

[5] Bitar H and Jakobsson B 2017 GDPR: securing personal data in compliance with new EU-regulations *Master's Thesis* Lulea University of Technology

[6] Bohr A and Memarzadeh K 2020 The rise of artificial intelligence in healthcare applications *Artificial Intelligence in Healthcare* (New York: Academic) pp 25–60

[7] Bonal X and González S 2020 The impact of lockdown on the learning gap: family and school divisions in times of crisis *Int. Rev. Educ.* **665** 635–55

[8] Ciampi M, Sicuranza M and Silvestri S 2022 A privacy-preserving and standard-based architecture for secondary use of clinical data *Information* **132** 87

[9] Coravos A, Doerr M, Goldsack J, Manta C, Shervey M, Woods B and Wood W A 2020 Modernizing and designing evaluation frameworks for connected sensor technologies in medicine *NPJ Digit. Med.* **31** 1–10

[10] Cowie M R, Blomster J I, Curtis L H, Duclaux S, Ford I, Fritz F and Zalewski A 2017 Electronic health records to facilitate clinical research *Clin. Res. Cardiol.* **1061** 1–9

[11] Elhoseny M, Abdelaziz A, Salama A S, Riad A M, Muhammad K and Sangaiah A K 2018 A hybrid model of internet of things and cloud computing to manage big data in health services applications *Future Gener. Comput. Syst.* **86** 1383–94

[12] Essén A, Scandurra I, Gerrits R, Humphrey G, Johansen M A, Kierkegaard P and Ancker J S 2018 Patient access to electronic health records: differences across ten countries *Health Policy Technol.* **71** 44–56

[13] European Data Protection Board 2020 Guidelines 05/2020 on consent under Regulation 2016/679

[14] Franklin J M and Schneeweiss S 2017 When and how can real-world data analyses substitute for randomized controlled trials? *Clin. Pharmacol. Ther.* **1026** 924–33

[15] Gemmen E, Rodriguez A M, Palmer A and Parmenter L 2018 Measuring treatment satisfaction with medication from patients' perspective: conceptual models and a review of measures *Value Health* **21** S54–5

[16] Jančiūtė L 2020 European data protection board: a nascent EU agency or an 'intergovernmental club'? *Int. Data Priv. Law* **101** 57–75

[17] Joseph S, Sempik J, Leu A and Becker S 2020 Young carers research, practice, and policy: an overview and critical perspective on possible future directions *Adolesc. Res. Rev.* **51** 77–89

[18] Jungkunz M, Köngeter A, Mehlis K, Winkler E C and Schickhardt C 2021 Secondary use of clinical data in data-gathering, non-interventional research or learning activities: definition, types, and a framework for risk assessment *J. Med. Internet Res.* **236** e26631

[19] Karvellas C J, Farhat M R, Sajjad I, Mogensen S S, Leung A A, Wald R and Bagshaw S M 2011 A comparison of early versus late initiation of renal replacement therapy in critically ill patients with acute kidney injury: a systematic review and meta-analysis *Crit. Care* **151** 1–10

[20] Katkade V B, Sanders K N and Zou K H 2018 Real-world data: an opportunity to supplement existing evidence for the use of long-established medicines in health care decision making *J. Multidiscip. Healthc.* **11** 295

[21] Kim H S, Lee S and Kim J H 2018 Real-world evidence versus randomized controlled trial: clinical research based on electronic medical records *J. Korean Med. Sci.* **33** e213

[22] Kitchin R 2014 *The Data Revolution: Big Data, Open Data, Data Infrastructures, and Their Consequences* (Thousand Oaks, CA: SAGE)

[23] Mealing N M, Banks E, Jorm L R, Steel D G, Clements M S and Rogers K D 2010 Investigation of relative risk estimates from studies of the same population with contrasting response rates and designs *BMC Med. Res. Method.* **101** 1–12

[24] Mette C, Zimmermann M, Grabemann M, Abdel-Hamid M, Uekermann J, Biskup C S and Kis B 2013 The impact of acute tryptophan depletion on attentional performance in adult patients with ADHD *Acta Psychiatr. Scand.* **1282** 124–32

[25] Mitrou L 2018 Data protection, artificial intelligence and cognitive services: is the general data protection regulation (GDPR) 'artificial intelligence-proof'? *SSRN* https://doi.org/10.2139/ssrn.3386914

[26] Moses H, Matheson D H, Cairns-Smith S, George B P, Palisch C and Dorsey E R 2015 The anatomy of medical research: US and international comparisons *JAMA* **3132** 174–89

[27] Patrick D L, Burke L B, Gwaltney C J, Leidy N K, Martin M L, Molsen E and Ring L 2011 Content validity—establishing and reporting the evidence in newly developed patient-reported outcomes PRO instruments for medical product evaluation: ISPOR PRO Good

Research Practices Task Force report: part 2—assessing respondent understanding *Value Health* **148** 978–88

[28] Piepoli M F, Corrà U, Adamopoulos S, Benzer W, Bjarnason-Wehrens B, Cupples M and Giannuzzi P 2014 Secondary prevention in the clinical management of patients with cardiovascular diseases. Core components, standards and outcome measures for referral and delivery: a policy statement from the cardiac rehabilitation section of the European Association for Cardiovascular Prevention and Rehabilitation Endorsed by the Committee for Practice Guidelines of the European Society of Cardiology *Eur. J. Prev. Cardiol.* **216** 664–81

[29] Raman S R, Curtis L H, Temple R, Andersson T, Ezekowitz J, Ford I and Hernandez A F 2018 Leveraging electronic health records for clinical research *Am. Heart J.* **202** 13–9

[30] Ristevski B and Chen M 2018 Big data analytics in medicine and healthcare *J. Integr. Bioinform.* **15** 20170030

[31] Rojas M I, Giles S S, Little M, Baron R, Livingston I, Dagenais T R and Rohwer F 2021 Swabbing the urban environment—a pipeline for sampling and detection of SARS-CoV-2 from environmental reservoirs *J. Vis. Exp.* **170** e62379

[32] Roski J, Bo-Linn G W and Andrews T A 2014 Creating value in health care through big data: opportunities and policy implications *Health Aff. (Millwood)* **337** 1115–22

[33] Sahama T, Stranieri A and Butler-Henderson K 2019 Patient-empowered electronic health records *Stud. Health Technol. Inform.* **264** 1765–6

[34] Valtysson B, Jørgensen R F and Munkholm J L 2021 Co-constitutive complexity *Nord. Rev.* **421** 124–40

[35] Wicks P, Stamford J, Grootenhuis M A, Haverman L and Ahmed S 2014 Innovations in e-health *Qual. Life Res.* **231** 195–203

Chapter 13

Internet of Things in biomedical system: significance, applications, and challenges

Ashish Tripathi, Arun Kumar Singh, Anand Bhushan Pandey, Arjun Chaudhary and Pushpa Choudhary

In recent years, it has been found that the Internet of Things (IoT) has played a significant role in various applications in biomedical systems like diagnosis, prevention, and real-time monitoring of various diseases. Internet of Medical Things (IoMT) is a well-known term that ensures the availability of medical services to patients on time. Thus, it ensures the health, wellness, and people care that requires real-time monitoring and processing of huge medical data, its storage, and on-demand availability. The medical data center as cloud storage plays a significant role in storing such data and its availability. As the medical data captured by IoMT devices are growing exponentially, this may be a major security and privacy concern for sensitive data. This mainly occurs either for stored data in the cloud or during the data transmission to the cloud. Integration of multiple IoT devices, data accuracy, and cost consideration are the other major concerns that cause obstacles to implementing IoT in biomedical systems. This chapter presents a detailed state-of-the-art survey on IoT and biomedical systems, followed by the major issues related to the implementation of IoT along with the significance and various applications of IoT in the biomedical system.

13.1 Introduction

The discovery of the internet is one of the key inventions in the computing world that has facilitated different services like communication, information sharing, and knowledge discovery from different places with an Internet connection. The first wide-area packet-switched network that implemented the TCP/IP protocol suite named 'Advanced Research Project Agency Network (ARPANET)' was coined in 1969 by the U.S. Military. This was the forerunner of modern internet technology. Before that, computers were used with limited functionalities and only for a few

doi:10.1088/978-0-7503-5311-3ch13

operations. But now, day by day, internet services are adding new functionalities and making our tasks as simple as possible. Now, the current computing scenario has been completely changed. Now, people are able to perform several tasks, i.e., watching movies, playing games, online photo editing, video conferencing, online chatting, banking transactions, online shopping, and so on by using the internet. To do all the tasks, it does not require that all data need to be present in the local system's storage area. This only needs an internet connection to access the data/to run any application stored in some other location around the world.

In IoT, 'things' means all physical devices with the ability to exchange data over the internet with other devices. These devices are embedded with unique components like sensors, software, and other required technologies to gather different kinds of data like humidity, sound, temperature, light, etc from the environment. IoT can be understood as a network of these things (physical devices) to connect, and exchange data with other compatible things over the internet.

IoT can be viewed as an embedded system that contains a group of connected devices and connected through the internet to establish communication with the human environment. In other words, IoT is a network of devices with embedded sensors, which are specially designed and programmed to do specific tasks. In the current scenario, the IoT presents the three-dimensional view of the internet, i.e., any device, any time, and any place. To strengthen this concept, cloud computing technology has played a crucial role in storing and processing the huge amount of data received from different IoT devices over the internet. This has helped IoT to be established as the next big thing after the internet. In recent years, the wide applicability of IoT can be seen in various fields such as finance, education, smart cities, biomedical, waste management, security and privacy, and agriculture. IoT is providing services to all fields in a real-time scenario for prediction as well as decision-making with minimal human interaction.

Biomedical systems include various IoT-based biomedical applications and it is an emerging area of research for IoT and its usage. Some examples of these applications include hospital management, waste management in hospitals, monitoring patients in remote locations, drug manufacturing and its supply, disease diagnosis, monitoring body through smartwatches, monitoring Parkinson's patients, etc.

In the current scenario, IoT is covering a large number of application areas in biomedical systems in a growing manner and due to this, it is affecting human lives on a daily basis. The IoT-enabled technologies ensure the health and wellness of patients through real-time monitoring and assistance. Also, these technologies support in the creation of disease specific tools for diagnosis, personalized treatment, empowering health through life supporting tools, sampling, medical-record keeping in a proper way, guidance through better training modules to medical students for disease detection and prevention.

The popularity of IoT is growing rapidly due to its several benefits such as higher accuracy in results, low-cost solutions, and better prediction ability in an efficient way. Further, several factors such as knowledge enhancement in terms of software, hardware and applications, upgraded availability of computer and mobile technologies, promotion and growth of the digital economy, and easy access to wireless technology are responsible for the rapid IoT revolution [1]. In a healthcare system, the IoT sensors are either used in wearable devices or embedded on the human body to collect physiological data such as body temperature, oxygen level, heartbeat, electrocardiogram (ECG), electromyogram (EMG), electroencephalogram (EEG), and so no [2]. These data are further used to understand the health condition of the patient based on the meaningful and precise result. In an IoT system, storage of data and its accessibility on time has a significant role in processing and getting meaningful information as a huge amount of data is gathered from diverse sources. The stored data is made available to different stakeholders such as doctors, health workers, drug manufacturers, researchers, and other authorized parties. Here, the data sharing with the healthcare personals through cloud storage allows quick access and diagnosis of disease as per requirement. Also, in the healthcare system, most of the IoT-enabled user interface allows a dashboard-like facility for the clinicians to care for patients through real-time data monitoring and performing user control. In recent years, many of the IoT systems have been discovered to monitor, provide security and privacy and control in healthcare [3].

In spite of the convenience of IoT-enabled devices and their applications in biomedical systems, new challenges are always arising when applying in real-time scenarios. The impact of such challenges may vary as per applicability. These challenges may include storage, management and analysis of data sensed by the devices, accuracy in the acquisition of signals from biomedical instruments, ensuring the comfort level of smart devices worn by the person, optimal energy efficiency and consumption of wearable devices, etc.

The chapter is divided into the following sections: Evolution of IoT in healthcare, Literature survey on IoT and biomedical systems; Significance of IoT for different stakeholders; Architecture, and role of IoT in healthcare; Role of IoT: a healthcare analytics; IoT in health and healthcare system; Challenges to IoT in healthcare; The future of IoT in healthcare; Conclusion.

13.2 Evolution of IoT in healthcare

In the last couple of years, IoT has evolved as a helping hand for medical practitioners, health workers, drug manufacturers, and patients in the healthcare sector. It has improved the quality of service with reduced cost. Due to this, IoT has emerged as a global interest for the stakeholders who are directly or indirectly related to the healthcare industry. However, the healthcare industry is leveraging the applicability of new healthcare devices, related services, and applications as per the current requirement. In this context, the IoT is supporting all aspects with endless applications to enhance the healthcare system.

The first interconnected appliance was developed by a computer science graduate of Carnegie Mellon University named David Nichols in 1982. He with his friends needed to buy a coke from a coke vending machine. They noticed that no indicator was available in the machine to show the presence and absence of coke and for that they were required to wait for a while for it to be refilled. To overcome this issue, they provided a solution by notifying of the availability/shortage of coke in the vending machine. They used a green light for the availability and a red light for the shortage of the coke. By this way, they remotely accessed the real-time availability of the content in the machine.

In 1988, 'Ubiquitous Concept' was introduced by Mark D Weiser, Chief Scientist, Xerox Park. This concept means that computing availability can be ensured in any device, at any location and in any format. This concept promoted devices to interconnect with each other through the internet. In result, it laid a base for the IoT concept.

Bill Joy, an inventor at Sun Microsystems and Berkeley Unix, presented the concept of the Device-to-Device web in 1999. This allowed connecting sensors within a network and made them able to establish direct communication between devices.

After that, in 1999, the term 'Internet of Things (IoT)' was coined by Kevin Ashton, Co-founder of Auto-ID Lab, MIT. According to him, the IoT can be described as the objects that are connected through the internet and use radio frequency identification (RFID) technology for encoding the digital data with meaningful labels, which is further handled by radio frequency for searching, identifying, tracking, and communicating with devices/people. Ashton's concept further helped computers and related technologies for gathering, tracking, storing, and processing data without human intervention. This concept has further evolved and been applied in various sectors with required updates as per users all over the world. Although, the foundation of IoT was laid by Ashton, other scientists and researchers have also contributed their effort to the evolution of IoT so far in different sectors.

In the last couple of years, IoT in healthcare is making its path and putting itself into practice among clinicians and patients by adding lots of potential services for the care of different patients as compared to the services available in the past decades. In the past decades, the healthcare suffered from several issues like costlier medical services, the aging of the global population, the severity of chronic disease, birth of new diseases, etc that became the major factor in losing faith in the healthcare sector. To overcome such issues, IoT has provided smart solutions that includes remote monitoring and expert advice to patients. IoT also includes monitoring of patients' bodies through smart wearable devices. Thus, IoT has provided accessible and low-cost services to patients that seemed like the stuff of dreams in the past decades.

13.3 Literature survey on IoT and biomedical systems

The basic objective of IoT is to establish communication among the things using the internet and sending and receiving of information conventionally available when used with 'electronic sensor' devices. In 2025, there will be 41.6 billion IoT devices, producing 79.4 zettabytes (ZB) of data, according to a prediction from International Data Corporation (IDC) [4]. Scientific charity claims that 'IoT' offers a variety of services. Continuity of contact is provided through mobile phone, NFC, Wi-Fi, GPS, etc. Contrary to software development, the major goal of IoT is to include organizations and automation. This section covers a detailed survey of IoT and its applications in the healthcare system.

Chowdary *et al* [5] created a wireless device that is used to compute the blood pressure, oxygen saturation, pulse rate, and temperature of a patient. Only the concerned doctor is granted access thanks to the fingerprint sensor attached to the microcontroller. The device obtains data from a Raspberry Pi, which serves as a sensor node of the given device, and is then sent to a web server for visualization. The real-time physiological parameters are adjusted every 20 s. The Raspberry Pi also has GSM connections and Zigbee modules. A mobile doctor receives an emergency SMS once the health data hits certain threshold values.

An AI system is implemented by Tan *et al* [6] to predict potential risks like diabetes, kidney-related problems, blood pressure, etc. The device keeps track of pulse rate, internal heat speed, and pulse that are the three fundamental signs of forecasting the risk. The front end layer of the system includes an interactive graphical user interface (GUI) that enables both doctors and patients to access and see the data and information stored. The back-end layer of the system places the outcome of the information acquisition system on the cloud data set. It also evaluates the prior information expertise. The developed model's accuracy for individuals with diabetes and kidney illness is 90.54% and 87.88%, respectively, compared to healthy humans.

A prototype that can only transmit electrocardiographic signals wirelessly over ZigBee was demonstrated by Nurdin *et al* [7]. They gathered a series of analog data by attaching several sensors to various body nodes, and then they created a web application to display the corresponding readings for the patients. Their application only supports 20 people at a time, and the data has various bandwidth problems that lead to mistakes in the suggested results.

By using heart rate and body fat percentage as her main components, Pereira *et al* [8] attempt to address the problem of wireless data transfer. They utilized an Arm 7 CPU for the suggested solution, which utilizes Wi-Fi for data transmission. Due to the usage of outdated technology that doesn't handle such long distance communication, the entire system appears to be constrained.

By keeping track of breathing rate, the status of the eyelids, and heartbeat, Tati Erlina *et al* [9] created a system that is focused on addressing the problem of monitoring the physiological condition of comatose patients. The entire system is designed to send data on the mobile through the android app and to display various measured readings. However, the solution failed to maintain system security and also put the security of the crucial data in danger.

Bansal *et al* [10] have created an IR sensor for a smart system to control the heart rate. By using Arduino Uno processes and filters, the heart rate signal values are constructed in the 1–3 Hz range. The Raspberry Pi is used as an IoT gateway to transport data between the Messaging Queuing Telemetry Transport (MQTT) protocol and the Node-Red cloud. A doctor or another registered person receives an SMS and email update via the cloud to remind them of the patient's heart rate. Things Peak allows users to see their heart rates in real-time.

Majumder *et al* [11] created a new tactile method by utilizing a smart IoT that received input from the sensor attached to the body in order to make early provisions for rapidly approaching heart failure. The purpose of the current effort is to develop a wisely coordinated IoT that utilizes a reduced power correspondence unit so that body pulses may subtly collect intrinsic heat levels employing a mobile phone without interfering with their regular daily activities.

The potential use of IoT and mobile devices in radiography for medical purposes has been mentioned by Gupta *et al* [12]. The diagnostic and medical industries have benefited from the incorporation of numerous radiological practices that are currently internet-based into the imaging workflow. Healthcare is undergoing a shift toward individualized healthcare systems thanks to portable wearables, smartphones, and IoT-enabled technology. They explore how mobile devices can be incorporated into radiology workflows, their impact on radiology-based imaging, and the importance of IoT in daily imaging workflow and future prospects.

In 2019, an IoT-based system for dental healthcare was developed by Liu *et al* [13]. This system makes use of deep learning, intelligent hardware, and a mobile terminal. This system has great potential to provide dental healthcare at home. The viability of its application in dental healthcare has been investigated by the authors. Their research points to a variety of IoT applications for dental disease screening and diagnosis. To carry out the task of acquiring images of teeth, they have developed a smart IoT-based dental device.

For the prediction and diagnosis of diabetes disease, a cloud and IoT-based technique is developed by Kumar *et al* [14]. In this technique, they have employed a fuzzy neural classifier for better result. They also proposed a novel classification method named Fuzzy Rule-based neural classifier to diagnose and determine the severity of the disease.

Nubenthan *et al* [15] proposed a system for WBAN. They provided a wireless interface for WBAN by applying IEEE 802.15.6 and IEEE 802.15.4j standards. They collected data from various sensors using Wi-Mon software to provide information about the severity level of the patient for disease such as dengue, malaria, etc. Collection of data in the form of different parameters such as pulse rate, oxygen saturation, ECG, and blood pressure is processed to monitor the health status. In this process, the Wi-Mon software supports with high accuracy.

13.4 Significance of IoT for different stakeholders

Real-time monitoring has a significant role for the better treatment of any disease. In the past years, before the invention of IoT, doctors communicated with patients through limited physical visits, text, and telephonic conversations. So, monitoring patients' health on a continuous basis and recommending required treatment accordingly on time became a major concern for the hospitals and doctors.

IoT-enabled devices have made remote monitoring possible in healthcare industry. Patients get excellent treatment as their remote monitoring provides real-time health updates to the doctors and the health staff [16]. IoT devices have simplified doctor–patient interactions, enhanced patient participation and hence their satisfaction. Additionally, long hospital stays and readmissions have been reduced by remote monitoring of the patients' health, causing reduction in healthcare expenses.

Thus, IoT has revolutionized the healthcare industry by device–people interaction in providing healthcare solutions. IoT applications in healthcare solutions are advantageous not only to the patients and the doctors but also to the patient's family members, the hospitals, and the insurance providers [17]. The details about how IoT facilitates different stakeholders are as follows.

13.4.1 Hospitals

There are numerous other applications for IoT devices in hospitals besides patient health monitoring. The real-time position of medical equipment like defibrillators, oxygen pumps, wheelchairs, nebulizers, and other monitoring equipment is tracked using IoT devices tagged with sensors. The placement of medical staff at various sites can also be monitored in real time using IoT-enabled systems.

The hygiene monitoring can also be done using IoT devices, which avoids infections. IoT devices are also used for managing pharmacy inventory, monitoring refrigerator temperatures and regulating the humidity and temperature of the environment.

13.4.2 Patients

Patients now have access to individualized care thanks to wearable gadgets such as wearable bands for monitoring fitness and other wirelessly connected equipment like glucometers and blood pressure and heart rate monitor cuffs. These gadgets can be programmed to notify the users about their blood pressure updates, appointments with their doctors etc.

People's lives have been completely changed by IoT, particularly elderly patients who find it very helpful as it continuously tracks their medical issues. It has significantly impacted the families and the individuals who live alone as its alarm mechanism alerts the family and the medical staff if any disruption or change happens in their regular activities.

13.4.3 Doctors/physicians

IoT-enabled home monitoring and wearables devices are used in monitoring patients' health by their physicians. They can monitor a patient's adherence to their treatment regimen or other medical needs. Healthcare staff may actively engage with their patients and be more and more attentive due to IoT. Data collected from an IoT device can help the doctors in choosing the better treatment for patients and getting the desired results.

13.4.4 Insurance companies in the health sector

IoT-connected intelligent gadgets present a wide range of prospects for health insurers. The underwriting and claims processes of insurance firms can benefit from the data collected by health monitoring devices. They can discover prospects for underwriting and spot fraudulent claims thanks to this data. In the operations of underwriting, processing claims, pricing, and risk evaluation, IoT devices provide clarity between clients and insurers. Customers will have sufficient visibility into the underlying reasoning behind each decision taken and the consequences of each operation process in view of IoT-captured data-driven judgments.

IoT devices produce health related data which is shared and utilized by the customers of the insurers and in return they may receive rewards. The customer who uses IoT devices for monitoring their regular activities, treatment programmes, and health precautions may also earn rewards. IoT devices may also be used by insurance firms to verify the claims and the data they collect.

13.5 Architecture and role of IoT in healthcare

Various things such as protocols, physical devices, gateways, sensors and actuators, cloud services, and protocols are the basic elements of IoT architecture. The architecture tells how the physical connectivity of the devices should be established to communicate, analyze, and monitor from remote locations. The devices in IoT are connected by a well-known internet protocol [18, 19]. Various research initiatives have been taken by researchers and companies, but till now no unique IoT architecture is accepted globally. Mostly, different architectures have been given by different researchers.

As per the researchers' point of view, the architecture of conventional IoT considers three layers, i.e., application layer, network layer, and perception layer [20, 21]. This architecture was introduced in the initial stages of research and it is called three-layer architecture, as shown in figure 13.1.

13.5.1 Three-layered IoT architecture

13.5.1.1 Application layer

Application layer is liable for giving the user application-specific services. This layer uses the processed data from cloud servers and serves as a bridge between cloud and IoT devices. Required tools to the developers are provided and solutions can be visualized and accessed by the end user through this layer. There are several application areas like smart health, smart homes, industry, health monitoring systems, entertainment, smart cities, etc, where IoT techniques can be deployed to deliver the related services. These techniques allow humans to conduct constant monitoring through accessibility and visualization of the data. Depending on the information the sensors gathered, the services offered in each region would change. Personal computers, mobile phones, laptops and other computing devices can be used by the users to access the data. To access such data, application layer protocols, i.e., FTP, SMTP, HTTP, and HTTPS are used through the browser.

Smartwatch is a perfect example for understanding the role of application layer. The sensors attached with the smartwatch, measure the pulse rate of the human body and display it on the smartwatch screen or the mobile app. By using Bluetooth technology, we can connect our smartphone to the app. The app can track both the

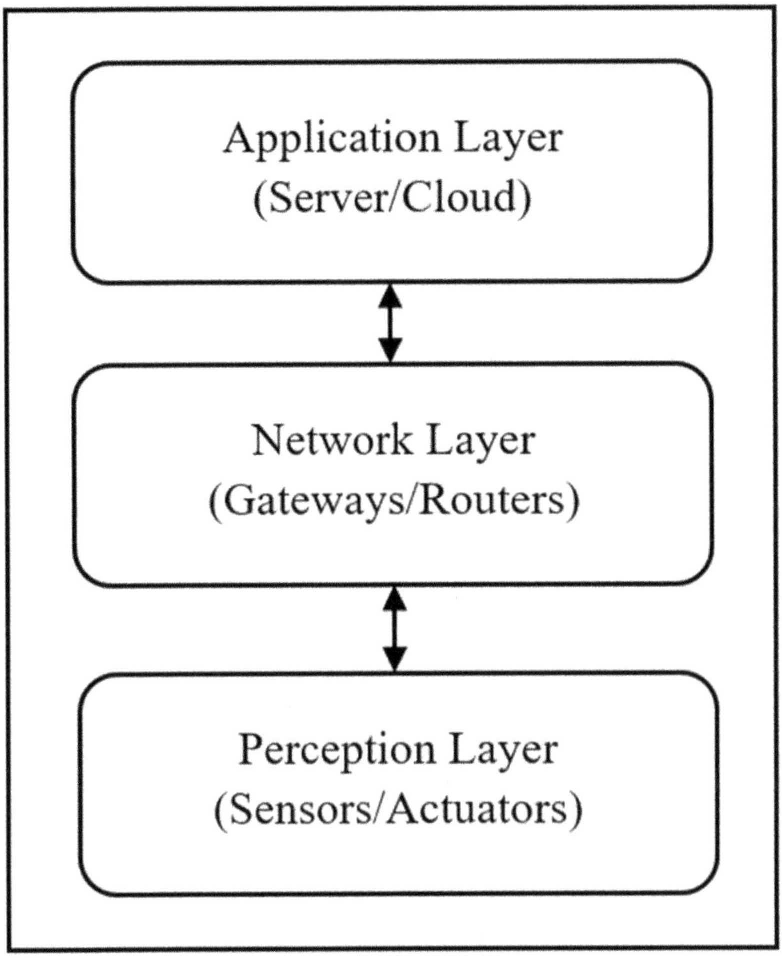

Figure 13.1. Three-layered IoT architecture.

past and the present data using a variety of visualization charts thanks to the data that is also present in the cloud.

13.5.1.2 Network layer

Secure data transfer from IoT devices to application users is the responsibility of the network layer. This layer connects network devices, and servers for transmitting and processing data sensed by the sensors. It is also known as a channel of communication for sending data from sensing layer to the storage platform. To establish communication among the network devices, this layer uses different kinds of communication protocols that are LPWAN, CoAP, MQTT, Zigbee, Z-Wave, NFC, RFID, Wi-Fi, Ethernet, Bluetooth, etc. Two types of data transmission, i.e., wired and wireless transmission are used in the network layer.

In the case of wired transmission, an ethernet cable is used by the network to establish connection. In turn, the network is connected to the Digital Subscriber Line (DSL) or network gateway. The wired networks are easy to implement and require only to plug into coaxial lines, phone lines, and power lines to establish connection.

On the other hand, due to the complexity and expensiveness of the wired network, wireless transmission is the best alternative. Set-up of wireless network is very easy and simple and overall running cost is less as compared to a wired network. Due to the advancement in the network technologies, we can see a variety of solutions like Wi-Fi, RFID, Bluetooth, Z-Wave, and ZigBee that are helpful in wireless transmission. Table 13.1 shows the comparison of wired and wireless transmission on different parameters.

13.5.1.3 Perception layer

It is the physical layer that uses sensors for collecting required information about the physical objects from the environment [22–24]. From the environment this layer is used to identify objects or physical parameters. Any physical object can be considered as a thing in IoT when it is linked to a sensor and actuator along with the further connection. Firstly, the device has a sensor which is used to detect and

Table 13.1. Comparison of wired and wireless transmission.

Parameters	Wired transmission	Wireless transmission
Cost	Cost is high. Following factors are involved: 1. Labour cost 2. Hardware cost 3. Wire cost 4. Replacement cost for any changes due to damage, and upgradation	Cost is low. Mainly, this cost includes configuration and running of the wireless network.
Scalability	Less scalable in terms of network set-up, and running, planning, and costing of network.	High scalable due to the following reasons: 1. No requirement of hardware installation 2. Less time is needed for its set-up and running 3. It requires only typical configuration
Speed/distance/ interference/ consistency	1. Fast 2. Insensitive to distance 3. Less effect of interference during transmission 4. Consistent data transmission	1. Slow 2. Highly sensitive to distance 3. High interference effect from other devices during transmission 4. Inconsistent data transmission

collect the data from external sources. The IoT sector's expansion is creating a number of opportunities for the use of sensor technology. RFID is the medical IoT sensor that is most frequently utilized in healthcare. The fundamental issues with RFID security are privacy and authentication.

In IoT architecture, the cognitive layer identifies the physical and sensory instruments. The perceptual layer sensor system identifies an item, detects it, and then gathers object data. Depending on the type of sensor, data can be gathered on things like temperature, movement, position, wetness, vibrations, distance, speed, chemical changes, etc. The following processing layer receives the information after that. The viewing layer uses the node to send the data it has gathered to the processing network layer.

13.5.2 Five-layered IoT architecture

Mainly the three factors like business aspects, technologies employed, and application domains are responsible for the changes and further improvement in the IoT architecture. For IoT devices, a variety of IoT architectures are available but five-layered architecture is recommended as the best architecture among the existing state-of-the-art architectures [23]. As the three-layered architecture mainly focuses on the core concept of the IoT, in the real world finer details of IoT are needed for better applicability in problem solving. Because of this, the literature has suggested a lot more layered architectures.

In five-layered architecture, the architecture of three layers, i.e., application, network, and perception are the same as we have seen in three-layered architecture. To these, processing, transport and business layers are included additionally. Figure 13.2 shows the five-layered architecture.

13.5.2.1 Transport layer

This layer works between processing layer and perception layer. It mainly transfers the data received from the sensor from perception to processing layer and vice-versa [24]. The transfer of such sensor data is executed through networks. These networks may include different networking technologies such as wireless, local area network (LAN), near field communication (NFC), RFID, Bluetooth, software-defined networking (SDN), and network functions virtualization (NFV).

13.5.2.2 Processing layer

This layer lies in the middle of the five-layered IoT architecture, so it is also named as middleware layer. It works on the data that comes from the transport layer. The work includes storing, analyzing, and processing of the data [22, 24]. It is capable of managing and giving the lower layers a wide range of services. It makes use of a variety of technologies, including big data processing modules, cloud computing, and databases.

13.5.2.3 Business layer

This is the top-most layer of the IoT architecture. The representation of the data and business model coming from the application layer is represented by this layer.

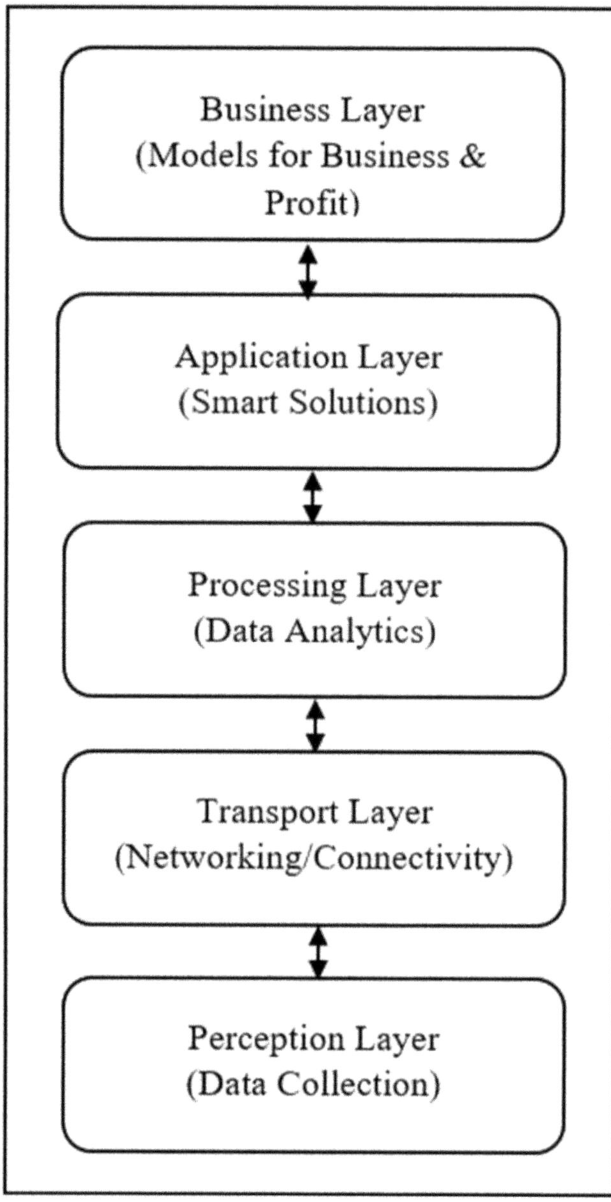

Figure 13.2. Five-layered IoT architecture.

The whole IoT system is managed by this layer. This includes the management of the user's privacy, applications, models related to business and profit, etc. This layer does several tasks for the betterment of the IoT devices. It entails creating graphs, outcomes analysis, flowcharts, and the device improvements, among other things [22].

13.6 Role of IoT: a healthcare analytics

IoT enables a real-time monitoring of the patient which helps in effective collection of patient data, tracking the patient and staff activities, etc, to ensure high quality healthcare services. IoT has drastically transformed healthcare in every dimension over the last several years and will continue to do so in years to come.

13.6.1 Benefits of Internet of Things

The benefits which the healthcare industry is experiencing from IoT devices are wide-ranging [25, 26]. Some of them are as follows.

13.6.1.1 Faster disease diagnosis, reporting and monitoring

IoT devices gather more and more data points regularly which helps in more accurate diagnosis. Remote health monitoring using connected IoT devices can save lives in case of a medical emergency such as diabetes, heart failure and asthma attacks, etc.

13.6.1.2 End-to-end connectivity and affordability

The patient care workflow can be automated with the help of healthcare mobility solution. The IoT enables interoperability, artificial intelligence, information exchange making healthcare service delivery more and more effective.

13.6.1.3 Data assortment and analysis

The huge amount of data that the healthcare IoT devices send in a very short time is hard to store and process. IoT devices can collect report and analyse the real-time data and minimize the requirement of storing the raw data.

13.6.1.4 Research activities

IoT in healthcare can be useful for research purposes as it helps us to collect a huge amount of data of patient's illness which would not have possible manually. This data can be used for statistical study which would ultimately help in medical research. The existing medical devices are also being updated by embedding chips in them.

13.6.1.5 Cost reduction and error reduction

The technology-driven set-up cuts down unnecessary visits and improves the allocation and planning process, i.e., the use of IoT connectivity helps in automation of hospitals and healthcare systems which ultimately reduces the cost. As IoT devices and the software automate the manual processes, there is less chance of human error.

13.6.1.6 Reduced hospital admissions and readmissions

An always-on IoT connection monitors the patient in real time, helping the healthcare providers to track and identify the problems and hence reducing the chances of hospitalization.

13.6.1.7 Better drug and equipment management

IoT devices make drug and equipment tracking very simple, which saves time spent in searching for what they actually need.

13.6.2 Applications of IoT devices in healthcare

Various IoT devices are available to monitor the health status of patients with different diseases [17, 27]. The details are as follows.

13.6.2.1 Glucose monitoring system (implantable)

Devices having sensors are implanted just below the skin of a patient suffering from diabetes. The sensors in the devices send notifications to the patient's mobile as soon as his/her glucose level is too low, and also records historical data.

13.6.2.2 Activity tracker (during cancer treatment)

Activity trackers are used to track the patient's fatigue levels, appetite, movements, etc, and the data collected prior to and after the treatment has started will help healthcare professionals to decide the adjustments needed in the recommended treatment plan.

13.6.2.3 Heart monitoring

These wearable devices monitor the patient's heart rate, which in turn can determine the blood pressure (high/low). Healthcare providers access the patient's heart monitor data during checkups and exams. The wearable devices may also alert when the patient is facing arrhythmias, strokes, palpitations, or full-blown heart attacks.

13.6.2.4 Medical alert system

These wearables are something which looks like jewelry but alerts the patient's family members in case of any emergency. For example, a medical alert bracelet will immediately notify the family members on their smartphones if the patient falls out of bed.

13.6.2.5 Ingestible sensor

These devices which look like pills are equipped with sensors and can be swallowed by the patients. These ingested sensors send information to the patient's mobile which helps them to follow the suitable dosages for medications. Some ingestible sensors are used to diagnose the patients with problems such as irritable bowel syndrome or colon cancer, etc.

13.6.2.6 Medication dispenser

These devices are implanted in a patient and dispense medication in steady doses. The patient will be alerted when there is a need to refill the medications. During routine visits, it can inform the doctor about any missed doses.

13.6.2.7 Wireless sensor

These are being used in laboratories and hospital refrigerators to monitor the temperature of blood samples, medications and other biomedical materials.

13.6.2.8 Trackable inhaler

IoT inhalers tell the patients/their physicians what they're experiencing that is causing asthma attacks to them and also remind the patients about their medications. A number of companies like Teva Pharmaceuticals and Propeller Health offer connected inhalers.

13.6.2.9 Wearables to fight depression

Apple has developed an app for its Apple Watch which will monitor cognitive and mood functions of manic depressive patients and help them cope with their depression.

13.6.2.10 Contact lenses

As of now, the connected contact lenses read glucose levels of diabetes patients but they'll be helping restore the eye's focus and improve vision in the near future.

13.6.2.11 Location services

Wheelchairs, defibrillators, nebulizers, or monitoring equipment are tagged with IoT sensors for medical staff to track them.

13.6.2.12 Moodables

These are head-mounted wearables which help in improving our mood by sending low-intensity current to the brain. Thync and Halo Neurosciences are working on this and have made substantial progress too.

13.6.2.13 Healthcare charting

IoT devices like Audemix reduce manual work done by the doctors during patient charting. This voice command powered device captures the patient's data.

13.7 IoT in health and healthcare system

There was a time when pen and paper were the only means to record a patient's information, and healthcare staff were required to monitor patient's conditions. But now IoT is handling such healthcare requirements in a better way [28, 29]. The healthcare areas and the major technology players working in those areas can be classified as follows.

13.7.1 IoT companies/systems in public health

As per the requirement of the patients, companies working in the healthcare sector have developed different systems which have directly benefited public health. Some of them are mentioned below [30].

13.7.1.1 Aclima (San Francisco, California)

Aclima studies 'how cities live and breathe' using its mobile sensing platform. Following a pilot programme in California, Google now equips all of its StreetView vehicles with Aclima sensors.

13.7.1.2 Nexleaf Analytics (Los Angeles, California)

Particularly in rural locations, its ColdTrace system offers wireless remote temperature monitoring for freezers storing vaccines. The company's StoveTrace technology is a similar cloud-based remote monitoring system for better cookstoves in rural regions.

13.7.1.3 SystemOne (Springfield, Massachusetts)

SystemOne transfers diagnostic data to healthcare works and clinicians in real time. It recently celebrated sending more than 10 million diagnostic results around the globe.

13.7.2 IoT companies/systems for chronic disease management

Some of the healthcare systems that are currently being used for chronic disease management are mentioned below.

13.7.2.1 Quio (Brooklyn, New York)

It provides a cloud platform with wireless connection to various therapeutic devices belonging to medications, health related activities, etc, for patients with chronic conditions.

13.7.2.2 Spry Health (Palo Alto, California)

This company's wearable Loop device offers 'hospital bed monitoring power in fitness tracker style.'

13.7.2.3 Pfizer (New York and Armonk, New York)

The real-time tracking of Parkinson's medication effectiveness and improved doctor–patient communication are two benefits of this Pfizer and IBM partnership.

13.7.3 IoT companies/systems for smart sleep

Following are the systems especially developed to offer an environment that helps in a sound sleep [30].

13.7.3.1 Eight (New York)

A mattress is connected to an environment and sleep sensing app called 'Eight,' which analyses the data it receives and transmits the analysis to a user's smartphone to find the perfect temperature for sleep.

13.7.3.2 Happiest Baby (Los Angeles, California)

The SNOO bassinet from Happiest Baby has a variety of features to promote deeper and safer sleep for young children. White noise, 'womb-like rocking,' a cry sensor that modifies sound and motion, and a 'SNOO Sack' that prevents rolling are all included.

13.7.3.3 Beddit (Espoo, Finland)

Apple-owned Beddit targets to enhance sleep quality by tracking heart rate, snoring, breathing, and sleep environment. The analysis of the collected data is used to determine the course of action to improve the experience.

13.7.4 IoT companies/systems for medication refills

Monitoring medication, doses, missed doses and refills is not an easy task. Some of the IoT systems developed to handle all these services are as follows.

13.7.4.1 AdhereTech (New York, New York)

AdhereTech smart pill bottle issues reminders regarding missed doses to patients and medication refills via text or phone.

13.7.4.2 Aeris Communications (Chicago, Illinois)

To ensure that patients follow medical recommendations, Aeris offers medical device manufacturers and healthcare practitioners a communication channel with the patients.

13.7.4.3 Otsuka America Pharmaceutical (Rockville, Maryland)

The Otsuka Abilify MyCite tablet contains an ingestible event marker (IEM) sensor that activates upon digestion and transmits data to the wearable MyCite Patch. The wearable MyCite Patch then transmits the data to a mobile app that enables the user to review 'medication ingestion data and activity level, as well as self-reported mood and quality of rest.'

13.7.5 IoT companies/systems to streamline hospice care

One of the most typical and crucial tasks in the healthcare field is the management of the resources and the services available. Some of the IoT automated environments currently imparting their services are [30] as follows.

13.7.5.1 GE Healthcare (New York, New York)

G.E.'s AutoBed platform monitors up to 1200 beds, processing 80 bed requests at a time, and tracks other patient needs such as nurse proximity.

13.7.5.2 Stanley Healthcare (Waltham, Massachusetts)

Provides a real-time location of the patient via wireless RFID.

13.7.5.3 Phillips (Andover, Massachusetts (North America))
It is used to monitor MRI performance. Philips's E-Alert has a sensor that measures environmental factors and compares them with a threshold value and triggers alerts if exceeded.

13.7.6 IoT companies/systems for remote care and monitoring

Remote care and monitoring is the problem which can be solved only by IoT-enabled healthcare systems.

13.7.6.1 Honeywell (Morris Plains, New Jersey)
Its Genesis Touch connects patients with remote care providers who receive transmitted biometrics data.

13.8 Challenges to IoT in healthcare

Every technological solution comes with a heap of challenges to it, which is the case with IoT healthcare as well. The IoT healthcare challenges can be classified under the following points [30, 31].

13.8.1 Data security and privacy

IoT devices collect and transfer data in real time but most of the IoT devices lack protocols and security needs, hence data security and privacy is one of the most significant challenges. Also, there is always a significant ambiguity regarding the ownership regulation of the data of electronic devices which makes the data highly susceptible to cybercriminals. Using a patient's health records, cybercriminals can create fake IDs for buying medical equipment and drugs; apart from this, they can also file a fake insurance claim in the name of the patient.

13.8.2 Integration (multiple devices and protocols)

IoT device manufacturers do not have any consensus regarding communication protocols and standards which may cause a hindrance in the integration of different devices. The scope of scalability is reduced and the processes slow down due to this non-uniformity of various connected devices' protocols.

13.8.3 Data overload and accuracy

Data aggregation is very difficult due to a variety of communication protocols and standards used by IoT devices. As more and more devices are connected, the amount of data will be so huge that deriving the insights from it will become extremely tough for doctors. This will be affecting the quality of their decision-making.

13.9 The future of IoT in healthcare

According to a report published by KPMG and the Organization of Pharmaceutical Producers of India (OPPI), 'about 75% of dispensaries, 60% of hospitals and 80% of doctors are working in urban areas, serving approximately 28% of Indian population' [32]. The IoT infrastructure requires reliable internet connectivity, cost effective IoT infrastructure, security and data analytics and India is picking up on all of these fronts. India has over 450 million smartphone users which can be very useful to build an IoT network and to aid healthcare workers in diagnosing, tracking and controlling disease.

Thus, in the field of healthcare, the future of IoT is very bright. An estimate published by Goldman Sachs says that healthcare IoT is going to save approximately $300 billion in the future [33]. IoT revenues related to healthcare are estimated to increase to $135 billion. According to 'Markets and Markets research', the market for IoT healthcare devices is predicted to reach as high as $94.2 billion by 2026, up from $26.5 billion in 2021.

13.10 Conclusion

There may be limitless predictions about the revolution that the IoT in healthcare can bring from increasing accessibility, enhancing the quality of healthcare to reducing the healthcare costs. From real-time health monitoring to virtual hospitals and labs, IoT has a dramatic impact on the healthcare systems available around the globe. Healthcare professionals irrespective of their disciplines are able to access and share the data with each other, to speed up the analysis. By virtue of a connected network of IoT devices one can imagine rural folk sitting in front of a screen, taking advice from a doctor sitting in a Metro hospital, or a city-based doctor examining a patient's chest x-ray and suggesting the next course of action. In developing countries like India, rural healthcare needs fresh impetus and IoT technology can deliver that booster shot to the healthcare systems of remote areas.

References

[1] Karthick R, Ramkumar R, Akram M and Kumar M V 2021 Overcome the challenges in bio-medical instruments using IOT—a review *Mater. Today Proc.* **45** 1614–9

[2] Peng H, Tian Y, Kurths J, Li L, Yang Y and Wang D 2017 Secure and energy-efficient data transmission system based on chaotic compressive sensing in body-to-body networks *IEEE Trans. Biomed. Circuits Syst.* **11** 558–73

[3] Gatouillat A, Badr Y, Massot B and Sejdić E 2018 Internet of medical things: a review of recent contributions dealing with cyber-physical systems in medicine *IEEE Internet Things J.* **5** 3810–22

[4] Dell Technologies: Internet of Things and data placement. https://infohub.delltechnologies.com/l/edge-to-core-and-the-internet-of-things-2/internet-of-things-and-data-placement

[5] Chowdary K C, Lokesh Krishna K, Prasad K L and Thejesh K 2019 An efficient wireless health monitoring system *Proc. Int. Conf. I-SMAC (IoT Soc. Mobile, Anal. Cloud), I-SMAC 2018* 373–7

[6] Tan E T and Halim Z A 2019 Health care monitoring system and analytics based on Internet of Things framework *IETE J. Res.* **65** 653–60

[7] Nurdin M R F, Hadiyoso S and Rizal A 2016 A low-cost Internet of Things (IoT) system for multi-patient ECG's monitoring *2016 Int. Conf. on Control, Electronics, Renewable Energy and Communications (ICCEREC) (September 2016)* (Piscataway, NJ: IEEE) 7–11

[8] Pereira M and Nagapriya K K 2017 A novel IoT based health monitoring system using LPC2129 *2017 2nd IEEE Int. Conf. on Recent Trends in Electronics, Information and Communication Technology (RTEICT) (May 2017)* (Piscataway, NJ: IEEE) 564–8

[9] Erlina T, Saputra M R and Putri R E 2018 A smart health system: monitoring comatose patient's physiological conditions remotely *2018 Int. Conf. on Information Technology Systems and Innovation (ICITSI) (October 2018)* (Piscataway, NJ: IEEE) 465–9

[10] Bansal P, Malik M and Kundu R 2018 Smart heart rate monitoring system *2018 IEEMA Engineer Infinite Conf. (eTechNxT) (March 2018)* (Piscataway, NJ: IEEE) 1–4

[11] Majumder A K M, ElSaadany Y A, Young R and Ucci D R 2019 An energy efficient wearable smart IoT system to predict cardiac arrest *Adv. Hum. Comput. Interact.* **2019** 1507465

[12] Gupta S, Johnson E M, Peacock J G, Jiang L, McBee M P, Sneider M B and Krupinski E A 2020 Radiology, mobile devices, and internet of things (IoT) *J. Digit. Imaging* **33** 735–46

[13] Liu L, Xu J, Huan Y, Zou Z, Yeh S C and Zheng L R 2019 A smart dental health-IoT platform based on intelligent hardware, deep learning, and mobile terminal *IEEE J. Biomed. Health Inform.* **24** 898–906

[14] Kumar P M, Lokesh S, Varatharajan R, Babu G C and Parthasarathy P 2018 Cloud and IoT based disease prediction and diagnosis system for healthcare using fuzzy neural classifier *Future Gener. Comput. Syst.* **86** 527–34

[15] Nubenthan S and Shalomy C 2017 A wireless continuous patient monitoring system for dengue: Wi-Mon *2017 6th National Conf. on Technology and Management (NCTM) (January 2017)* (Piscataway, NJ: IEEE) 23–7

[16] Mendonça M, Jerónimo T, Julião M, Santos J, Pombo N and Silva B 2019 An IoT-based healthcare ecosystem for home intelligent assistant services in smart homes *EAI Int. Conf. on IoT Technologies for HealthCare (December 2019)* (Berlin: Springer) 142–55

[17] Pradhan B, Bhattacharyya S and Pal K 2021 IoT-based applications in healthcare devices *J. Healthc. Eng.* **2021** 6632599

[18] Silva B N, Khan M and Han K 2018 Internet of things: a comprehensive review of enabling technologies, architecture, and challenges *IETE Tech. Rev.* **35** 205–20

[19] Liu Y and Zhou G 2012 Key technologies and applications of internet of things *2012 5th Int. Conf. on Intelligent Computation Technology and Automation (January 2012)* (Piscataway, NJ: IEEE) 197–200

[20] Ngu A H, Gutierrez M, Metsis V, Nepal S and Sheng Q Z 2016 IoT middleware: a survey on issues and enabling technologies *IEEE Internet Things J.* **4** 1–20

[21] Lin J, Yu W, Zhang N, Yang X, Zhang H and Zhao W 2017 A survey on internet of things: architecture, enabling technologies, security and privacy, and applications *IEEE Internet Things J.* **4** 1125–42

[22] Kassab W A and Darabkh K A 2020 A–Z survey of Internet of Things: architectures, protocols, applications, recent advances, future directions and recommendations *J. Netw. Comput. Appl.* **163** 102663

[23] Kumar R P and Smys S 2018 A novel report on architecture, protocols and applications in Internet of Things (IoT) *2018 2nd Int. Conf. on Inventive Systems and control (ICISC) (January 2018)* (Piscataway, NJ: IEEE) 1156–61

[24] Firouzi F, Farahani B, Weinberger M, DePace G and Aliee F S 2020 IoT fundamentals: definitions, architectures, challenges, and promises *Intelligent Internet of Things* (Cham: Springer) pp 3–50

[25] De Michele R and Furini M 2019 IoT healthcare: benefits, issues and challenges *Proc. 5th EAI Int. Conf. on Smart Objects and Technologies Forsocial Good (September 2019)* 160–4
[26] Joyia G J, Liaqat R M, Farooq A and Rehman S 2017 Internet of Medical Things (IoMT): applications, benefits and future challenges in healthcare domain *J. Commun.* **12** 240–7
[27] Sayrafian K *et al* 2021 IoT for healthcare applications *Inclusive Radio Communications for 5G and Beyond* (New York: Academic) pp 221–52
[28] Elhoseny M, Ramírez-González G, Abu-Elnasr O M, Shawkat S A, Arunkumar N and Farouk A 2018 Secure medical data transmission model for IoT-based healthcaresystems *IEEE Access* **6** 20596–608
[29] Huifeng W, Kadry S N and Raj E D 2020 Continuous health monitoring of sports-personusing IoT devices based wearable technology *Comput. Commun.* **160** 588–95
[30] How IoT helps improve healthcare https://builtin.com/internet-things/iot-in-healthcare
[31] Knickerbocker J U *et al* 2018 Heterogeneous integration technology demonstrations for future healthcare, IoT, and AI computing solutions *2018 IEEE 68th Electronic Components and Technology Conf. (ECTC) (May 2018)* (Piscataway, NJ: IEEE) 1519–28
[32] Selvaraj S and Sundaravaradhan S 2020 Challenges and opportunities in IoT healthcare systems: a systematic review *SN Appl. Sci.* **2** 1–8
[33] Krishnamoorthy S, Dua A and Gupta S 2021 Role of emerging technologies in future IoT-driven Healthcare 4.0 technologies: a survey, current challenges and future directions *J. Ambient Intell. Humaniz. Comput.* **14** 361–407

IOP Publishing

Internet of Things in Biomedical Sciences
Challenges and applications
Varun Bajaj and Irshad Ahmad Ansari

Chapter 14

Automated IoT-based detection of periodic leg movement using optimal wavelet-based entropy features

Manish Sharma, Mohammad Arif and Kushagra Asthana

Periodic leg movements (PLMs) are involuntary, repetitive movements induced by specific muscular contractions during the sleep cycle and analyzed using polysomnography (PSG) recordings. Leg movements (LMs) can be accompanied by waking or sleep disruption. The PLM index reflects the severity of motor symptoms and their impact on sleep structure. A high PLM index may lead to other health-related problems and significantly affect personal well-being. This condition can be assessed by developing an automated PLM detector. The proposed study presents an automatic detection of LM and PLM by developing a model based on machine learning and signal processing techniques. In this study, the Wisconsin sleep cohort (WSC), which is a publicly available database on national sleep research resource (NSRR), is used to develop the model. A total of 2565 subjects were employed in this study. For automated PLM detection, wavelet-based entropy features, namely Tsallis entropy, wavelet entropy, and sample entropy, are extracted from single-channel electromyography (EMG) epochs. The features so obtained are applied to various supervised ML algorithms. Our proposed model achieved an overall accuracy of 82.2% and 81.5% for LMs and PLMs classification, respectively, using an ensemble bagged trees classifier with a 10-fold cross-validation technique.

The suggested model is efficient and dependable and appears to be a candidate that can be installed in a cloud-based clinical system. An IoT-based system can be developed containing EMG sensors and connected to the internet. The EMG data from the IoT-based hardware can be moved to the cloud. The data can be used on the cloud to detect LM and PLM using our model.

doi:10.1088/978-0-7503-5311-3ch14

14.1 Introduction

Sleep is an essential biological cycle that helps people conserve energy and survive [22]. Also, it is widely recognized as a significant contributor to physical and mental health in people. Sleep is equally required for critical functions such as memory, learning, emotions, cardiovascular and metabolic activities, and cellular toxin removal [7, 13, 39], for which a healthy sleep is required that involves good quality, sufficient time, proper scheduling and regularity, and the absence of sleep disruptions or disorders [14]. Periodic leg movements (PLMs) are generally accompanied by complete awakenings, as described by Rechtschaen and Kales in 1968, or by EEG arousal signals such as alpha activity, spindles, K-alpha, K-complexes, and K-spindle activities [21]. Further, the findings of Karadeniz *et al* [15] suggested that leg movements are a symptom of an underlying arousal issue and that the number of awakenings was much higher following leg movements than concurrently. Altogether, the research associated with PLM and sleep disorders [31, 34] argues that our public health community and society as a whole should take sleep [11, 26, 28, 30, 34, 35] and its related disorders [27, 32, 35] more seriously.

Leg movements are the most often occurring events during sleep. These moments are involuntary jerks in leg muscles that can often disrupt sleep. They are scored in nocturnal polysomnography. According to the American academy of sleep medicine (AASM) [5] manual for the scoring of sleep and associated events, a leg movement (LM) event is stored if the minimum duration of the LM event is 0.5 s and the maximum duration of LM event is 10 s. An LM event has a minimum amplitude of an 8 μV rise in EMG voltage above resting EMG. Electromyograph comprises two electrodes placed on the left and right anterior tibialis. EMG measures muscle response or electrical activity in response to stimulation of nerves of the muscle. When the aforementioned leg movements occur periodically, it is called periodic leg movement (PLM). A PLM series comprises a minimum of four leg movements with inter-movement intervals of 5–90 s. The movement resembles twitching, kicking, and jerking the lower extremities of the leg during sleep. These movements are repetitive, episodic, and not in one's control. PLMs are most significant during non-rapid eye movement (NREM) stages 1 and 2. These movements occur less often during NREM-3 and rapid eye movements (REM) sleep stage. AASM manual for sleep scoring and related events has detailed the guidelines for scoring PLMs. Defining a PLM series requires a minimum of four consecutive LM epochs.

LM that fulfills AASM criteria can be included in a PLM series; that is, the minimum time between two consecutive LMs (defined as the duration between onsets of successive LMs) should be 5 s, and the maximum period length between LMs (defined as the duration between onsets of successive LMs) should not be more than 90 s. In contrast, the leg muscles of two different legs separated by less than 5 s are considered a single leg movement. PLMs are expressed as an index comprising the number of PLMs per hour of sleep. This index is known as the periodic leg movement index (PLMI) [3]. Although the PLM is just a normal sleep phenomenon, an increased PLMI has adverse consequences on a person's health. It is often categorized as a disorder. A PLMI of more than five and less than 25 is considered mild; PLMI of >25 and <50 is considered moderate, and >50 is severe [20]. The primary symptoms of periodic leg movement disorder (PLMD) comprise poor sleep, daytime sleepiness, frequent awakenings, tiredness, and fatigue in the morning [2]. The primary cause of PLMD is still unknown. In most cases, the subject is unaware if such a disorder exists. It is often taken for insomnia. Medications and comorbidities like antidopaminergics, antidepressants and antihistaminergics, kidney diseases, heart diseases, and iron deficiency anemia have been reported to either cause PLMD in normal subjects or worsen it in existing PLMD subjects [10]. PLMD is often reported to disrupt sleep and co-occur with other sleep disorders like restless leg syndrome (RLS) and narcolepsy. Culpepper *et al* investigated two patterns of periodic leg movement syndrome (PLMS) activity [8]. It was observed in the first pattern that PLM was high at the beginning of the sleep and decreased slowly till the end. The second pattern had a more evenly distributed activity with somewhat more significant activity in the middle of the night.

Although there were no apparent factors segregating the two patterns, some researchers have concluded that younger patients were more likely to show the second pattern [8]. Moreover, it was studied that insomnia patients exhibited the first pattern activity while narcoleptic patients exhibited the second pattern activity [4]. Another study concluded that the first pattern was more prevalent in patients with idiopathic PLM or RLS. The second pattern occurs in patients with sleep disorders such as sleep apnea and narcolepsy [1]. Dauvilliers *et al* [9] studied the prevalence of PLM in narcoleptic subjects. 169 patients with narcolepsy and 119 normal patients were compared for the presence of PLM. It was found that a high PLMI was observed in both REM and NREM sleep in narcoleptic patients. PLMs were significantly higher in REM sleep compared to NREM sleep. This suggests that PLM is a dominant symptom of narcolepsy. Mendelson *et al* [17] studied the occurrence of PLM in insomniac patients. Many researchers have claimed that PLM directly impacts the ability to sleep. However, no significant proof has been investigated to accept this claim. In this study, all the patients had complaints about the inability to sleep well. Also, the subjects had varied PLMIs. It can be concluded that the PLMI is not a significant factor in complaints about the inability to sleep. RLS is defined as the uncontrollable urge to move one's leg. It is often associated with PLM. Although PLM is an involuntary movement, RLS is the urge to jerk one's leg. The majority of subjects with PLM also suffer from RLS. Since RLS is a voluntary activity, it does disrupt sleep and is a potential cause of insomnia. Mucsi *et al* [19] investigated the relationship between RLS and specific insomnia symptoms. It was concluded that RLS patients were more prone to having insomnia compared to healthy patients. Despite PLM not being a significant cause of insomnia, PLMs are associated with RLS. There have been many attempts to design and validate automated PLM detectors. The gold standard is Stanford PLM automatic detector (S-PLMAD) [18]. The Stanford detector utilized the Wisconsin Sleep Cohort (WSC) ($n = 1076$) to design and the Stanford Sleep Cohort ($n = 760$) to validate. This detector incorporated adaptive noise cancellation to suppress cardiac interference. The correlation between visually scored PLMS and automated detected was obtained to be 0.97. Ferri *et al* [12] validated visually scored PLMS against automatically detected PLMS using sleep analysis software Hypnolab 1.2 (SWS

Soft, Italy). 30 (15 normal and 15 RLS) subjects were part of this study. The EMG signals were digitally bandpass filtered with an additional notch filter. The correlation factor between the visually scored and computer detected PLMS was obtained to be 0.94. Sharma *et al* [27] proposed an automated PLM detector using EOG and EMG signals on 108 subjects. A biorthogonal filter bank was used for wavelet decomposition along with Hjorth Parameters. The detector classified the PLM subjects against normal healthy subjects with 97.5% accuracy.

14.2 Material used

WSC is a longitudinal study (involving repeated observations of the same variables) of causes, consequences, and the biological history of sleep disorders. A mailed questionnaire surveyed subjects aged 30–60 who worked for four large state agencies regarding their sleep cycle and other characteristics. The responses to these questionnaires were also included in the dataset. For each subject, the following files were available in the dataset. EDF files contain the PSG data. Table 14.1 describes available files in the grass and twin comet systems.

LMs were scored using leg EMG in the dataset. PLMs were scored based on the criteria mentioned above. PLMI is calculated for each subject and shown as a percentage of all subjects. A higher PLMI corresponds to a higher degree of PLMD. Subjects have been categorized as normal if PLMI < 5, mild if PLMI > 5 and PLMI < 25, moderate if PLMI > 25 and PLMI < 50, severe if PLMI > 50.

$$\mathrm{PLMI} = \frac{\text{total number of periodic leg movement}}{\text{sleep duration in hours}}. \tag{14.1}$$

PLMI in insomniac and healthy subjects were compared in table 14.2.

Table 14.1. Description of available files in the cohort.

Sl. No.	File extension	Description
1	.edf	Contains raw PSG data from 16 channels
2	.sco.txt	WSC respiratory event scoring for grass system
3	.stg.txt	WSC sleep staging for grass system
4	.log.txt	WSC bio-calibrations and light indicators for grass system
5	.allscore.txt	WSC staging and respiratory event scoring for the twin comet system

Table 14.2. PLMD in insomniac and non-insomniac subjects.

Subjects type	Normal	Mild	Moderate	Severe
Insomniac	22.1%	18%	7.6%	1.1%
Healthy	22%	19.6%	7.7%	1.4%
Overall	44.2%	37.7%	15.4%	2.6%

14.3 Methodology

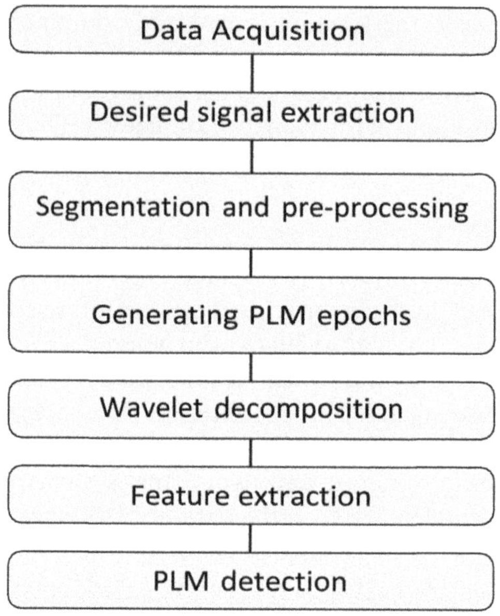

14.3.1 Data acquisition

The sleep laboratory of Wisconsin University contributed the data to NSRR [40, 41]. NSRR furnished the dataset for this project. The total number of epochs across 2565 subjects is 2632 081. The normal epochs are 1458 100, and PLM epochs are 17 148. These epochs were used to design and validate our detector. Per our knowledge, this is one of the most extensive training sets for designing and validating our PLM detector.

14.3.2 Desired signal extraction

This study's two particular channels were of concern: chin EMG and leg EMG. Chin EMG was rejected because the probe placement on the chin was less (almost negligibly) susceptible to leg movements. Leg EMG was identified for further processing.

14.3.3 Segmentation and pre-processing

The EMG signal in WSC is sampled at two different frequencies. The signals were initially sampled at 100 Hz collected from 2000 to 2009. later, the signals were sampled at 200 Hz frequency from 2009 to 2016 in the grass and twin comet systems, respectively. The continuous time-series leg EMG signal has been segmented into 30 s epochs. The number of samples in an epoch is computed as the frequency times epoch duration. The computed samples constitute one epoch. 'LM' events were scored along with their timestamps in the annotations.

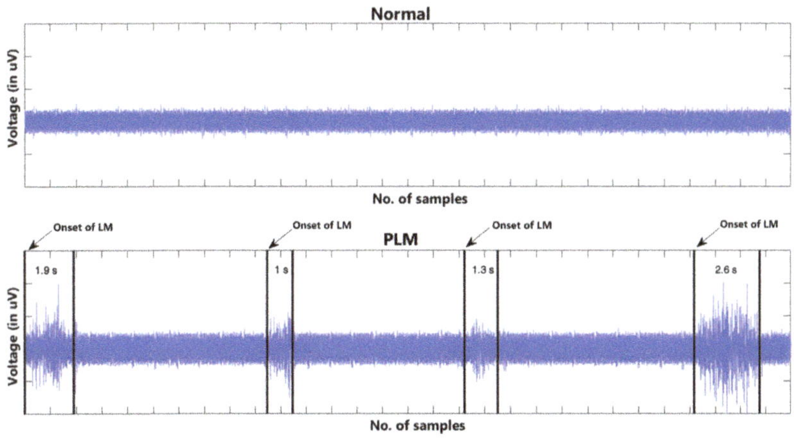

Figure 14.1. Comparison between normal and PLM event.

Along with LM events, arousal, hypopnea, mixed apnea, central apnea, obstructive apnea, and desaturation events were also scored. The epochs that contain one or more LM events were labeled as LM epochs. The epochs that do not contain any of the events mentioned above were labeled as 'normal' epochs.

The use of Fourier transform for the decomposition of signals fails as it cannot obtain time localization information [6]. While the capacity to assess transient signals in both the time and frequency domains makes the wavelet domain favorable for its applications in various communication and signal processing applications [16, 27]. In the proposed study, we employed an optimal biorthogonal wavelet filter. With joint bandwidth duration localization, the objective function is a convex quadratic function of pass-band and stop-band errors; while employing a half-band analysis filter, we used a linear phase optimal biorthogonal wavelet filter bank (OBWFB). Figure 14.1 shows the application of OBWFB on a single leg movement epoch.

14.3.4 Generating PLM epochs

In the dataset, leg movements were annotated in the files '.sco.txt' in the grass system and 'allscore.txt' in the twin comet system. The LM events were scored along with their respective timestamps. The EMG signal was divided into 30 s epochs. The epochs that contain one or more leg movements were labeled as LM epochs. AASM criteria [5] states that four or more consecutive LMs with inter-movement interval of 5–90 s constitute a PLM. Following this criterion, all the LM events that satisfy the above-mentioned requirement were marked as PLM series. The epochs in which the LMs of the PLM series fell were labeled as PLM epochs. It can be fairly concluded that PLM epochs are a subset of LM epochs. The epochs in which there were no scored events were labeled as normal epochs. Our detector classified the PLM epochs against the normal epochs. The plot below clearly distinguishes a PLM epoch from a normal epoch.

14.3.5 Wavelet decomposition

The EMG is non-stationary; hence wavelets are frequently utilized to give excellent duration-frequency localization when decomposing the signal [29]. We used the wavelet decomposition technique to break down the signal into sub-bands. The number of decomposition levels and sub-bands is crucial to preserving the significant frequency parts of the signal classification. In this study, we utilized five-level wavelet decomposition techniques to decompose EMG signals into six sub-bands (figure 14.2). The first band (SB1) is called the approximate band, while other sub-bands (SB2–SB6) are called the detailed band [24, 25, 33].

14.3.6 Feature extraction

The collected information in the EMG signal was converted into a smaller set of data or features. We extracted different features from the sub-bands obtained after the epoch decomposition. Extracted features for classifying sleep into five different classes are stated below:

Tsallis entropy: Tsallis entropy is essentially a Boltzmann–Gibbs theory generalization [37]. The benefit of the Tsallis entropy is that it can quantify the uncertainty of generalized systems. It can also be utilized to explain systems with multifractal space–time constraints and non-stationary nature. Moreover, the summation part in the mathematical formula of Tsallis entropy allows it to take less computation time as compared to other methods. EMG signals are non-stationary and have non-extensivity. Hence, Tsallis entropy appears to be a better choice for this study. It is defined as,

$$S_q = \frac{n}{q - 1}\left(1 - \sum_i z_i^q\right).$$

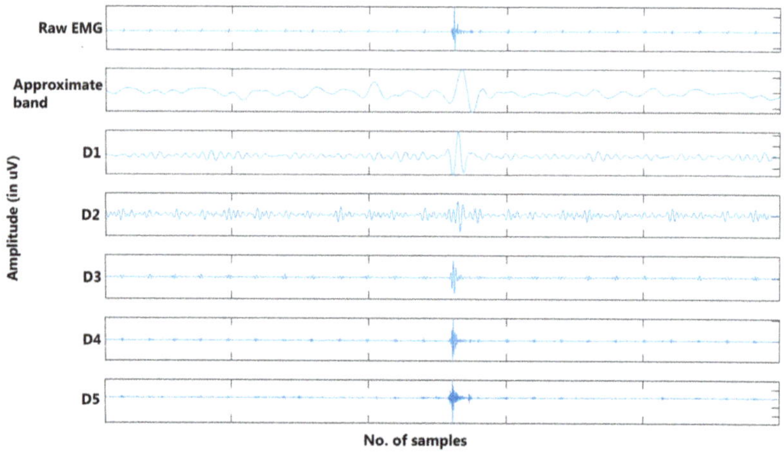

Figure 14.2. Sub-bands obtained after wavelet decomposition of LM.

Here n is a positive constant, q is the Tsallis parameter, and z_i is a discrete collection of probabilities with the condition:

$$\sum_i z^i = 1.$$

Wavelet entropy: Wavelet entropy (WE) [23] is a one-of-a-kind technique for analyzing the transitory features of non-stationary signals in both the temporal and frequency domains. It has been beneficial in obtaining vital clinical information from physiological signals such as ECG, EEG, EMG, and intracranial pressure recordings.

For a discrete random variable T, with possible outcomes $t_1, t_2, \ldots, t_n$ that corresponds to the probability of $P(t_1), P(t_2), \ldots, P(t_n)$. The entropy of T is as follows:

$$H(T) = -\sum_{i=1}^{n} P(t_i)\log P(t_i).$$

Sample entropy: Sample entropy (SampEn) is an updated form of approximation entropy (ApEn) that is used to analyze the complexity of time-series physiological signals data. Similar to approximate entropy, it is also a measure of complexity, but unlike approximation entropy, it eliminates self-similar patterns. Assuming the length of time-series data = $a_1, a_2, \ldots, a_n$ with a constant time interval T, the vector of length z is taken as $X_z(i) = x_1, x_2, \ldots, x_{i+z-1}$ and the distance function of Chebyshev distance is defined as $d[X_z(m), X_z(n)]$ provided $m \neq n$. Then the sample entropy is defined as:

$$\text{SampEn} = -\ln\frac{U}{V}$$

where, $U = d[X_{z+1}(m), X_{z+1}(n)] < r$ and $V = d[X_{z+}(m), X_{z+}(n)] < r$. In general, the value of z is taken as 2, and r is given by 0.2 × *standard deviations*.

14.3.7 Classification

The classification is performed after the extraction of the following features as mentioned above, Tsallis entropy, wavelet entropy, and sample entropy from all the six sub-bands of each epoch of the leg EMG signal. The ranked features are fed to several classifiers like support vector machine (SVM) [28], k-nearest neighbors (KNN) [13], decision trees [28, 30], ensembled bagged trees (EBT) [34], ensembled boosted trees, logistic regression [26], for classification of PLM epochs from normal epochs. The classifiers utilized supervised machine learning techniques for automated classification. For validation, we used a ten-fold cross-validation technique. This technique works by dividing the dataset into 90:10 split. 90 process was repeated ten times until the complete dataset was exhausted. The main advantage of this technique is that all the available dataset is used for validation and in training the model. Since the process is repeated ten times, it assures good accuracy.

Higher fold classification produced similar results with much slower processing speed; hence we selected 10-fold cross-validation.

14.3.8 Results

In this study, the EBT classifier produced the best results as compared to all the other available classifiers in the classification learner app in MATLAB version 2020. All the results obtained after classification utilizing different features and their combinations with the overall accuracy and Cohens kappa value are represented in the confusion matrices below (tables 14.3–14.5).

14.3.8.1 LM classification

14.3.8.2 PLM classification

As seen from table 14.5, the proposed model yielded the best results for the classification of PLM events when all three features, namely Tsallis, wavelet, and sample entropy, were jointly used, that is 81.5%. The model also produced a kappa value of 0.629 041.

Table 14.3. Confusion matrix of leg EMG channel using all three features combined.

Accuracy = 79.6% kappa = 0.592 30			
	Predicted class		
True class	Normal	LM	*F*1 score
Normal	308 409	74 198	0.80
LM	81 819	300 934	0.79

Table 14.4. Confusion matrix of leg EMG channel using the Tsallis and wavelet combined.

Accuracy = 82.2% kappa = 0.643 462			
	Predicted class		
True class	Normal	LM	*F*1 score
Normal	304 328	78 352	0.80
LM	58 088	324 592	0.79

Table 14.5. Confusion matrix of leg EMG channel using all features combined.

Accuracy = 81.5% kappa = 0.629 041			
	Predicted class		
True class	Normal	PLM	*F*1 score
Normal	172 302	45 490	0.81
PLM	35 302	182 490	0.82

14.4 Discussion

This study intended to design and validate a PLM detector. Many studies have been taken up in the past to design a PLM detector. The first attempt at a PLM detector was made by Tauchmann *et al* [36] in 1996. The need for a reliable, accurate PLM detector is very pressing. Earlier, LMs were scored by a sleep technician. A sleep diary was maintained where the sleep technicians would manually score all the events. It was a cumbersome process and was prone to human errors. If we talk about PLM, it is even more complex. In due course, many types of scoring software were used for manual scoring. This software solved the problem to some extent but was still prone to human errors. The need for a reliable automated detector has long intrigued researchers.

We were able to design and validate an automated PLM detector with good accuracy. The raw EMG signal has a significant noise component. The biorthogonal filter used reduces noise and makes the features significant. Wavelet decomposition decomposes the signal into six sub-bands to preserve the signal's dominating frequency components. We used the following entropy-based features, Tsallis entropy, wavelet entropy, and sample entropy.

Moreover, we combined the features mentioned above in order to increase the overall accuracy of the proposed model. For classification, we experimented with multiple machine learning-based classifiers. EBT classifier produced the best results of all.

To the best of our knowledge, this is the first longitudinal study to utilize the whole WSC dataset for the detection of LM and PLM events. The proposed work successfully classifies LM and PLM events with good accuracy. For the classification of LM events, three different entropy-based features were extracted. The classification accuracy (CA) achieved after extracting the Tsallis entropy is 79.6%. A combination of Tsallis and wavelet entropy is finally extracted to increase the overall accuracy of our model, achieving a CA of 82.2%. In order to reach the final objective of our work, that is, to detect the PLM events, Tsallis, wavelet, and sample entropies are extracted from the leg EMG signal. We used Tsallis, wavelet, and sample entropy combined to achieve the best results and finally attained a CA of 81.5% from the proposed model. We compared our results to other remarkable detectors. All the detectors were based on the WSC in table 14.6.

Table 14.6. Comparison of similar detectors.

Detector	PLM count	Accuracy (%)
Tauchmann *et al* [36]	1436	97
Ferri *et al* [12]	7237	94.3
Wetter *et al* [38]	11 160	99
S-PLMAD [18]	3443	98
Proposed work	17 148	81.5

Tauchmann *et al* [36] worked on the first PLM detector in 1996. A split of 1671 and 1740 PLMs was used for optimizing and validating, respectively. Simply thresholding the rectified EMG was used to detect the PLMs. Ferri *et al* [12] modified this algorithm to include a bandpass filter and two thresholds for detecting PLMs. It was a significant improvement. Wetter [38] took a different approach. He focused on detecting burst spikes recurring at a high repetition rate, referred to as burst density. Burst density was thresholded to detect PLM. This significantly reduced false detection. S-PLMAD [18] is considered the gold standard in automated PLM detection methods. Significant effort has been made to suppress noise. ECG interference from EMG was also removed. An advanced algorithm for signal-to-noise ratio enhancement and adaptive noise cancellation was also incorporated. One important point to note here is that this is the most extensive set of subjects used for designing and validating a PLM detector to the best of our knowledge. The subjects were not filtered by any means. Subjects were varied based on their anthropological features, sleep health, mental health, etc. This fact has undoubtedly contributed to the difficulty in classification. Although, using such a large subject set paves the way for a very accurate and reliable PLM detector in the future. If we had only utilized RLS patients, insomniac patients, narcoleptic patients, or any other sub-group of patients where PLM is more prevalent, we would have been able to classify it with better accuracy.

There are certain significant limitations with our PLM detector, of which one is an attempt at classifying a broad spectrum of subjects. Although we could detect PLM with good correlation, such systems cannot be used for clinical diagnosis. PLMD and RLS are commonly observed in patients who complain about sleep. However, these are not the only factors that affect sleep quality. Our detector is not perfect because of a large number of false detections of PLM. In diagnosis, false detection of PLM or RLS can lead to ignoring other factors affecting the patient's sleep.

Notwithstanding, this study creates a strong foundation for further research and development of sleep disorder detectors. Many steps can be undertaken to improve this research. This can show a direction for further research. One is to limit the number of subjects and utilize similar controls. By similar controls, we mean that patients with higher PLMI are easily classified from normal patients compared to patients with low PLMI. Another approach could be using convolutional neural networks. Learning in neural networks happens, similar to the human brain. They

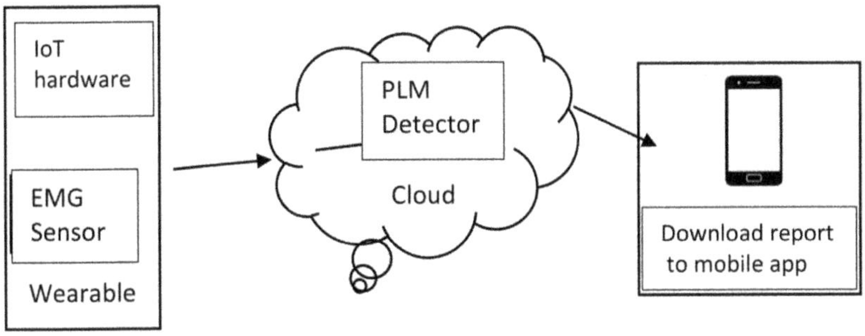

Figure 14.3. IoT based hardware architecture for PLM detector.

consist of an artificial network of parameters, which helps the computer learn and optimize itself by analyzing new data.

Another important application of this detector could be deploying it in IoT-based hardware. The hardware may be an internet-connected wearable with onboard EMG sensors. The IoT device will record the EMG signal and push it to the cloud. The signal can be fed into this detector, and a report can be generated the next morning on PLM prevalence (figure 14.3).

14.5 Conclusion

PLM is a very common disorder. However, it is not critical until the PLMI is high. A high PLMI is a natural cause and/or implication of many other sleep disorders. Visual detection of PLM events is a tedious task and is also prone to human errors. Hence, a model for the automatic detection of LM as well as PLM events is developed using wavelet-based entropy features, namely Tsallis, wavelet, and sample entropy. Our model is developed using the WSC dataset, which according to our knowledge, is the largest dataset (2565 subjects) used to detect PLM events. For the detailed study of the EMG signal, we utilized five-level wavelet decomposition, which resulted in six sub-bands, the features extracted from these sub-bands were input to machine learning-based classifiers.

It was found that the best classification accuracy was achieved with all three entropies combined. Among the machine learning-based classifiers in the development of the proposed model, the EBT classifier yielded the best results of 82.2% and 81.5% for LM and PLM classification, respectively. We incorporated 10-fold cross-validation. The proposed model is fast as well as simple to use. This research could be a basis to advance methods of sleep disorder diagnosis. PLM is a matter of concern for many patients and sleep-doctors. We hope that our research positively contributes to academia and industry.

References

[1] Metman L V and Kompoliti K 2010 Periodic limb movements *Encyclopedia of Movement Disorders* (Oxford: Academic) pp 444–9

[2] Aikens J E, Vanable P A, Tadimeti L, Caruana-Montaldo B and Mendelson W B 1999 Differential rates of psychopathology symptoms in periodic limb movement disorder, obstructive sleep apnea, psychophysiological insomnia, and insomnia with psychiatric disorder *Sleep* **22** 775–80

[3] Alessandria M and Provini F 2013 Periodic limb movements during sleep: a new sleeprelated cardiovascular risk factor? *Frontiers Neurol.* **4** 116

[4] Baker H and Hesla P E 1991 Características de los movimientos periódicos durante el dormir (mioclonia nocturna). estudio en un centro de trastornos del dormir *Salud Ment.* **14** 44–8

[5] Berry R B, Budhiraja R, Gottlieb D J, Gozal D, Iber C, Kapur V K, Mar-cus C L, Mehra R, Parthasarathy S and Quan S F *et al* 2012 Rules for scoring respiratory events in sleep: update of the 2007 AASM manual for the scoring of sleep and associated events: deliberations of the sleep apnea definitions task force of the american academy of sleep medicine *J. Clin. Sleep Med.* **8** 597–619

[6] Chen J and Li G 2014 Tsallis wavelet entropy and its application in power signal analysis *Entropy* **16** 3009–25

[7] Cincin A, Sari I, Oğuz M, Sert S, Bozbay M, Ataş H, Ozben B, Tigen K and Basaran Y 2015 Effect of acute sleep deprivation on heart rate recovery in healthy young adults *Sleep Breath.* **19** 631–6

[8] Culpepper W J, Badia P and Shaffer J I 1992 Time-of-night patterns in plms activity *Sleep* **15** 306–11

[9] Dauvilliers Y, Pennestri M H, Petit D, Dang-Vu T, Lavigne G and Montplaisir J 2007 Periodic leg movements during sleep and wakefulness in narcolepsy *J. Sleep Res.* **16** 333–9

[10] DelRosso L M, Mogavero M P and Ferri R 2021 Restless sleep disorder, restless legs syndrome, and periodic limb movement disorder—sleep in motion! *Pediatr. Pulmonol.* **57** 1879–86

[11] Dhok S, Pimpalkhute V, Chandurkar A, Bhurane A A, Sharma M and Acharya U R 2020 Automated phase classification in cyclic alternating patterns in sleep stages using Wigner–Ville distribution based features *Comput. Biol. Med.* **119** 103691

[12] Ferri R, Zucconi M, Manconi M, Bruni O, Miano S, Plazzi G and Ferini-Strambi L 2005 Computer-assisted detection of nocturnal leg motor activity in patients with restless legs syndrome and periodic leg movements during sleep *Sleep* **28** 998–1004

[13] Frank E, Sidor M M, Gamble K L, Cirelli C, Sharkey K M, Hoyle N, Tikotzky L, Talbot L S, McCarthy M J and Hasler B P 2013 Circadian clocks, brain function, and development *Ann. N.Y. Acad. Sci.* **1306** 43–67

[14] Gruber R, Carrey N, Weiss S K, Frappier J Y, Rourke L, Brouillette R T and Wise M S 2014 Position statement on pediatric sleep for psychiatrists *J. Can. Acad. Child Adolesc. Psychiatry* **23** 174

[15] Karadeniz D, Ondze B, Besset A and Billiard M 2000 EEG arousals and awakenings in relation with periodic leg movements during sleep *J. Sleep Res.* **9** 273–7

[16] Li B, Zhang P, Liang S and Ren G 2008 Feature extraction and selection for fault diagnosis of gear using wavelet entropy and mutual information *2008 9th Int. Conf. on Signal Processing* (Piscataway, NJ: IEEE) 2846–50

[17] Mendelson W B 1996 Are periodic leg movements associated with clinical sleep disturbance? *Sleep* **19** 219–23

[18] Moore H IV, Leary E, Lee S Y, Carrillo O, Stubbs R, Peppard P, Young T, Widrow B and Mignot E 2014 Design and validation of a periodic leg movement detector *PLoS One* **9** e114565

[19] Mucsi I, Molnar M Z, Ambrus C, Szeifert L, Kovacs A Z, Zoller R, Barotfi S, Remport A and Novak M 2005 Restless legs syndrome, insomnia and quality of life in patients on maintenance dialysis *Nephrol. Dial. Transplant.* **20** 571–7

[20] Natarajan R *et al* 2010 Review of periodic limb movement and restless leg syndrome *J. Postgrad. Med.* **56** 157

[21] Kales A and Rechtschaffen A 1968 *A Manual of Standardized Terminology, Techniques and Scoring System for Sleep Stages in Human Subjects* (U. S. National Institute of Neurological Diseases and Blindness, Neurological Information Network)

[22] Rechtschaffen A, Bergmann B M, Everson C A, Kushida C A and Gilliland M A 1989 Sleep deprivation in the rat: X. Integration and discussion of the findings *Sleep* **12** 68–87

[23] Rosso O A, Blanco S, Yordanova J, Kolev V, Figliola A, Schürmann M and Başar E 2001 Wavelet entropy: a new tool for analysis of short duration brain electrical signals *J. Neurosci. Methods* **105** 65–75

[24] Sharma M and Acharya U R 2018 Analysis of knee-joint vibroarthographic signals using bandwidth-duration localized three-channel filter bank *Comput. Electr. Eng.* **72** 191–202

[25] Sharma M, Achuth P, Deb D, Puthankattil S D and Acharya U R 2018 An automated diagnosis of depression using three-channel bandwidth-duration localized wavelet filter bank with eeg signals *Cogn. Syst. Res.* **52** 508–20

[26] Sharma M, Bhurane A A and Acharya U R 2022 An expert system for automated classification of phases in cyclic alternating patterns of sleep using optimal wavelet-based entropy features *Expert Syst.* e12939

[27] Sharma M, Darji J, Thakrar M and Acharya U R 2022 Automated identification of sleep disorders using wavelet-based features extracted from electrooculogram and electromyogram signals *Comput. Biol. Med.* **143** 105224

[28] Sharma M, Goyal D, Achuth P and Acharya U R 2018 An accurate sleep stages classification system using a new class of optimally time–frequency localized three-band wavelet filter bank *Comput. Biol. Med.* **98** 58–75

[29] Sharma M, Kolte R, Patwardhan P and Gadre V 2010 Time–frequency localization optimized biorthogonal wavelets *2010 Int. Conf. on Signal Processing and Communications (SPCOM)* (Piscataway, NJ: IEEE) 1–5

[30] Sharma M, Patel S, Choudhary S and Acharya U R 2020 Automated detection of sleep stages using energy-localized orthogonal wavelet filter banks *Arab. J. Sci. Eng.* **45** 2531–44

[31] Sharma M, Patel V, Tiwari J and Acharya U R 2021 Automated characterization of cyclic alternating pattern using wavelet-based features and ensemble learning techniques with EEG signals *Diagnostics* **11** 1380

[32] Sharma M, Raval M and Acharya U R 2019 A new approach to identify obstructive sleep apnea using an optimal orthogonal wavelet filter bank with ECG signals *Inform. Med. Unlocked* **16** 100170

[33] Sharma M, Sharma P, Pachori R B and Acharya U R 2018 Dual-tree complex wavelet transform-based features for automated alcoholism identification *Int. J. Fuzzy Syst.* **20** 1297–308

[34] Sharma M, Tiwari J and Acharya U R 2021 Automatic sleep-stage scoring in healthy and sleep disorder patients using optimal wavelet filter bank technique with EEG signals *Int. J. Environ. Res. Public Health* **18** 3087

[35] Sharma M, Tiwari J, Patel V and Acharya U R 2021 Automated identification of sleep disorder types using triplet half-band filter and ensemble machine learning techniques with EEG signals *Electronics* **10** 1531

[36] Tauchmann N and Pollmacher T 1996 Automatic detection of periodic leg movements (PLM) *J. Sleep Res.* **5** 273–5

[37] Tsallis C 1988 Possible generalization of Boltzmann–Gibbs statistics *J. Stat. Phys.* **52** 479–87

[38] Wetter T C, Dirlich G, Streit J, Trenkwalder C, Schuld A and Pollmächer T 2004 An automatic method for scoring leg movements in polygraphic sleep recordings and its validity in comparison to visual scoring *Sleep* **27** 324–8

[39] Xie L *et al* 2013 Sleep drives metabolite clearance from the adult brain *Science* **342** 373–7

[40] Young T, Palta M, Dempsey J, Peppard P E, Nieto F J and Hla K M 2009 Burden of sleep apnea: rationale, design, and major findings of the Wisconsin sleep cohort study *WMJ* **108** 246

[41] Zhang G Q, Cui L, Mueller R, Tao S, Kim M, Rueschman M, Mariani S, Mobley D and Redline S 2018 The national sleep research resource: towards a sleep data commons *J. Am. Med. Inform. Assoc.* **25** 1351–8

www.ingramcontent.com/pod-product-compliance
Ingram Content Group UK Ltd.
Pitfield, Milton Keynes, MK11 3LW, UK
UKHW051902100926
8556IPUK00005B/739

9 780750 353090